Nursing and social change

Nursing and Social Change is essential reading for all students of nursing who wish to understand how their profession has developed in a historical context from its earliest beginnings to the present day. Now in its third edition, the book has been completely revised to take into account the challenges facing nurses today.

The first half of the book covers the history of nursing and includes the latest research findings on the life and work of Florence Nightingale and new references for further reading. The second half of the book reflects the profound changes which have affected the profession over the years since the book's second edition in 1980. Ten new chapters include contributions from senior members of the nursing profession who have been closely involved in the most recent health service reorganisation and the radical changes to nurse education. Topics covered include:

- nurse education and Project 2000
- nursing and care in the community
- nursing outside the NHS
- nurses as managers
- economic change and industrial relations
- international and inter-regional organisation
- health problems of the world

Offering a unique combination of scholarship and readability, *Nursing and Social Change* provides students and teachers with a comprehensive and up-to-date source of reference.

Contributors:
June Clark, Professor of Nursing, University of Middlesex; **Val Cowie**, formerly Director of the Labour Relations and Legal Department, Royal College of Nursing; **Margaret Green**, Visiting Professor, Exeter College of Nursing; **Paul Lloyd**, RCN Adviser in Occupational Health Nursing; **Shelagh Murphy**, International Secretary, The Royal College of Nursing; **Peter Nolan**, Senior Lecturer, Department of Nursing Studies, University of Birmingham; **Muriel Skeet**, Consultant, World Health Organisation.

Monica E. Baly, formerly a Regional Nursing Officer of the Royal College of Nursing, is now editor of the *History of Nursing Journal*.

Nursing and social change

Third edition

Monica E. Baly

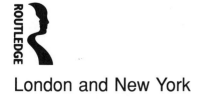

London and New York

First edition published 1973
Second edition published 1980
by William Heinemann Medical Books Ltd

Third edition published 1995
by Routledge
11 New Fetter Lane, London EC4P 4EE

Simultaneously published in the USA and Canada
by Routledge
29 West 35th Street, New York, NY 10001

Typeset in Times by Florencetype Ltd, Kewstoke, Avon
Printed and bound in Great Britain by
Biddles Ltd, Guildford and King's Lynn

British Library Cataloguing in Publication Data
A catalogue record for this book is available from the
British Library.

Library of Congress Cataloging in Publication Data
Baly, Monica E. (Monica Eileen)
    Nursing and social change/Monica E. Baly. – 3rd ed.
        p. cm.
    Includes bibliographical references and index.
    1. Nursing – History.   2. Nursing – Social aspects –
History.
    I. Title.
    [DNLM: 1. History of Nursing.   2. Social change.   WY
11.1 B198na 1994]
RT31.B34 1994
610.73'09–dc20
DNLM/DLC
for Library of Congress   94–10724
                                                            CIP

ISBN 0–415–10197–2 (hbk)
ISBN 0–415–10198–0 (pbk)

Contents

List of illustrations

Contributors

Monica E. Baly, formerly lecturer for the Diploma in Nursing and Regional Officer of the Royal College of Nursing.

June Clark, Professor of Nursing Studies, University of Middlesex.

Val Cowie, formerly Director of the Labour Relations and Legal Department of the Royal College of Nursing.

Mavis Gordon, Principal Occupational Health Tutor, Royal College of Nursing.

Margaret Green, formerly Director of Education, Royal College of Nursing, Visiting Professor, Exeter College of Nursing.

Paul Lloyd, Adviser in Occupational Health Nursing, Royal College of Nursing.

Shelagh Murphy, International Secretary, Royal College of Nursing.

Peter Nolan, Senior Lecturer, Department of Nursing Studies, University of Birmingham.

Muriel Skeet, Consultant, World Health Organisation.

Acknowledgements

Acknowledgement is gratefully expressed to the following:

Plates pp.76–9: Bath Reference Library.

Chapter 1, Fig. 1.1: M. G. A. Wilson, *Population Geography*, Thomas Nelson Australia Pty Ltd. Figs. 1.2 and 1.3: *District Nursing*, Heinemann.

Chapter 5, Fig. 5.1: G. Talbot Griffith, *Population Problems of the Age of Malthus*, Cambridge University Press.

Chapter 8, Fig. 8.1: HMSO (Crown copyright).

Chapter 15, Fig. 15.1: T. McKeown and C. R. Lowe, *Introduction to Social Medicine*, Blackwell, 1966.

Chapter 18, Figs. 18.1, 18.2 and 18.3: HMSO (Crown copyright); Fig. 18.4: HMSO (Crown copyright); Table 18.3: Pre-registration nursing, figures supplied by the English National Board, March 1992; Table 18.4: DHSS, Aug. 1993, published by *Nursing Standard*.

Chapter 21, Fig. 21.1: Open University.

Chapter 22, Figs. 22.1 and 22.2: June Clark.

Chapter 25, Fig. 25.1: NAHAT (1993), *NHS Handbook, 1993–4*, Figs. 25.2 and 25.3: OECD, Paris.

Chapter 28, Fig. 28.1: OECD, Paris.

Setting out on the voyage to Ithaca
You must pray that the way be long ...
Many be the summer mornings
When with what pleasure, with what delight
You enter harbours never seen before.

Do not hurry the journey at all.
Better that it should last many years;
Be quite old when you anchor at the island,
Rich with all you have gained on the way,
Not expecting Ithaca to give you riches.
Ithaca has given you your lovely journey –
Without Ithaca you would not have set out.

Ithaca has no more to give you now.
Poor though you find it, Ithaca has not cheated you.
Wise as you have become, with all your experience,
You will have understood the meaning of an Ithaca.

Cavafy, 1911

Preface to the third edition

It is twenty years since the first edition of *Nursing and Social Change* was published. It was designed to supplement lectures for students doing Part A of the Diploma in Nursing, as the syllabus was at that time. The expanded second edition, published thirteen years ago, was designed to meet the defects of the first and to meet the needs of a wider group of post-registration students. If a week is a long time in politics, thirteen years is an aeon in the National Health Service at the present time and inevitably some of the later material is out of date. In order to meet this need, Routledge have agreed to publish an updated third edition of the book originally published by Heinemann.

The scheme of the book, which traced social change in each period and the new health needs it produced, then examined how these needs were met and is still valid. Students need to keep a historical perspective or they are in danger of what E. P. Thompson describes as 'the enormous condescension of posterity'. With the exception of the chapter on Florence Nightingale, which has been rewritten in the light of new research, the first half of the book has been left more or less intact.

It is the second half that presents the challenge. To quote from the first edition:

> the development of nursing is like weaving a cloth with social change as the warp and, running to and fro with the weft is the shuttle of care . . . only by tracing the threads to their historical origin can we begin to understand the confusion and profusion of the health services in the twentieth century.

In the past thirteen years the shuttle has moved faster than ever and we have been subjected to more change than we can comfortably tolerate. Because change has been so profound, we have recruited other contributors to deal with specialised areas. It is hoped that with a comprehensive basic training students will cease to think about nursing in separate compartments, but some specialisation is inevitable and this book is designed to cover the needs of post-registration students.

In consultation with the publishers it was agreed to drop the appendices, which took up 18 per cent of the book; as new material is added, it is necessary to keep the size of the book within bounds and it is impossible to include everything. Moreover, change is continuous and everything is in the state of flux and, like Heraclitus's river, you cannot step into the same place twice.

I am grateful to my colleagues who have contributed to the third edition. 'Mental health nursing' was written by Dr Peter Nolan, assisted by Professor David Sines on 'people with learning difficulties' and reflects the upheavals in that service as it moves into the community. 'Health at work' was written by Paul Lloyd and Mavis Gordon of the Royal College of Nursing and is a reminder of nursing outside the National Health Service. 'Nurses as managers' and 'The road to reorganisation' was undertaken by Professor June Clark, who has advised on the book throughout and was associated with the second edition. Professor Clark has also updated the chapter on research.

One of the most important changes in the last decade has been the change in nursing education, the culmination of fifty years of reports, and who better to deal with it than Professor Margaret Green, herself the chairman of the Project 2000 Group Committee and the committee on PREP? Another area of confusing change has been in economic change and industrial relations, and we are grateful to Val Cowie, latterly of the Labour Relations Department of the Royal College of Nursing for bringing the chapter up to date. 'Health problems of the world', a depressing reassessment, was written by Muriel Skeet, a World Health Organisation consultant and an authority on the subject. Shelagh Murphy, secretary to the International Department of the Royal College of Nursing, undertook the revision of International and Inter-regional Organisations and the difficult task of dealing with the European Economic Community regulations. With the advice of Wendy Laughlin, Tutor, Bath and Swindon College of Nursing, I have revised the chapter on 'New problems for old in the community'. We are grateful to the team at Routledge for their help and suggestions in the revision of this book and for their patience with what has been a complicated undertaking.

Although over one-third of the book is new, it is worth looking back to see how many of our present problems have their precursors in the past. So often we have been here before. The Elizabethans chased up putative fathers with the object of making them responsible for their offspring, sturdy beggars were offered workfare, there was a prices and incomes scale and lone mothers were supported by the parish. Later the Speenhamland Scale was a method of income support.

The Victorians worried about rising claims for benefit and sought to find a solution in the workhouse test. They argued as fiercely about the cost of the Poor Rate as we do about the health service, and they eventually conceded that poverty led to ill health and unemployment which was itself a drain on the economy. Spurred on by Adam Smith they debated passionately about the extent to which the state should intervene in welfare and the labour market, and vacillated between *laissez-faire* and control.

Since the foundation of the Nightingale School we have continually discussed the composition and training of the nursing team. The idea of multiskilling is not new. Since the inception of the National Health Service, conferences and reports have advocated giving the patient more information and making hospitals more user-friendly. The organisation of the health service has gone from hospitals springing up at whim and in competition with one another, through an unbelievable saga of unification, organisation and reorganisation until the wheel has come full circle back to competition. In history it happens earlier than you think.

Today's students of nursing take a broad view of the health services, and they are more likely to look at the historical perspective and realise that if they do not know where they have come from they will not know where they are going, and, if they do not understand the past, they will be destined for ever to repeat its mistakes.

Bath, 1994

Chapter 1

Social change and attitudes to care

Not to know what took place before you were born is to remain forever a child.

Cicero

Nursing has developed as a response to changing social needs. As the structure of society alters, so new demands for health care arise; new habits and customs alter the disease pattern while changes in the size and composition of the population create fresh problems for sanitation and community living. These changes are continuous and tend to accelerate as knowledge accumulates, but they are not only perpetual, they are also erratic. In some periods development seems so slow that variations in the structure of society are almost imperceptible, at other times circumstances combine to produce change so quickly that the whole social basis of society alters in one generation, and with these rapid changes come new ideas about 'rights' and responsibilities, and indeed the whole social purpose. It was not coincidental that the ideas of the so-called Enlightenment, the precursor of the French Revolution, should have occurred in the same broad spectrum of time as American independence, Thomas Paine's *Rights of Man* and the change in much of Europe from an agrarian to an industrial society.

There is considerable controversy among social scientists about what is crucial to, and above all what initiates, social change. Marxists believe the key factor to be the technology of production, and Marx himself argued that productivity was the primary determinant of all social organisation and that the philosophical, religious and political ideas and values by which men have interpreted society were secondary and derivative – a theory Marx described as 'the material conception of history'. However, other sociologists such as Max Weber have denied the purely Marxian dialectic and have argued that ideas, particularly religious ideas, have had profound consequences for social change. Weber himself and other historians confidently asserted that there was a strong relationship between seventeenth-century Puritanism and the rise of capitalism,[1] while Halévy claimed that in the late eighteenth century working-class conversions to Methodism saved England from a revolution similar to that in France.[2]

Within these two schools of thought, the economic and the history of ideas, there are many sub-divisions, and, depending on their bias, sociologists stress different aspects in what they believe to be the most significant force for fostering change. Some emphasise the importance of changes in communications and the far-reaching effects of printing in the fifteenth century, or the fact that the 'take-off into growth'[3] occurred when man could at last travel faster than a horse. Again, demographic change is always linked in a complicated way with social and economic change; sometimes as with the depopulation of much of Europe in the late fourteenth century it seems to cause economic change, whereas at other times, as in the nineteenth century, it appears to be both a cause and a consequence of social change.

Other candidates for social change are the scientific revolution, war and racial conflict, the use and abuse of power, the effect of the mass media in moulding public opinion and the power of pollsters and sociologists to bring about change by self-fulfilling prophecies and what is sometimes known as 'the definition of the situation'.[4] If sociologists announce that nurses leave because of harsh discipline there is a tendency for nurses, and their relatives, to look for harsh discipline and see it even in the simple restraints required for communal living. In the study of history it is important to remember that what men *believe* to be true is often as significant as what *is* true.

Although opinions differ as to what is fundamental to social change there is no doubt that the pattern of society changes, and as it does so it produces new health needs in the community. Whether society attempts to meet these new health needs and whether it meets them with any degree of success depends on a variety of factors which include religious attitudes and beliefs, cultural patterns, economic resource together with population change, the state of knowledge and the way in which health care is organised and delivered.

RELIGIOUS ATTITUDES AND BELIEFS

Primitive belief

Primitive man attributed disease and epidemic to evil spirits, which he sought to drive out by means of magic. The early myths about the birth of Asclepius and his connection with snakes and the underworld and the fact that worshippers who sacrificed at his shrine would be cured through the agency of dreams has an obvious psychological significance in what Freud called 'the collective mind'.[5] Often illness and misfortune were thought to be due to the breaking of a taboo or the failure to perform a ritual, and this could only be expiated by the correct sacrifice, and in many parts of the world there are still taboos and rituals about pregnancy, childbirth and death, indicating our debt to the collective unconscious.

Particularly important in the study of mental ill health is the age-old idea of suffering as a result of sin; moreover, as in the Oedipus myth, the gods could inflict punishment even when the sin was not consciously committed. Linked with this was the idea of symbolic appeasement, where the sins of the community could be laid on a sacrificial animal, usually the goat, who became the 'scapegoat',[6] or in Christian symbolism, the lamb. Other societies and cults believed that evil could be transferred to an animate or inanimate object of which the effigy was the most familiar, including a model of the afflicted part of the body. By burning the image, or sticking pins in it, the 'evil' was destroyed. The apparent ability of some persons to assist in this transference of evil led to witchcraft, devil doctors and sorcerers who ran a profitable trade until the Church in its endeavour to root out heresy connoted witches with the devil himself and ordered their burning.

Anthropomorphic religion

This was the stepping-stone between primitive magic and the monotheistic religions. With social growth men moved away from primitive belief and animism, and in the more sophisticated societies these spirits were translated into anthropomorphic gods and goddesses. Now, as Frazer suggests, 'more thoughtful men were looking for a truer theory of nature and were questioning the efficacy of magic'.[7] In Greece the period is strikingly illustrated by Homer and the early classical playwrights; but while the Olympian hierarchy brought some order to the chaos of primitive belief, because it incorporated so much primeval superstition it became impossibly complicated. Behind every sophisticated Greek myth there lies an older, darker and deeper configuration. Confusion led to questioning, for while it was possible to blame disaster on vague spirits, it was less easy for intelligent men to accept the irrational behaviour of personalised gods who threw thunderbolts at will. By the fourth century BC the observant had begun to notice a causal relationship between disaster and physical phenomena, and some, like Aristophanes, began to ridicule the Olympians and their deeds. It was this same spirit of questioning and scepticism that produced the new approach to disease exemplified by Hippocrates and Aristotle (see Chapter 2). At the same time Socrates (469–399 BC) and his disciple, Plato (427–348 BC), were laying the foundations of logical thought and encouraging deductive reasoning. Plato, by connecting knowledge with ideas of virtue and love, and in his new conception of 'God' and the relationship of religion with morality, exercised a great influence on subsequent philosophers and paved the way for Christianity, which in some ways he helped to shape.

Christianity

By the time Paul and Barnabas brought Christian teaching to Asia Minor in the first century AD there was already fertile soil for the seed. Christianity appealed to the philosophers in the Greek tradition as a rational system of thought, and at the same time commended itself to the poor and humble-minded. With its roots in older Hebrew and Hellenistic thought it had, as Gilbert Murray pointed out, 'a strange subterranean power with a new humanity and intense feeling of brotherhood and incessant care for the, poor'.[8]

Christianity was an important influence on attitudes to suffering soon manifest in new movements for the care of the sick, such as the appointment of deacons and deaconesses to administer charity and to visit the sick in their homes, a movement many subsequent reformers sought to emulate. Much of the Gospel is about attitudes to the poor, the sick and the disabled, and the Good Samaritan who bound up the wounds is the ideal for the Christian to copy. Curiously enough, however, the early Church was ambivalent in its attitude to suffering; the early Christians had a profound Messianic faith which meant that they viewed this transitory life as of little consequence and only to be endured as a passport to the life and the world to come. Did not Lazarus, whose sores were licked by the dogs, rest on the bosom of Father Abraham? Not only did this engender a passive attitude to sickness, it was also antipathetic to any enquiry into the cause of disease, and as the Church put forward more extreme dogma, enquiry became equated with heresy, a sin calling for excommunication. Moreover, it must be remembered that cure in the Gospels was always apparently achieved by a miracle; cure therefore was in the hands of God, and all men could do was to assist by faith and prayer. So it came about that the first religion to be based on compassion and brotherly love discouraged scientific understanding, and while ideals of care were promoted their effect was hampered by the lack of knowledge.

The Reformation and the evangelical revival

However, attitudes to care and 'good works' may vary within a major religion, and Christianity in its chequered path has produced a wide range of beliefs, dogmas and schisms which have at times resulted in bitter controversy and war. In the sixteenth century two main faiths emerged, each determined to conquer the Christian world, and in the terrible conflict that followed many of the attitudes of compassion fostered by the earlier Church passed into oblivion – a sad characteristic of religious and ideological warfare. As the strife subsided the philosophies of the different faiths showed themselves in different attitudes to care. The Catholic Reformation, with its doctrine based on faith and works, saw an upsurge in corporate care and the founding of a number of new orders with practical concerns in the world, many of which were concerned with nursing the sick. The Protestants, on the other hand, with their insistence on 'justification by faith alone' and personal 'election' tended to emphasise individual and family duty, and there arose what has been described by sociologists as the Protestant ethic, where, it is alleged, there is a congruence between the ascetic Protestant and the value attitudes this produces in certain personalities. Although the pattern of behaviour has its roots in religious belief, it is in fact acted out in attitudes to work, wealth and philanthropy, and this is seen as underlying many of the charitable endeavours of the eighteenth century, including the endowing of hospitals.

As the more extreme attitudes of Calvinistic predestination and dissent modified in the eighteenth century, many Protestants adopted new attitudes based on evangelical teaching, and groups like the Wesleyans and the Quakers with their human and social concerns began to flourish. These attitudes coincided with the scientific thought of the period, which was largely engendered by the Nonconformists, who, because they were excluded from the universities by the Test Act, had established their own superior schools which had a bias towards the practical and to industry, in which so many eminent Nonconformists were interested. Thus, Protestant philanthropy, yoked to science and rational thought, paved the way for a new attitude to illness which was to come to fulfilment in the following century.

Islam

By contrast with Christianity, Islam, also a religion based on the duty of man to God and his neighbour, exhorted man to enquire. Islam, in turn, produced a number of sects and mystical philosophies many of which reflected what it had absorbed from its conquered territories, including the Greek medical writings from the library at Alexandria. For a few centuries after the death of the prophet, Mohammed (AD 632), Islam led the world in medical knowledge. Adopting the methods of Hippocrates and Galen, the Arabs advanced the idea of disease entities and organised a hospital system where treatment was free and patients were nursed according to their different ailments by attendants under the supervision of a physician. Two of these physicians, Avicenna (980–1036) and Averroes (1126–98) have earned themselves places in the history of medicine and philosophy. Both wrote commentaries on, and translated the works of, Aristotle, and as these works were translated into Latin new versions entered the corpus of western European medicine. Having been written in Greek and subsequently filtered through Arabic and Latin to the vernacular of the practising physician, it is small wonder that medieval medicine bore little resemblance to the Greek original.

Eventually war and economic decline disrupted the Islamic world and its medical practice, and teaching deteriorated. However, before the light went out much of the Arabic progressive thought, and its dubious translations, had passed via travellers to the growing universities of Europe, of which some – such as Salerno, Bologna and Paris – specialised in training physicians.

CULTURAL PATTERNS

The cultural pattern of a society, although enduring, is always changing, and these changes affect attitudes to life, death and sickness. Provided they do not conflict with fundamental tenets new ideas are absorbed by what is known as 'syncretisation'; new concepts are more easily accepted if they in some way relate to old ideas; for example, societies with ritual washing procedures accept notions of hygiene more readily than those who have no such tradition. Syncretisation is easier with ethnic groups and cultures which have already been exposed to scientific ideas, but too rapid absorption may produce conflict and the disruption will exacerbate the difference between old and new groups and between the generations. In societies where women are kept at home and not exposed to new influences, rapid change may exaggerate the difference in the rate of adaptation between men and women and make the cultural shock all the greater when it does come.

Cultural attitudes to care are often bound up with religious practice and sanction. Many pagan societies left the weak and the deformed on the hillside to perish – Oedipus being the classic example. Other societies controlled their populations by infanticide, and McKeown and others have pointed out that this was more widespread in England in the eighteenth century than we care to believe.[9] Primitive societies had, and still have in many parts of the world, a number of ways of keeping their populations within their capacity to feed them. Cultural patterns about abortion, infanticide, a prolonged post-natal period and homosexuality may well be conditioned by whether the society in question is aggressive and wishes to expand, or whether it is static and concerned with the threat of over-population. The polarisation of these concerns affects not only attitudes to infant care and the protection of child life, but also customs about betrothal, marriage, the age of marriage, monogamy and a whole range of kinship patterns.

However, not only are there cultural differences to care between races and different historical periods, there are also differences between occupational classes which seem to have a certain periodicity. Examples are the limitation of family size and the higher divorce rates of the upper classes at the beginning of the century, which have now spread to all classes. Until the interest in child psychology, the higher income groups turned out their offspring to boarding schools at a tender age; now the middle classes read Dr Spock and working-class mothers leave their children in the crèche all day. As the population profile alters, so do the traditional attitudes to the older generation. The nuclear family has replaced the old extended family, and at the same time pensions and retirement attitudes have changed the accepted life style of older people, who are more independent and active than previously. This is not because the young care less but because attitudes to age are changing.

POPULATION PATTERNS AND ECONOMIC RESOURCE

Population changes and economic fluctuations were in the past always interrelated and interdependent. Although records before the nineteenth century are scarce, evidence suggests that in subsistence societies there is a set pattern of births and deaths; death rates range from 35 to 55 per thousand population while the birth rate remains slightly higher to give a growth rate of 0.5 to 1 per cent. Even this growth would be too much for resources, but the ecological balance is maintained by the historical tendency of the death rate to produce dramatic peaks. Apart from war, the main reason for these peaks is the propensity of population aggregations to outstrip food supplies and in their under-nourished state to become prey to pathological micro-organisms. Pestilence and famine, the twin fears of subsistence communities, keep the population roughly in balance.

However, it takes little to change this balance; a little more food or the elimination of the plague for a few years makes all the difference. During the early years of the eighteenth century the death rate was high in most of Europe, then the population began to increase dramatically, although at different speeds in different areas. The reasons for this increase are complicated and still the subject of debate; McKeown and the medical demographers favour the idea that there was a fall in mortality due to better nutrition and marginally better hygiene, while other historians suggest that there was a rise in fertility. Whatever the cause, there was a period when the death rate was falling and the birth rate remained comparatively high; this is known as demographic transition (see Figure 1.1), and it is crucial, not only to the understanding of the problem of the nineteenth century, but to an understanding of the health problems facing the rapidly developing countries. Eventually the 'transition' moves into stage three, because as it becomes clear that fewer children are needed for replacement and child labour no longer has significance, the birth rate tends to fall; but the population continues to grow, although now more slowly because people are living longer – the shape of the population profile has changed (see Figure 1.2).

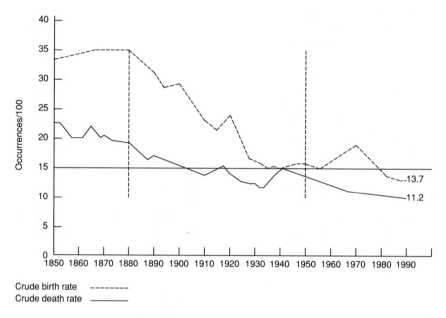

Crude birth rate   ‑ ‑ ‑ ‑ ‑ ‑ ‑ ‑
Crude death rate   ——————

Figure 1.1 The demographic transition in England and Wales

This demographic transition is perhaps the most dramatic factor in determining attitudes to care. Within a single life time the infant mortality rate fell from 154 per thousand live births to 17 per thousand, and the major concern of the health services has changed from child care to geriatric care.

Population growth, industrialisation and urbanisation are intrinsically linked, although the extent to which population pressure creates technological change and innovation is arguable. Some historians believe that rapid population growth delays innovation because, while there is a pool of cheap labour, there is no need to find new methods; this argument is supported by the long delay in taking weaving into the factories – the weavers were earning less and less and, while they turned out cheap cloth, why spend money on a factory? However this is by no means the whole story: population pressure also creates a growing market. Although industrialisation and urbanisation create new health hazards, countries that industrialise also increase their gross national product and are able to offer health programmes undreamed of in agrarian societies.

THE STATE OF KNOWLEDGE

From Galen to Harvey in the seventeenth century there was little advance in medical knowledge. Moreover, even after Harvey's discovery of the

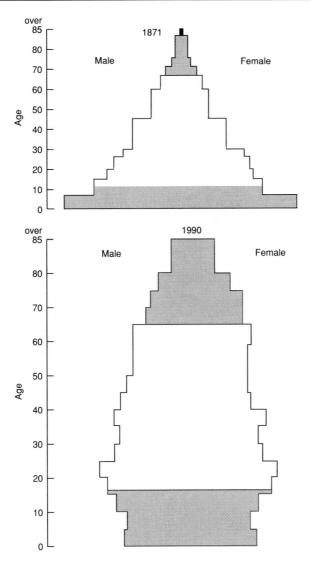

Figure 1.2 Population profiles, 1871 and 1990
Note: Shaded areas indicate dependent population (children and elderly population)

circulation of the blood and the so-called scientific revolution following Newton's *Principia Mathematica* (1687), the new knowledge made little difference to the health of the population. The impressive array of medical treatises were largely academic, and although Edward Jenner's discovery of a vaccine against smallpox in 1796 might have been a breakthrough, it was not effective until vaccination was made compulsory in 1853 – by which time smallpox was declining. Indeed, it is doubtful if medicine was any significant benefit to mankind until the late nineteenth century; improvements in health – and the growth of the population – resulted from better feeding, housing and, above all, sanitation.

At the end of the nineteenth century, after the discoveries of men like Pasteur and Koch, it suddenly appeared as if the millennium was in sight; as each successive micro-organism yielded up its secret all diseases seemed preventable or curable. However, it must be remembered that these developments were linked to, and interdependent with, the upheavals in society, and paradoxically some of these new discoveries related to the diseases that had been fanned by industrialisation and urbanisation. But the fact that doctors could now *cure* created a new attitude to medicine; now people began to have different expectations of doctors and of a health service. This concept of scientific medicine able to cure coincided with the reformation of nursing and the idea of nursing as a profession, and profoundly affected its development in the next century. Nurses, particularly hospital nurses, were seen as auxiliaries to the doctors who would provide cure. As they caught the reflected glory of scientific doctors – the Sir Patrick Cullens of Shaw's *The Doctor's Dilemma* who discoursed on phagocytes – the nurses became 'scientific' and attached to the new technology.

However, increasing scientific and technical knowledge has brought a number of problems, not least of which is increased specialisation and fragmentation to the detriment of total care. Furthermore, by curing and preventing bacterial disease more non-pathological illness has been uncovered, and this is just as disabling, but is less likely to yield to the advances of scientific knowledge. Recent critics, like Illich, have pointed out that disease cannot be considered 'as an isolated entity; it takes place in the context of the patient's total environment of which only the patient himself is aware', and 'effective care is dependent on self care'.[10] But, paradoxically, the vast increase in medical knowledge during the twentieth century has created a gap between the patient and the medical élite with whom the ordinary citizen feels he cannot compete. To quote Thomas Szasz, 'Life itself is now viewed as an illness which begins with conception and ends with death, requiring at every step along the way the skilful assistance of physicians, especially mental health professionals.'

There is no denying that the incredible burst of medical knowledge in the twentieth century has both prolonged life and often improved its quality. It comes as a shock to read of eminent Victorians and to realise how much of their lives were spent in illness and disability, often apparently due to chronic bacterial infection. But the bacteria have been largely conquered and people are still ill; now much ill health arises from the way people live, and since the present determinants of health again lie outside scientific medicine, health workers must extend their studies to a number of related fields including psychology, sociology and the behavioural sciences.

THE ORGANISATION OF THE HEALTH SERVICES

Economic advance, scientific knowledge and compassionate attitudes do not of themselves ensure that the demands for health care are met. Improved health standards also depend on how wealth is distributed and medical care organised. In the integrated, corporate life of the Middle Ages most organised care came through the agency of religion; then, in more secular times this was replaced by the parish and by private philanthropy. But as medicine advanced and the demand for care grew, the problems of providing care became beyond the scope of private charity, and increasingly it has become the concern of the state or large insurance schemes. Throughout the western world, and much of the developing world, there are many variations on state and insurance schemes, from countries like Britain where the state is the main provider, to the United States where care is largely provided through insurance schemes. But although the developed countries spend marginally different proportions of their gross national product on health care, the results in terms of life expectancy, infant mortality and morbidity rates are more than marginally disparate. Finding a yardstick for measuring health care is notoriously difficult, but one thing is certain: measurement must be concerned with the general quality of life as well as the more spectacular advances in prolonging life. Unless all members of society are equally valued in an integrated community there will always be gaps in health care.

REFERENCES

1 Weber, M. (1930) *The Protestant Ethic and the Rise of Capitalism* trans. Talcott Parsons, London: Allen & Unwin; also Tawney, R. (1938) *Religion and the Rise of Capitalism*, London: Penguin Books.
2 Halévy, Elie (1913–23), *History of the English People*, London: Benn; 7 volumes reissued in translations published 1947–52.
3 Rostow, W. W. (1960) *The Stages of Economic Growth*, London: Cambridge University Press.
4 Thomas, W. I. (1923) *The Unadjusted Girl*, Boston: Little Brown.
5 Freud, S. (1938) *The Psychopathology of Everyday Life*, London: Penguin Books, p. 232; see also Freud (1950), *Totem and Taboo* London: Routledge.
6 Frazer, J. G. (1950) *The Golden Bough*, London: Macmillan, chs 55–8.
7 Ibid., chs 4–6.
8 Murray, G. (1935) *Five Stages of Greek Religion*, London: Watts, ch. 5.
9 McKeown, T. (1976) *The Modern Rise of Population*, London: Arnold.
10 Illich, I. (1975) *Medical Nemesis*, London: Calder & Boyars Ltd; see also Szasz, T. (1973) *Ideology and Insanity*, London: Penguin Books.

FURTHER READING

Cipolla, C. (1974) *The Economic History of World Population*, London: Penguin Books.
McKeown, T. and Lowe, C. R. (1966) *An Introduction to Social Medicine*, 2nd edn. 1974, Oxford, London: Blackwell Scientific Publications.
Mills, C. Wright (1962) *The Marxists*, London: Penguin Books.

Chapter 2

Change and care before the Reformation

Over 10,000 years ago predatory man, probably aided by climatic change, discovered the use of domestic animals and agriculture, thus bringing about the first agricultural revolution. Then, some time before 3000 BC men began to explore the possibilities of working metal, and eventually with the use of iron for tools they gained a new ascendancy over the environment. The greater control of the biological converters, plants and animals, led to a larger and more dependable food supply, so that populations increased and people began to live together in ports and cities.

Of the peoples of the Near East and the Mediterranean the Greeks exploited these changes most fully. Ionia was the meeting point for earlier cultures, and the Greeks, untrammelled by traditions of earlier ages, were able to synthesise old ideas and graft on new ones. The long coastline and the seafaring tradition gave opportunities for trade and the exchange of ideas, while pressure from the tribes in the north forced expansion and emigration. Greek progressive thought lasted over 600 years until the first century after Christ, during which time advances were made in the study of mathematics, physics and astronomy; there was a flowering of philosophy and scholarship, and works of art became more realistic. In this atmosphere of enquiry men began to look afresh at the causes of disease and ill health. New problems had arisen, the crowding of people into towns made them more vulnerable, and there were now difficulties in public water supply and sanitation; moreover, the effect of an epidemic in a town was easily observable and, with the advance of literacy, these effects were recorded. A striking example of this is the account of the 'plague' during the Peloponnesian war in Athens in 429 BC by the historian Thucydides, who, as he says, for the sake of posterity, left a detailed description of the signs and symptoms, but for all his lucidity and the tracing of the epidemic to its source in Ethiopia, the diagnosis of this particular outbreak has continued to elude medical historians. However, Thucydides makes the important point that the infection spread rapidly because the port of Piraeus and the city of Athens were crowded with refugees from the war, many of whom were already under-nourished, and that there were many houses 'where people perished through lack of attention'. When people did visit the sick they often caught the infection and lost their own lives, and while compassion was not a particular Greek characteristic, visiting the sick at risk to yourself was obviously considered to be a point of honour.[1]

THE BEGINNING OF SCIENTIFIC MEDICINE

There gradually evolved three approaches to disease. With its roots in the primitive past, temple medicine still flourished and sufferers came to the sanctuaries of Asclepius to be cured through their dreams or by the sacred serpents. Snakes in primitive mythology were considered symbols of rejuvenescence and healing because of their ability to slough their skins, it is therefore a little ironical that this symbol of superstition should still provide the emblem for scientific medical journals.

The second approach was through the various schools of philosophy. By the fifth century BC philosophy meant the endeavour to understand and to teach men how to live wisely and well, and this involved holding the right opinions about God, the world, man and virtue, and because of this, the later philosophers began to be interested in the practical problems of everyday behaviour that destroyed the peace of mind of individuals. These various philosophical schools added to the theories about health but took no part in medical practice. The third approach was the rational school of medicine, and this made the greatest contribution to medical knowledge and had far-reaching effects. The rational schools had many disciples and Greek physicians were famed over the Graeco-Roman world, but three men stand out, whose work, often mistranslated and misunderstood, dominated much of medicine for the next 1,500 years.

Hippocrates

Hippocrates (c. 460 BC) is often considered the father of medicine. Born on the island of Cos he was the son of a physician and is important because he left us a picture of what a physician ought to be: kind, observant, calm, courteous and, above all, incorruptible. Hippocrates' code of ethics and the oath associated with his name are still acceptable, and although the oath is no longer administered it is still worth recalling when considering whether patients' notes are confidential.

The other great Hippocratic contribution was the method. In his 'Airs, waters and places' Hippocrates uses methods of observation and recording that enabled him to develop the concept of disease entities where, although each patient was different, there were sufficient common characteristics to justify a special name for the disease, and much medical nomenclature derives from this source. Observation was based on bedside care; κλινικος means 'to do with beds' and denotes the clinical situation, a term now misused to describe situations and places that have nothing to do with bedside care. The 'Collection of aphorisms' gives some perspicacious descriptions and observations, many of which have remained in the literature to the present century; tuberculosis, malaria and mumps are described with accuracy and for the first time epilepsy is seen as having a natural rather than a supernatural cause. The aphorisms and the body of knowledge collected by the Hippocratic School comprised a whole library and was eventually handed down to future generations through the famous medical library of Alexandria.

Aristotle

Aristotle (382–322 BC) was also the son of a physician and, at an early age, a pupil of Plato to whom he gave twenty years of devoted discipleship although later he dissented from much of Plato's teaching. His varied life included lecturing and writing, and he was a tutor to Alexander the Great and ran a school of philosophy in Athens. Like Hippocrates, his systematic and catalogued library eventually came down to posterity through many viscissitudes and exerted great influence. To the Middle Ages he was 'the Philosopher' and this led to some strange results because he was venerated on the two subjects on which he went farthest astray – astronomy and medicine. Apart from this he was famed for his system of deductive logic in which he explored the science of reasoning, and for his works on ethics, metaphysics and politics.

In astronomy Aristotle believed that the earth was a solid, stationary ball at the centre of the universe; between the earth and the outer ring of fixed stars lay concentric crystalline spheres upon which were embedded the sun, moon and planets. Aristotelian physics proceed from the assumption that there are two kinds of motion, natural and unnatural. On earth, beneath the moon's orbit, things moved in straight lines, stones fell down, sparks flew up; everything moved to its proper place. Above the lunar sphere were the incorruptible heavenly bodies whose motion was always circular, which was to medieval man the perfect movement and the circle the perfect shape. This idea persisted until the seventeenth century when Newton showed that the physical laws of the earth apply throughout the universe. The advantage of the Aristotelian system was that it was immediately comprehensible, the earth does appear stationary, and it all dovetailed neatly into conventional Christianity with man at the centre of the universe. However, the other outcome was that man was related firmly within the cosmological system and to the planets, whose movements governed his life and often his sickness and health: theories of health and disease were therefore bound up with astrology, it was 'what the stars foretell' with a vengeance.

Another aspect of Artistotle's teaching which had a profound effect on medieval medicine was his misunderstanding of the circulatory system and his theory of the four humours: blood, water, yellow bile and black bile. Excess of these was thought to correspond with the main temperaments of man; that is, sanguine, phlegmatic, choleric and melancholic. The importance of the correction of these 'imbalances' dominated much medieval medicine and accounts for the fact that treatment was often based on purging, starving and blood-letting until well into the nineteenth century, with leeches still around in the twentieth. That Aristotle strode the medieval world like a Colossus can be seen in the wealth of Aristotelian allusions and imagery, both cosmological and medical, to be found in sixteenth and seventeenth century literature, of which Shakespeare, Marlowe and Jonson provide a rich harvest.

Galen of Pergamon

Galen of Pergamon (AD 129–199) is perhaps a figure more sympathetic to modern thought and philosophy, still much influenced by Platonic ideas, though he lived 400 years later. He was a Stoic, but at odds with that philosophy because of his insistence that the body had been formed for a known and intelligible purpose by a Creator, and for this reason his theories appealed to Christians and Muslims alike. Galen, like Aristotle, advanced the study of anatomy, leaving accurate descriptions of bones and pioneer work on muscles – he dissected Rhesus monkeys and showed the detailed insertions and functioning; he based his physiology on the 'pneumo' – the breath of life drawn from a world spirit, and from the idea that the main vessels carried both air and blood. Although his system bears some relationship to the main vessels and organs because he had no knowledge of the chemistry of the blood or the gaseous exchange, he completely misinterpreted the respiratory and circulatory systems, an error that remained until Harvey in the seventeenth century.

In AD 161 Galen went to Rome and became physician to Marcus Aurelius; here he demonstrated anatomy and practised medicine, and, amid professional jealousy and acrimony, left his picture of the philosopher doctor in a treatise that has strong Platonic overtones.[2] Much of Galen's work has a modern ring; in writing of the effect of occupation on health he says, 'the life of many men is in the involved business of their occupation, and it is inevitable that they should be harmed by what they do and that it should be impossible to change it.'[3] Although Galen maintained that health was a condition of perfect equilibrium, he was prepared to overlook small ailments and excluded from ill health 'all conditions and lack of vigour which are the natural accompaniment of old age' – a precept which might with profit be reinstated. However, it is in the concept of population disease occurrence that Galen made his greatest contribution; he postulated that epidemics depended on three main factors, the atmosphere and the environment, the susceptibility of members of the population and the fact that certain kinds of behaviour had an effect on the genesis of disease. In other words, the predisposing factors were environment, susceptibility or immunity and modes of behaviour.

Although the Greek physicians did not understand the causes of infectious disease they realised from observation there was a link between hygiene and health and therefore took steps to improve civic sanitation. Physicians were appointed to administer health matters in towns and to care for people unable to afford a fee. Attempts were made to ensure clean water, proper burial facilities and the drainage of marshes, the atmosphere from which was thought to induce malaria – the scourge of the Graeco-Roman world. The other main Greek contribution was the emphasis on positive health; physical and mental health were seen as related, and general education included physical training in the gymnasia and baths, and under the dictum of 'moderation in all things' harmony in healthy living was encouraged.

THE COMING OF CHRISTIANITY

Galen had been a friend of the Emperor Marcus Aurelius and his writing influenced Roman medicine; the Romans, although they did not rate physicians highly, valued public health and the Greek tradition of *mens sana in corpore sano*. When the Roman Empire declined and the tribes from the north overran Rome, most of this tradition was lost. However, as the Christian Church slowly ousted paganism it absorbed some of the knowledge of the Greek and Roman schools which it preserved in the various institutions it set up across Europe.

In the first century the Church organised women called deaconesses to visit the sick and needy, and Paul himself, although misogynic in outlook with no high opinion of the constancy of women, did commend women to 'good works', and in the Epistle to the Romans praised Phoebe who held office in the congregation at Cenchrea and who was 'the good friend to many'. After the official recognition of Christianity in AD 335, the Christian deaconesses inspired a number of converts to take up the nursing of the sick. For a short period nursing seems to have had a vogue among disillusioned upper-class Roman women who, as the temporal world of Rome fell about them, tried to find salvation through works of charity. St Jerome (AD 340–420), also by no means predisposed towards women, has left us a picture of how Fabiola (d. AD 399) cared for and carried the sick and 'washed their putrid matter that others could not bear to look on'. Paula, another ardent Christian accompanied St Jerome to Bethlehem, and founded three convents for women over which she herself presided and which carried on the tradition of giving care to the sick. However, as Christianity became official, devout men and women, fearing material corruption, began to move into isolation. At first they were eremites, then later monasteries were established and the early Christian tradition of nursing the sick in their own homes was lost, a tradition to which in later centuries reformers like Pastor Fliedner sought to return.

Although the early monasteries had withdrawn from the world, the monks remained the custodians of much medical writing, which they put into practice not for the benefit of ordinary people but on behalf of their sick brethren. As time passed some orders, particularly those of St Benedict (480–544) – the first of the great western Church orders – and later the rule of St Augustine, extended their ministrations to care for the sick who lived nearby. Care was now given to pilgrims and later monasteries began to provide buildings called *nosokomeions* – from the Greek *nosos* meaning disease – the remains of which can occasionally be seen in the ruins of dissolved monasteries. Although these houses gave some care and treatment, the understanding of illness was deterred because of the attitude of the Church to suffering; for the most part the unfortunate sufferers were washed and fed, purged and bled, prayed over, and prepared for the life and the world to come.

As the Church became more concerned with dogma there were times when there was a reversion to primitive belief and superstition. St Augustine of Hippo (345–430), who came to Christianity through a dual theology of God and Satan, was very influential, and in fact his writings inspired both Luther and Calvin some 1,200 years later. He firmly pronounced that 'All diseases are to be ascribed to demons'. This belief that illnesses were caused by evil spirits and that cure was in the hands of God alone had an important bearing on subsequent attempts at establishing a rational system of care; any endeavour to treat illness was bedevilled with a certain ambivalence of purpose.

SOCIAL AND ECONOMIC CHANGE IN EUROPE

With the spread of Christianity the sphere of influence shifted northwards, and during the eleventh and twelfth centuries there was comparative stability and economic growth; the population increased and trade prospered in what is sometimes known as the 'commercial revolution'. Throughout Europe extensive tracts of land owned by lay and ecclesiastical lords were let to lesser lords and freemen in return for service; land tenure was built on a complicated system of duties, rights and responsibilities varying from place to place. The serf or bondsman was governed by the demands of the lord's land, his own allotment and the observances required by the Church, whose ceremonies dominated men's lives from birth to death. The life of medieval man was probably as the philosopher Thomas Hobbes (1588–1679) described much later, 'poor, nasty, brutish and short'.[4] Short it may have been, but his other epithet, 'solitary', it was not. Between the guilds, the manor, the Church and the occasional excitements of miracle plays and the mummers with their vivid allegories, the life of medieval man was corporate and communal, a fact that had an important bearing on the meeting of his needs in time of want, but it also accounts for much of the anxiety suffered by sixteenth-century men when that corporate world was lost after the Reformation.

Unfortunately, this period of prosperity and growth was disturbed by population pressure. While the growing population had unused land easily exploitable there was no great problem, but without roads and transport, and with the constant fear of robbers, there was a limit to colonisation. In the absence of scientific knowledge about fertilisation the soil became impoverished and productivity fell, with the situation exacerbated by climatic disasters and a series of bad harvests. In 1315 torrential rains ruined harvests from the Pyrenees to Russia, and in the great famine that followed men were reduced to eating dogs. By the middle of the fourteenth century Europe was suffering from the weight of a population that had out-grown its strength; in places the peasantry faced starvation. Unwilling, or unable, to find new land further afield many of these starvelings sought employment in the towns which were growing in size throughout western Christendom. The crowded towns were insalubrious and the population of Europe was physically and mentally ill-equipped to withstand infection, for, although medieval man knew little about disease his spiritual mentors made sure that he regarded it as an affliction of the Almighty incurred because of the wickedness of man.

THE ILLS OF THE MEDIEVAL WORLD

Medieval man prayed to be delivered from those twin captains of death – famine and pestilence; when their prayers apparently received no answer they despaired, or turned to millenarianism, or looked to the stars or the supernatural for explanation. Here, Aristotelian cosmology conveniently came to their aid in the form of a comet or some unexplained planetary movement.

'Pestilence' was the term used to describe a variety of acute fevers, but the greatest scourge of the Middle Ages was undoubtedly the bubonic plague caused by *B. pestis* and transmitted by rats and fleas which had increased in number in parts of Europe. The great epidemic of 1348, after-wards known as the Black Death, came from the East and took hold of the ports of Genoa, Venice and Messina from which it appears to have spread with terrifying rapidity across Europe, leaving a trail of death and destruction unequalled in the annals. In the absence of reliable population records it is impossible to say how many people died; some estimates suggest that the population fell by one third, but this is a matter of contro-versy; what we do know is that the effects were uneven. We have Boccaccio's account of how Florence was devastated, but Venice seems to have escaped lightly; areas in the south of England were badly effected but the north east was almost free. Moreover, there is considerable debate over the medieval transition from feudalism and what caused the economic decline; most historians would now agree that the depopulation of the late fourteenth century was due to the previous over-population, and there had been economic decline before the successive waves of the plague hastened the restoration of population balance to what the land would support.

However, plague was not the only disease to spread from the East to scourge the debilitated population. Leprosy, a disease of antiquity, probably brought to Europe by infected crusaders, ravaged practically the whole continent; the incidence is not known because it was often used as a generic term to include such skin conditions as scrofula, lupus, yaws, scabies, psoriaris and skin cancer. Lepers were outlawed and 'declared dead' and kept in isolation in special leprosia, of which there were some 19,000 in Christendom. The lazars are interesting because they seem to have appealed to the highest-minded for charity and care, presumably because of their biblical connection, and secondly, because medieval doctors adopted the Hebrew ritual of making lepers outcasts and thus established that certain groups of patients – often those with rashes – should be isolated. Sometimes the right thing was done for the wrong reason.

Two other prevalent diseases were smallpox and syphilis; the 'small' and the 'great' poxes. 'Pox' was a collective term like 'plague' and was often used loosely or as an expletive. Smallpox came to Europe from Egypt via Spain in the twelfth century, its transmission probably assisted by the then fashionable pilgrimages to Compostela; it spread northwards and, until a policy of vaccination was established in the nineteenth century, it was one of the main causes of death in Europe, attacking rich and poor alike and at times altering the dynastic rule and even the balance of power.

The history of syphilis is more obscure; it may have come from the New World in the fifteenth century, or a new strain may have been added from another source; whatever the reason, there was an upsurge in the fifteenth century when it became widespread but imperfectly understood; in 1579 it was alleged that 15 out of every 20 patients attending St Bartholomew's hospital had the 'pox'. Gonorrhoea, on the other hand, had been described by the Greeks and the Arabs and was omnipresent, and was probably responsible for a good deal of blindness.

The Rickettsial diseases were commonplace and often referred to as 'fevers'; they were associated with rodents and lice and war and famine were their harbingers, they decimated armies and were prevalent in gaols, hospitals and asylums and were one of the reasons why care in institutions was a refuge of last resort.

For those who escaped death from plague, smallpox, typhus or violence there was always tuberculosis, which is probably the oldest known disease and was pandemic in Europe; its death rate is unknown but it is likely that inter-current infections claimed many tubercular victims; contrary to popular belief tuberculosis was probably declining in the first decades of the nineteenth century.[5] Apart from the bacterial and virus diseases there must have been much ill health due to malnutrition leading to a reduction in manpower, which in turn would lead to lowered productivity and a poorer supply of food; avitaminosis, scurvy and rickets undermined the health of a large section of the population until the agrarian reforms of the eighteenth century.

MEETING THE NEED FOR CARE IN THE MIDDLE AGES

The basic needs of men in the Middle Ages were for more and different food and better shelter; in the absence of these life was full of peril and could only be coped with by a faith that was strong enough to comprehend all ills as the will of God. Medieval man saw the Church, the saints and God as working together for his salvation and his physical and spiritual healing and protection, and it would be vain to look for separate categories of care in the modern manner. The integrated society was the hallmark of the age of faith, where mind, body and estate – temporal and spiritual welfare – were all as one, and for those who died well, holding the true faith, there was the certainty of the life hereafter.

In the twelfth and early thirteenth centuries Christendom was still an open society, with fluid frontiers and Latin the common language for the educated, with life dominated by the international trade routes and their Fairs, pilgrimages, the interchange of craftsmen and the intermarriage of the aristocracy. With the men away at the Crusades it was a period when women played an important part in society; they managed estates and even kingdoms, and with the foundation of so many nunneries it was the period of distinguished abbesses, some of whom, like Hildegarde of Bingen, had a strongly feminist attitude and urged women to start a *muliebre tempus*, an era of women, and rescue the failing Church from the weak hands of men. A spiritual revival with an emphasis on good works again made nursing fashionable; nobly born women were inspired to found hospitals and queens both founded institutions and nursed in them. In 1198, Pope Innocent III built the hospital of Santa Spirito for the poor in Rome, an example which led to further endowments; hospices like the *hôtels-Dieu* on the pilgrim routes were re-endowed, two English examples being St Bartholomew's (1123) on the northern route into London, and St Thomas's (1215) at Southwark. Another example was the transfer of St Mary's of Bethlehem, after the fourth Crusade, to Bishopsgate in London where later it specialised in giving protection to the insane.

However, what has been seen as an 'early Renaissance' was short-lived; the depopulation of the fourteenth century, the effect of the prolonged

wars in France, the economic decline and the attitude of the Church itself
in the conflict between the secular and spiritual leaders for dominance led
to a more closed society. National antagonisms arose and the foundations
were laid the division between east and west that still exist today, and for
the rise of Brandenburg and Habsburg Austria – in fact, most modern
political problems were prefigured at this stage.

Before this, Christendom had received its leadership from the monastic
orders. Man's highest duty was to lead a holy life but this could not be
achieved in a world of sin; for most men, therefore, perfection had to come
vicariously, and prayers centred on the monasteries that they would obtain
the necessary sanctity for salvation. But as time went by each group
seemed to fail: the ascetic became worldly, or the unworldly became too
far removed from the common touch, and there were constant calls for
'reform' by bishops, princes and laymen. It is this reforming movement
which is the connecting thread through the medieval Church and which
accounts for changes in attitudes towards the sick and suffering and good
works in the world.

The regular orders

The early monks of St Benedict and the rule ascribed to St Augustine, as
they proliferated, tended to live in the world, sharing the lives of the
common people and their daily needs. However, worldly involvement led
to the risk of contamination, for some in these circumstances sanctity
seemed impossible and there was a retreat to the cloisters. From time to
time monastic houses were reorganised with changes of emphasis on
contemplation or on good works; then in the twelfth century, with the
blessing of the papacy, there was a wave of new foundations created specifically for reform which included the Cluniacs, Carthusians and Cistercians,
who, turning their backs on the towns, sought solitude in the mountains
and on the moorlands. In England, the ruins of their once great buildings
still stand majestically on the Yorkshire moors or at places like Tintern.
Ironically, however, by the time most of these buildings were complete the
depopulation and the pessimism of the fourteenth century had set in and
there was little enthusiasm for the monastic ideal.

The secular clergy

Besides the monasteries there were the ordinary clergy of the parishes
within the various dioceses who generally had their episcopal sees in the
main cities. The cathedrals and large churches were specially endowed with
lands and revenues which supported colleges of priests, only some of whom
would be resident. Those of good education, the bishops or prebends,
would often hold key positions in the administration of the Church and

state and would be away from the diocese; the better parochial rectories were served by vicars and curates whose duties lay in serving the people in their parish. Apart from the parish clergy, there were other priests who were hired by individuals to say mass and perform other duties; the clerical section was, as Chaucer indicates, very large.

Popular religion and the uncloistered orders

Much popular religion was a mixture of folk religion and the inheritance from pre-Christian communities, but the early Church had tolerated this and managed to fuse them into a lively whole. How people cared for their sick reflected this synthesis of Christian faith and pagan superstition. But as time went by, with the monasteries becoming isolated, with the best of the secular clergy removed to administration, the mass in a language people did not understand and the Bible forbidden, men and women, seized with the spirit and convinced that Christ came in poverty and not in power, started various popular movements. Some of these appeared almost by accident, but in southern Europe there was a spate of sects like the Cathars, the Albigensians and the Waldensians, while in the Netherlands a group of women, following the priest Begue and later known as 'Beguines', tried to follow a religious life by helping the poor and the sick in the community but without taking vows, an undertaking that was immediately suspect.

Now instead of tolerating diversity the Church began to demand conformity. The Inquisition was set up in 1215, and Innocent III approved the Dominican order for the express purpose of converting heretics; when disputation failed the Dominicans and the authorities took more drastic action and thus began the great heresy hunt which was to darken the later part of the thirteenth century. Men and women whose only desire was to help mankind but to live a religious life without taking vows often found themselves denounced, and perished in the flames.

Some popular movements did escape; the Beguines were protected by the Dominicans, but not their brothers the Begards. St Francis of Assisi (1182–1226) did not intend to found an order, but as he and his followers begged and preached their way across Europe they drew under their wing a wide range of dissidents, including a number of women who were seeking a religious life outside the cloisters; for these, with the help of Clare of Assisi, St Francis founded the Poor Clares, who, as the 'Little Sisters' or the 'Minoresses', founded houses for the poor all over Europe. Although St Francis intended his brethren to be *humiliati* and to live in poverty, the new friars did in fact amass wealth and by 1282 the Franciscan order possessed 1,583 houses in Europe and, as Chaucer makes clear in the *Canterbury Tales*, they were soon subject to the same strictures as the monks before them. Other foundations of mendicant friars were the

Carmelites and the Austin Friars; the friars are important because they provided most of the organised care for the sick in England in the fourteenth century, and their hospitals sometimes became the basis of later foundations, for example, Grey Friar's Hospital for Foundlings after the dissolution of the monasteries was refounded as Christ's Hospital for poor children and later became a famous public school for boys. The friars are also important because their itinerant preaching and condemnation of wealth in the Church led to much debate and provided a curtain-raiser to the Reformation.

Unfortunately, antagonism developed between the regular clergy and the uncloistered orders and sometimes between both and the secular clergy; moreover, there were tensions between the right and left wings of the various orders and as this mounted groups were denounced as heretics, sometimes with bitter results as with the Hussites in Bohemia. Finally, in most countries in northern Europe both the regulars and the uncloistered orders lost their property as for one reason or another the monasteries were dissolved.

Military orders

In the middle of the eleventh century a hospice for pilgrims was built in Jerusalem and run by a group calling itself 'the order of St John'. During the Crusades (1095–1271) the order cared for a number of knights, and from the generous donations they received reconstituted themselves as the Knights of St John or the Knights Hospitallers. Apart from the order of St John there were the Templars, whose financial operations and arrogance eventually led to their tragic downfall in 1312, but whose mother house at Bethlehem was removed to London. The third order, the Teutonic Knights, were subsequently destined to play an important role in eastern Europe and in Baltic trade.

The Knights of St John were the true hospitallers; their concern was not with the poor but with the valuable lives of the crusaders. The Knights took a vow of obedience, chastity and poverty, but while they were strong on the first part they were somewhat weak on the other two parts. Although the Knights were renowned for their high standard of medical care and bravery they often struck Europeans as half pagan because they had become so acclimatised in dress and custom to the Near East; furthermore, the record of their personal quarrels and egotism suggests that the various 'langues' were more competitive than co-operative. Nevertheless, the examples of the Knights' hospitals remaining in Rhodes and Malta bear witness to their standards of excellence, and records in Rhodes suggest that the coverage on night duty in a ward might well be envied by a modern hospital. However, while the mobility and education of the Knights led them to be able to absorb new ideas about treatment and medicine –

especially those culled from the Arabs with whom they were in contact –
the same mobility led to the dissemination of disease and the gains made
were probably more than offset by the effect of disastrous new epidemics.

Village nursing

For the most part the sick were cared for in their own homes, which, in
spite of the prevalence of rats and other animal vectors of disease in their
daub and wattle dwellings, were probably the safest places. When the
family failed, as must have often been the case in the time of epidemic,
then there were neighbours, quacks, wise women, the midwife and witches
with their charms, simples, herbal remedies and concoctions that were
often neither simple nor herbal. Some gave care for a fixed fee, but the
offer to 'cure' was fraught with danger since it might be construed as black
magic and denounced; others gave help because succouring the sick was
clearly Christian duty. However, the expected life span was about twenty
years and only the fit survived childhood; death came most frequently from
violence, virulent infection and starvation, and for women the great hazard
was childbirth. In these circumstances it was probably of little moment
whether medieval man received medical or nursing care and for the most
part he expected neither. But, in the age of faith what he did expect was
the resurrection to eternal life and that 'vile bodies would be changed into
a glorious body'.

THE UNIVERSITIES

Until the twelfth century the monks, assisted by the barbers, performed
surgery, then in 1139, the second Lateran Council, in an attempt to reform
the Church, forbade the monks the letting of blood. Medieval doctrine held
that every man's body was in the image of Christ, and to wound a body or
to dissect a dead body was both impious and inhuman. This interdict left
the field clear for the barbers; those who practised surgery began to draw
away and formed themselves into guilds of surgeons, appointing masters
and taking on apprentices. Such advances in surgery as there were, were
mainly made by army surgeons, and in 1252 Bruno de Longoburgo
published the *Chirugia Magna* in Padua, but little progress was made until
the fifteenth century when men began to dissect animals and, like
Leonardo da Vinci (1452–1519), record their findings.

In England the Guilds of Surgeons and Barbers were separate; within
each there were different grades and they charged different fees accordingly. The fees caused friction and eventually, to overcome this, the guilds
were united by Henry VIII in the charter of 1540.

The medieval university was another aspect of the corporate life of the
times where students and scholars met for their mutual benefit. Learning

was based on the trivium and the quadrivium, which were the seven liberal arts – literally the skills appropriate to free men. It so happened that Italy, in contact with the classical world and the Arab and Byzantine cultures, placed a high premium on literacy; it is alleged that over 60 per cent of the children in Florence were attending school in 1338. Italy therefore attracted scholars to various centres and medicine was taught as an academic subject in the School of Salerno from the tenth century. From Salerno similar medical 'Schools' grew up in the growing universities in such places as Bologna, Padua, Paris, Oxford and St Andrews in Scotland. As with the Greeks, philosophy and medicine were closely linked, and the fundamental authorities were Aristotle and Galen and other classical writers who dealt with aspects of health. Medicine as such then was part of the liberal arts and viewed as a purely academic subject; those who graduated were licensed to teach by the conferment of the *Licentia docenda* and thus, physicians trained in universities became *doctors*.

In spite of what seems to have been academic study, the universities offered professional training. The Master of Arts corresponded with the master craftsman in other walks of life and was the training and qualification considered appropriate for theologians and physicians as well as for civil and canon lawyers, civil servants and the administrators who were to form the backbone of the public service in countries advancing to nationhood.

REFERENCES

1 Thucydides, *The Peloponnesian War*, translated by Rex Warner, London: Penguin Classics, Bk II ch. V, pp. 123–9.
2 Galen (AD 157) *Hygiene* quoted by Frazer Brockington in *World Health* (1958), London: Pelican Books, p. 161.
4 Hobbes, T. *The Leviathan*, Everyman Library (1914), London: Dent, Part I, ch. 13.
5 McKeown, T. and Lowe, C. R. *An Introduction to Social Medicine*, London: Blackwell Scientific Publications, p.8.

FURTHER READING

Heer, F. (1962) *The Medieval World*, London: Weidenfeld & Nicolson.
Inglis, B. (1965) *A History of Medicine*, London: Weidenfeld & Nicolson.
Leff, S. and V. (1956) *From Witchcraft to World Health*, London: Lawrence & Wishart.
Singer, C. and Underwood, E. A. (1962) *A Short History of Medicine*, London: Oxford University Press.
Webster, C. (ed.) (1979) *Health, Medicine and Mortality in the Sixteenth Century*, Cambridge: Cambridge University Press.
Ziegler, P. (1969) *The Black Death*, London: Collins.

Chapter 3

The sixteenth-century transition

The consequences of the fall in the population in the fourteenth century were far-reaching: there was profound despair as the epidemics became endemic and men either turned their faces to the wall or looked for salvation in arcane cults like millenarianism or astrology, neither of which was conducive to the return to normal life. Nevertheless, as the survivors took up the threads of life again there were a number of gains. Since the twelfth century there had been a tendency to commute rents in kind for money services, landlords found paid labour cheaper and more efficient and now the process was accelerated and villein holdings increased. At the same time instead of over-population, the demand for labour exceeded supply, and by the operation of the market mechanism, labourers claimed higher wages and in some cases these doubled. Attempts were made to curb the wage–price spiral but the Statute of Labourers 1349 and similar medieval efforts at prices and incomes control were unsuccessful because of the competition for labour. But the peasants' gain was often the landlords' loss. In order to make good the losses many made their farms less labour-intensive, or, taking advantage of the new purchasing power of the peasants, diversified and grew crops like hops, which caused the chroniclers to inveigh against the fact that the labourers would now only drink 'the best brown ale'.[1] However, the landlords who turned to sheep-farming were the most likely to recoup their fortunes for, as the crisis receded, the demand for clothing increased and, thanks to royal encouragement, there was an improvement in English cloth and more labour was attracted away from the land – never to return. The woolsack had become the symbol of wealth.

This accelerated emancipation replaced the old relationship between the lord and the villein with a new contractual relationship; there was now a growing landless class and, as Max Weber put it, 'the peasants were freed from the land and the land from the peasants'. The change from subsistence farming to producing for the market led to the growth of towns and the nucleus of what was to become an urban proletariat; depopulation and changes in farming laid the foundation for what some historians have claimed to be an early industrial revolution.[2]

These changes, the break-up of the feudal system and the high death rate had an important effect on the Church. The Church had suffered disproportionately from the plague; nearly half the beneficed clergy perished and some religious houses were obliterated. New recruits were trained but there were complaints that they lacked the educational and spiritual calibre of their predecessors, fewer were able to teach in French or Latin and this gave rise to the use of the vernacular as a means of communication, a change that was to be intensified by the invention of printing by Johan Gutenberg about 1453. Although printing had been known in China for centuries it had had little relevance for Europe, but now with a growing educated laity there was a new demand for books. The new process spread rapidly from Germany to Italy and then all over Europe; although printing did not of itself promote new ideas, it hastened the circulation of the existing ones and played an important role in spreading the ideas of the Renaissance and the Reformation.

THE NEW LEARNING AND THE RENAISSANCE

The rebirth or revival of ancient learning in Europe in the fourteenth to the sixteenth centuries was not a sudden break with the past, but circumstances combined to quicken change and break the pattern of medieval thought. European society became more secular, although still religious; more individual, although still dominated by institutions; and, although still held together by religious faith, more questioning.

Scholars attempted to rediscover the ideas and styles of the Greek and Roman civilisations. Those who recovered the linguistic skills and ideas were nicknamed 'humanists' because they concentrated on practical concerns like the art of speaking and writing and the political and social facets of life, rather than the old abstract medieval philosophy which was so often concerned with useless abstract disputation – a definition which should not be confused with the modern misuse of the term 'humanist'. Desiderus Erasmus, Colet and Sir Thomas More were all men of this 'new learning', and they and others like them were to be the inspiration for the new style of grammar school which was to be such a force in shaping European thought in the next few centuries.

New classical studies, together with the changed social and economic climate, led thinking members of society to place a new emphasis on the individuality of man and man's attitude to his uniqueness which manifested itself in the literature of the age, of which Shakespeare is the supreme example; in Shakespeare each character is an individual, superbly drawn with a clearly recognisable personality and psychological characteristics, and this is a far call from the symbolic figures of 'good' and 'evil' in the morality plays of a century earlier.

Change was also hastened by technological advance, and as occurred in the late eighteenth century, change fostered change. The development of the compass and the lateen rig aided exploration and colonisation, which in turn opened up new ideas about the nature of the world and led men to question the old authorities. The development of gunpowder and artillery not only changed the nature of war but the possibility of man's ascendancy over man, and this was particularly true in the field of colonisation where a few Europeans could subdue a whole indigenous population.

Technological change was contemporaneous with scientific discoveries that could not be fitted into the old medieval 'world view'. In 1530, Copernicus (1473–1543) put forward a theory that the sun was the centre of the universe around which other heavenly bodies moved, an idea that conflicted with the Aristotelian concept of the stationary world and the fixed heavens which constituted the very core of medieval philosophy – itself tied in with theories about sickness and health. Later, Galileo (1564–1642) made his important observations about velocity, which brought him into contact with the Inquisition, and in 1623 he was forced to recant his adherence to the Copernican theory. Nevertheless, in spite of these advances the Renaissance cannot be considered as a period of scientific advance, and for this reason there is little progress in medical knowledge, but the questioning, and the progress in the understanding of anatomy, laid the foundations for the scientific revolution of the seventeenth century.

One of the most important aspects of the Renaissance is that educated men and women truly believed that they were living in a period of great change and they felt themselves to be different from the Middle Ages, which they regarded as barbarous.[3] Perhaps this is best seen by looking at an altar piece of the fourteenth century and comparing it with a religious painting depicting the same subject by Raphael or Leonardo, which shows how quickly men moved away from symbolism to representing men and women as they really were.

THE REFORMATION

For some time men like John Wycliffe in England (1330–84) and John Hus in Bohemia (1373–1415) had attacked the corruption of the Church and had emphasised the importance of the Bible and its teachings, and to some extent this wave of anti-clericalism was bound up with the nationalistic and political aspirations of countries turning away from the old concept of Christendom and the universalist policies of the Holy Roman Empire – aspirations that were the bedrock of the Reformation. In the early sixteenth century the Church was attacked by scholars who were advocates of the new learning; Colet, Erasmus and other humanists tried to goad the

Church to reform from within – rather as the Franciscans had done two centuries earlier, and when they failed the denunciations became more outspoken and bitter. Further attacks came from Saxony where, in 1517, Martin Luther (1483–1546) nailed his ninety-five theses for debate on the door of the Castle church at Wittenberg. Luther, who was a monk and a theologian, and his friends were soon forced into a more radical argument at Worms, and in the Confessions of Augsburg in 1530 the 'reformed' doctrine was set out. This derived from the epistles of St Paul and the conviction that man's bridge to God was by faith alone and from this stemmed the idea of the 'priesthood of all believers' and the denial of the Catholic system of priestly intermediaries, the sacraments and supernatural aids such as intercession. 'Reform' now meant not only the reform of corrupt practice but a fundamental change in doctrine.

Apart from the dynamism of Luther himself there were other changes that accelerated 'reformation'. Of paramount importance was the invention of printing, for now the Bible was available to all; moreover, printing coincided with economic recovery and there was a growth in urbanisation and commerce and, whether or not there was a relationship between the 'Protestant ethic' and capitalism,[4] it is undeniable that the new faith had a greater appeal to townsmen. At the same time vernacular literature, dissidence in religious matters and vigorous national courts were fostering a growth in national feeling and the reformed faiths tended to become national, a development which was to have tragic consequences in the next century. Too late did the humanists now draw back; the Lutheran doctrinal message meant the break-up of the Catholic Church and the sundering of the unity of Christendom.

The fact that Europe was now divided into two aggressive faiths – Protestant and Catholic, each with its sub-divisions and each determined to conquer the Christian world – had profound consequences for the care of the sick. It was not because the monasteries were dissolved – as far as the sick were concerned they had long since ceased to have relevance – but that the challenge to the Catholic Church came together with the ideas of the Renaissance, and the old certainties about faith, duty and knowledge were gone for ever. Henceforth man was on a quest for new certainties which continually evaded him; knowledge overturned more knowledge, and of all the uncertainties the cause, meaning and the solution of social evils was the most elusive.

THE DISSOLUTION OF THE MONASTERIES

In England after the legal quibbles about the annulment of his marriage to Catherine of Aragon, in 1534 Henry VIII broke with the Pope and declared himself Supreme Head of the Church in England. As wealth had been dissipated by war and the troubles in Ireland, Henry and his advisers took advantage of the anti-clerical sentiments and looked to the monasteries as a way of replenishing the coffers, but Henry was, and remained, a Catholic. Dissolution was not a new idea; the monasteries were now out of step with the ideals of the Renaissance and the Church's landholding was so enormous that it had been attacked by social reformers of all shades. The Commissioners under Thomas Cromwell visited the monasteries to assess their wealth; then, as the financial situation grew more urgent, a statute was passed ordering the suppression of the smaller monasteries. About 40 per cent of the monks decided to leave the cloister and the rest were transferred. However, the need for money was still urgent and in 1539 the dissolution of the larger houses was ordered.

The plate and movables were transferred to the royal treasury and the sites of land sold off, with many districts still bearing the traces of their former ownership in their present name, a good indication of how much was owned by 'bishops', 'abbots', 'monks', 'canons', 'friars' and other clerics. The cathedral churches survived since they were part of Henry's plan for reorganisation, and in these there was considerable continuity of personnel. About 10,000 monks and nuns were displaced, but many heads of houses received bishoprics and others were absorbed into the parish system. The remainder were given pensions that were for the most part adequate and occasionally handsome – some were linked to the cost of living; a wise precaution with Tudor inflation. But while the monks often found employment either in or outside the Church, the nuns did less well, their dowers were meagre, and many must have suffered hardship when thrown into an indifferent and changed world.

The question remains why the men of the Renaissance made such efforts, often remarkably successfully, to replace the monastic education, scholarship, music, libraries and almsgiving with secular institutions but did apparently nothing for the sick, and why there was no hospital system to parallel the new grammar schools of Edward VI. The answer lies partly in the attitude to illness. The reformed Church in its various sects and the new Church of England, no less than the Catholic, held suffering to be the will of God; indeed, the extreme Protestants with their ideas about 'predestination' were in some ways more fatalistic. Cranmer (1489–1556), for all his devotion to the new learning and his connection with advanced thought in Europe, in his collects continually urges the endurance of things temporal that we may attain to the life eternal, and his prayer for deliverance from the plague and other common sickness which starts, 'O Lord God, who has punished us for our sins and consumed us for our transgressions by thy late and dreadful visitation . . .' shows little change from the medieval attitude. Secondly, in spite of the advances in the study of anatomy by men like Andreas Vesalius and Leonardo da Vinci, there was no advance about the causation of disease; Renaissance man was as far from the truth in this respect as his medieval predecessors. Thirdly, society was still predominately rural, living for the most part in closely knit village communities where the social, physical and welfare needs, so often interrelated, were dealt with within the family circle.

TUDOR INFLATION AND THE ENCLOSURES

Although people were still debilitated by infection in the early sixteenth century, the decline in numbers had been checked and the population was increasing. Throughout Europe labour shortages had already produced changes in agricultural policy, and now, as the population rose, there was unemployment. To make matters worse, there were violent fluctuations in prices, which rose by about 3 per cent a year, and by 1600 the price of grain was five times what it had been in 1500, in fact until the present post-war inflation, the Tudor price rises were considered to be inflation *par excellence*. The reasons are complex; first there was increased 'demand', because there were more people; then for the first time men came to realise the correlation between the supply of silver and prices – more money in circulation means higher prices, and in Tudor times there was an influx of new metal from America. Because of inflation real wages fell; for example during the century the wages of building workers doubled but food prices rose fivefold over the 1500 level. Although this was partly offset by the fact that some commodities remained cheap because of low wages, the labourer was clearly worse off at the end of the century due to circumstances beyond his control.[5] The increasing population also affected the price of wool, which rose sharply; it was therefore more profitable to turn to sheep-farming and enclose the common land. The Tudor enclosures, rather like mechanisation in the nineteenth century and automation in the twentieth century, were seen as the root of all social immiseration – they were the banner for the Tudor protesters. Sir Thomas More (1478–1535), a humanist and scholar of wide repute, wrote, 'Your sheep that were wont to be so meek and tame, and so small eaters ... now swallow down very men themselves.'[6] In fact, not more than 3 per cent of the arable land was enclosed, and towards the end of the century, because of a fall in the price of wool, there was a return to arable farming, but this of course only made for more uncertainty. With prices fluctuating some people made money and there was a good deal of social mobility, which is evident from the ease with which the monastic lands were sold off and the number of new 'manor' houses put up by the thrusting newly rich soon to establish themselves as country gentlemen, a process to be repeated in the nineteenth century. Money made in the town was spent in the country.

THE ELIZABETHAN POOR LAWS

The price revolution, the discharging of soldiers and monastic servants and unemployment led to fears of social unrest and a breakdown of law and order, and although the stories of sturdy beggars and the bogey rhymes about the 'the beggars coming to town' are probably exaggerated, these prompted action. As early as 1388, after the Black Death, there had been an attempt to control the mobility of labour and vagrancy by a Poor Law Act designed to keep the poor in their own parishes and from pushing up wages. Then, during the reign of Henry VIII people began to consider how they could separate the two great categories of poor – the 'impotent' and the able-bodied unemployed. In 1536, William Marshall, in a draft for a Poor Law Act listed seven main causes of poverty, of which one was: 'Also others old, sick, lame, feeble and impotent persons not able to labour for their living but are driven of necessity to procure alms and charity of the people.' Some of these, Marshall points out, have fallen into poverty only through 'the visitation of God through sickness'. On the other hand there were 'a great multitude of strong and valiant beggars, vagabonds and idle persons of both kinds, men and women, which though they might labour for a living if they would put themselves to it as divers others do, but give themselves to live idly by begging and procuring alms'. Every age, it seems, accuses the workers of being work-shy, but most periods have more workers than there are jobs.

In 1552, under Edward VI, the Justices of the Peace were encouraged to provide for the impotent poor by building and maintaining almshouses by what might be described as a system of voluntary planned giving. Then in 1576 the first Elizabethan Poor Relief Act instructed Justices to provide materials like hemp and set the able-bodied applicants to work; if they did not work there would be no relief. In both cases there was a certain parochial reluctance to lay out money and the problem continued. At the end of the century after considerable debate in the Privy Council the Poor Law Act 1601 codified the previous legislation in what has become known as 'the 43rd Elizabeth' – the basis of all social policy for the next 300 years.

The Act gave Justices of the Peace the power to control wages and prices, to appoint Overseers of the Poor and collect a compulsory poor rate from the parishioners. Basically there were four main groups of parish poor and each called for a different solution. There were the 'impotent' poor who included the old, the sick, the crippled and the insane, then 'the labouring poor' generally known as the able-bodied and thirdly, as a sub-division, the rogues and vagabonds who would not work, and finally the illegitimate parish children.

The impotent had been the traditional recipients of upper-class poor relief since medieval times when the Church encouraged almsgiving as beneficial for the donor's soul. Almshouses and hospitals for the poor proliferated until well into the seventeenth century, and many are still standing as a memorial to the Tudor parish welfare. However, the numbers of the impotent were comparatively small and not a great problem partly because the Poor Laws laid down that parents and children must maintain one another, and the Overseers, with one eye on the rates, made sure that they did. This group were overshadowed by the labouring poor, the landless day workers who were particularly vulnerable to poor harvest, harsh winters and adverse trade conditions, and to these could be added discharged sailors and soldiers and their dependants, and sometimes their deserted dependants. For these the parish was to hold a stock of materials such as wool, thread and iron on which they could be put to work, either in 'work houses' or more often as outdoor relief; in return the applicants were, as the Overseers recorded, 'given relief'. However, for the recalcitrant and those who broke the parish bounds there were 'houses of correction' and, because this is how the palace of Bridewell in London was used, these houses were often later known as 'Bridewells'. Finally, there were the orphans and the unwanted bastards; many a putative father married his lass when she proved fertile, but some did not and it was the duty of the Overseers to see that children without parents were apprenticed, and the Statute of Artificers 1563 was designed to make sure the young were kept under the control of a master. Only when they were 23 years old could they marry and set up in business on their own.

Every parish was responsible for its own poor; it was therefore essential that no responsibility be accepted for vagabonds from other parishes, and much time and effort was spent in getting wanderers back to their parish of 'settlement', which was either the parish in which the vagrant was born or, if that were not known, where he had resided for a year. The Act of Settlement of 1662 allowed settlement rights to be obtained by marriage, inheritance or apprenticeship, but in spite of some relaxation in the rules, until well into the nineteenth century the Overseers' records show litigation between parishes about responsibility and money paid out to send paupers back to their own parish. The settlement laws meant that sick paupers could not travel and look for treatment in places that had hospitals. When Bath, in the eighteenth century, decided to build a 'national' hospital so that cripples from all over the country could use its healing waters, it was inaugurated by an Act of Parliament and special arrangements had to be made to get round the settlement laws; the same exemption applied to the 'Bedlam Beggars'.

The way Tudor paternalism attempted to solve the problems of poverty, chronic sickness and unemployment is important because it is an example of what once had been considered the responsibility of the Church being taken over by a secular activity; this secularisation not only had the blessing of the reformed Church, it was also on the road to a national social policy.

Although the Elizabethan Poor Law was later criticised as clumsy, paternalistic, demoralising and a burden on the rates, it did attempt to deal with the main social needs of the day by measures which at the time appeared appropriate to each different category; furthermore, each locality was free to adapt the measures as they thought fit. As Dr Frazer puts it, with each parish a sort of petty kingdom with its own sovereign will, the Poor Law became the nationally combined rationalisation of accumulated local custom. Indeed the student of Poor Law history is well advised to accept as a first premise that the story of poor relief is but dimly (and often not at all) told through the pages of national legislation.[7]

Some parishes preferred outdoor relief, some were obviously harsh, but others were indulgent. Nevertheless, the chronic sick and the old were housed, the able-bodied unemployed given some work – albeit, often unpleasant, but at least they were kept above subsistence level, the children were apprenticed and the recidivists locked up.

Many of the problems are still with us: apart from in total war or a totalitarian society, there is always some unemployment and argument as to how it should be relieved. The Elizabethans had their vagrants and the twentieth century its 'dropouts', and like the elderly sick with no one to care for them, they still defy a satisfactory solution. But whatever its merits or demerits, the fact remains that 'the 43rd of Elizabeth' lasted for over 200 years during which time, in spite of civil and international strife and domestic upheavals, the rural poor, wretchedly depressed though they often were, never suffered the same deprivations as the peasantry on the Continent, and although the parish poor relief system was not the only reason for this difference it was an important factor.

THE ROYAL HOSPITALS

After the dissolution there were petitions that some of the confiscated property and money be used to deal with the social evils of the day, with the result that some earlier hospitals were refounded. Although their purpose tended to change, they were no longer primarily for pilgrims and travellers. The five 'Royal' hospitals endowed by Henry VIII and Edward VI were St Bartholomew's, St Thomas's, Bethlehem, Bridewell and Christ's Hospital. St Bartholomew's was opened as a hospital again because there were complaints about the sick on the streets around Smithfield; St Thomas's was rededicated to St Thomas the Apostle – Becket the Martyr was hardly a saint congenial to Henry VIII – and continued to deal with the sick at Southwark, the busy southern end of London Bridge. The Bethlehem Hospital at Bishopsgate, the old hospice of the Templars, was now refounded and continued to give service to 'persons fallen out of their wits'; ex-patients were known as 'Poor Toms' and were allowed to beg without being picked up by the Vagrancy laws. Shakespeare in *King Lear*, written in 1606, makes Edgar disguise himself as a 'Poor Tom' with antics that must have been familiar to his audience. Bridewell had also once belonged to the Knights Hospitallers and was on the estate of St Bride's Well on the banks of the Thames at the mouth of the Fleet. On this Henry built a palace in which to entertain Charles V; Edward VI, with no such pretensions, gave it to the City as a hospital but it was soon used to deal with sturdy beggars, and thus, the name became synonymous with 'reformatory' or 'prison'. It was intended that Christ's Hospital should continue as a hospital for foundlings but infection was rife and most of the babies died so it eventually became a school for poor children.

The Protestant faith emphasised man's personal relationship with God and the Renaissance his individuality, so although illness was still seen as coming from God there was a tendency to see it in a more secular and matter-of-fact light. With the move away from the corporate life the idea of a 'nursing order' smacked of Catholicism and, with the nuns expelled and the aristocratic interest withdrawn, the nursing staff in the refounded hospitals changed their character. The City authorities engaged and paid local women to run them; the matron replaced the mother superior and the women of Smithfield or Southwark the nursing nuns. The new matrons were responsible for the work of the nurses whose duties were often largely domestic, and from some accounts they seem to have had little contact with their patients. However, it must be remembered that the patients were not necessarily the physically ill but the main social casualties of the day whose needs of 'mind, body and estate' were so often interrelated. Meanwhile, the Elizabethan era was drawing to a close and, as methods of government and the different Christian doctrines came into sharper relief, the stage was set for the religious and civil wars of the seventeenth century.

REFERENCES

1 Langland, W., *The Vision Concerning Piers Plowman*, quoted in M. Abram, *The Life and Manner of the Middle Ages* (1913), London: Routledge.
2 Nef U. (1950) *The Progress of Technology*, Russell & Russell.
3 Vasari, G. *The Lives of the Artists*, trans George Bull, Penguin Classics (1965), London: Penguin Books, pp. 38 ff.
4 Tawney, R. H. (1926) *Religion and the Rise of Capitalism*, reprinted 1938, London: Penguin.
5 Koenigsberger, H. and Mosse, G. L. (1968) *Europe in the Sixteenth Century*, London: Longman, p. 36.
6 More, Sir Thomas (first publ. 1516) *Utopia*, Bk I, Penguin Classics, London: Penguin Books.
7 Frazer, D. (1973) *The Evolution of the British Welfare State*, London: Macmillan.

FURTHER READING

Chadwick, O. (1964) *The Reformation (The Pelican History of the Church, 3)* London: Penguin Books.
Elton, G. R. (1953) *The Tudor Revolution in Government*, Cambridge: Cambridge University Press.

Gilmore, M. P. (1952) *The World of Humanism 1453–1517*, New York: Harper & Row.

Slack, P. (1985) *The Impact of the Plague in Tudor and Stuart England*, London: Routledge.

Webb, S. and B. (1911) *English Poor Law History, Part I* (reprinted 1963), London: Cass.

Chapter 4

New approaches to care

The Reformation came not because Europe was irreligious but because it was religious.

Owen Chadwick, *The Reformation*

From the sixteenth to the nineteenth century attitudes to care derived mainly from the different religious groups, and it is this diversity of religious belief and philosophy that provides the matrix on which the present mosaic of European health care is set. Most of these attitudes and philosophies have their origins in two main streams, the Protestant Church with its variety of different sects, and the reformed Catholic Church with its many new orders.

THE PROTESTANT CHURCH

Both Luther and Calvin knew that if the authority of the Pope were taken away, unless it was replaced by a civil authority anarchy would ensue. The magistrates and the Reformed Church had therefore to work together in a concept of 'throne and altar', a suggestion not unacceptable to many of the princes of Europe who saw it as a release from the dominance of the Pope and Emperor. This view was not shared by all reformers, especially the 'spirituals' like the Anabaptists, and this led to the first main schism in the Protestant movement.

Luther saw that if 'the priesthood of all believers' was to be a reality the community must take over some of the functions of the Church, and this was to have far-reaching consequences. First, in education Luther advocated a compulsory universal system that gave practical as well as religious instruction; it was this 'practical' element that gave Protestant education its science bias in the next century and thus its especial appeal to the rising, and practical, middle classes. Second, Luther had to find a way of dealing with the poor and the sick. In 1523 he laid down model regulations for the Saxon town of Leisnig which, although they were never put fully into effect, show the Protestant emphasis on total community responsibility.

The parish was to elect ten guardians from its parishioners and these, with the councillors, were to look after the communal treasury and the care of the poor and the sick. The guardians were also to buy up wheat when it was cheap and sell it to the community as relief in hard times. Although the main tenet of the Protestant faith was 'justification through faith alone', faith through the love of God meant loving one's neighbour and this emphasised the Christian's duty in the community. Since there was a considerable exchange between the reformers in Germany and in England, particularly during the Marian persecutions, it seems likely that the 'Leisniger Ordung' influenced the drafters of the Poor Law with its accent on parish responsibility.

The Church of Calvin, on the other hand, was more systematised and less democratic, with the Elders concerned more with morals than with the physical and economic needs of the community, a dichotomy that some-times led to a conflict of aims – for example, punishment for moral delinquency, like being absent from the sermon, might override claims of sickness. Other Protestant sects, as they developed, produced their own rules, but the emphasis was always on individual responsibility in the community with a particular stress on family unity and responsibility – another characteristic of the Elizabethan Poor Law.

THE CATHOLIC REFORMATION

The moves towards Catholic reform began prior to, and independently of, the Lutheran revolt, but after 1521 it took on a new urgency. Although the Council of Trent (1545–63), which was set up to deal with the criticisms of the 'reformers', came too late to prevent schism and in the end merely refuted the doctrines Calvin had set out in his Institutes of Religion in 1536, nevertheless many individuals in all walks of life were already helping to reinvigorate the Catholic Church with a new spirit. There was a renewal in the life of the religious orders who had been so much a part of the Catholic Church and which, once imbued with a reforming spirit, became part of the new movement. In Italy teaching and pastoral care was in the hands of the Friars, the Franciscans, Dominicans and the Augustinians, who had devel-oped their own internal 'reform movement': the 'Observants', in other words, those who wished to observe the strict rule of their founders. These reformers were now encouraged, and although it was once thought that the monastic movement would be swept away as the humanists wished, the upsurge of piety was such that a number of new orders were established.

At the same time there was a revival among the regulars with the founding of new orders like the Capuchins, the Theatines, the Oratorians and, the most influential of all, the Jesuits. There were similar reforms among orders for women, typical of which were the Ursulines, founded in 1535 by St Angeli Merci, who played a leading role in the education of women.

Both the 'reformed' and the new orders were fired with missionary zeal and some were instrumental in helping the conquistadores bring Catholicism to Central and South America, but as well as its proselytising mission, there was in the Catholic Church a wide diffusion of the theory and practice of meditative prayer and with this meditation went a new stress on charitable activity. Typical of the period were the Spanish mystics like St Teresa of Avila (1515–82) and St John of the Cross, whose lives, writings and reforming activities were to have an influence on Miss Nightingale and other nineteenth-century reformers. The idea of systematic meditation, coupled with a drive towards charitable works in the world, produced a devotional ideal not only for the clergy but for devout men and women everywhere and was inspirational in the development of the services to the sick in Catholic countries.

Thus, while the Protestant sects were developing the idea of the parish as a vehicle for care and the concept of individual responsibility, the Catholic Church was encouraging new orders who were to have the responsibility for the giving of care. Unfortunately during the period of bitter religious antagonism that followed the Reformation, these two approaches were often seen as mutually exclusive and as representing the two irreconcilable attitudes of the two main Christian faiths.

THE RELIGIOUS WARS AND THE WITCH CRAZE

The original demands of Luther were moderate, but the replies, like the replies to many demands for reform since, were too little and too late. The situation was exacerbated by the rising tide of nationalism, the increasing power of monarchs and the conflict between the temporal and spiritual heads of the Catholic Church; the religious issues were therefore entangled with *Realpolitik*. As the reformers defended their theological and ecclesiological positions more rigidly, each trying to give their respective Churches a firmer structure, so they took up stances from which it was difficult to retreat; thus compromise and the ecumenical approach rapidly became impossible. In an age of intense religious feeling holding the right faith was seen as the prerequisite to salvation and, for some at least, it was better to burn for a few minutes in this world than for ever in Hell. God-fearing men on both sides accepted that they must defend their faith with the sword, and less God-fearing men used the religious issue for political, economic and even personal ends. For the best part of the first half of the seventeenth century Europe was torn with religious strife, of which the Thirty Years War (1616–48) and the Civil War in England (1642–46) – which was by no means only a religious issue – were the most outstanding.

Although international war may at times enlarge medical knowledge because of exchange of ideas, as in the Crusades, or because of the need to experiment, as with the treatment of gunshot wounds in the Hundred

Years War, civil and religious wars assume a different character, and as they become fanatical, as Thucydides reminds us in a passage that could well apply to Northern Ireland, 'words change their meaning' and compassion is obscured.[1] In this situation in the seventeenth century there was a recrudescence of the mania of witch-hunting which operated against the giving of care outside the family circle and left its mark on country superstition for many years to come and had a bearing on some of the subsequent attitudes to mental illness. Originally rooted in the medieval 'devil doctrines', it became an excuse to hunt out heretics on both sides. Luther burned witches with as much conviction as the Inquisition, and as the mania increased and the trials multiplied denunciations began to include not only the deformed and the mentally and physically aberrant, but educated men and women. Although all figures on the subject must be treated with caution it has been estimated over 5 million people were either burned or drowned in the various 'crazes' in Europe. There were undoubtedly numbers who confessed to being in league with the devil, to practising black magic and who genuinely believed themselves to be witches, but leaving aside the confessions extracted by the revolting methods set out in *Malleus Maleficans* ('The hammer of witches') some confessions seem to have been spontaneous and even ecstatic. There has been much speculation as to why this mass hysteria and unbridled sadism should have gripped Europe and, like the rise of Nazism with which parallels have been drawn, no completely satisfactory answer has been found. Once the hysteria started it gave opportunities for personal revenge, for getting rid of unwanted relations and, as in twentieth-century Germany, fear bred fear, which was heightened by the horror-inspiring sermons of the times and by perverted sexuality and frustration. There was, however, another possible factor: it has been suggested that the use of hallucinatory drugs was rife and that concoctions of mandrake, hemlock, henbane and aconite were the basis of some of the 'visions' and the confessions. Certainly, Shakespeare and the Renaissance poets are full of stories of drugs, poisons and charms with magical effects, of which *A Midsummer Night's Dream* and *Romeo and Juliet* are good examples. Some of these concoctions may have been given for innocent purposes without under-standing the consequences: a recurring failure in drug administration down the ages.

In these circumstances the village nurse or midwife could be in danger; 'black magic' calls on a diabolical agency to inflict harm, 'white magic' on benevolent spirits to do good often with the aid of herbs and charms; white magic and healing were therefore closely related. But the Church, 'reformed' or otherwise, insisted that healing was from God and, in the tensions of the times, black and white magic were soon confused. Although the men of the Renaissance had questioned the assumptions of Aristotelian cosmology and the Protestant Church had rejected the idea of cure by miracles, nevertheless the Protestant king still 'touched' to cure the King's Evil, and both Protestant and Catholic doctors believed in alchemy and astrology. The Reformation, the Renaissance and the scientific revolution of the seventeenth century each had, as Professor Trevor-Roper points out, 'its Janus-face'.[2] This dark underside is a warning, if one were needed, against regarding history as a continual progression towards the light.

ST VINCENT DE PAUL (1581–1660)

Vincent de Paul was a typical figure of the Catholic Reformation, and, of the many saints and reformers the movement was to produce, he had the greatest influence on nursing. Born the son of a farmer in Pouy in Gascony, he became the protégé of a rich attorney and was trained for the priesthood at the Franciscan College at Dax. After eventful early years, which included capture by pirates and being a slave in Tunis, he came to Paris under the directorship of Pierre de Bérulle, who had introduced the Oratory to France and who was a fervent worker for the Catholic Reformation. In 1611, St Vincent accepted the position as a poor curé at Clichy near Paris and at the same time became tutor to the Gondi family where Phillipe Gondi, a friend of Bérulle, was the general of the royal galleys. In 1617, Madame Gondi asked St Vincent to join a preaching mission in Picardy, and here he found his true vocation, preaching and appealing to the people. Accepting a small parish at Bresse, he established his first charitable institution, 'The Association of Charity of the Servants of the Poor'. Madame Gondi then made available money for missions on her own estates, and having failed to get the Jesuits, Vincent organised this himself, establishing 'Charities' in each village. Always good at appealing to the charitable instincts of women, he was often overwhelmed with offers, and from these he developed 'Sisterhoods' with their own hierarchy and organisation. The rules which were drawn up by St Vincent stressed that the Sister was to take food to the sick and to see that the patient was washed and made comfortable *before* the meal, and she was encouraged to stay with those who were alone and to watch over the dying.

In 1619 St Vincent became chaplain to the royal galleys and Superior of the 'Order of Visitation' founded by St Jane Frances de Chantal who had been guided by St Francis de Sales. St Jane Frances had founded her own order where the sisters were expected to exercise their apostolate outside the convent, visiting the poor, tending the sick and comforting the dying. This reformed pattern was being fostered by devout, wealthy intellectuals of whom Madame Gondi was one and Mademoiselle Le Gras (Louise de Marillac, 1561–1660) was another. Le Gras had been a friend of Bérulle, and when he died Louise chose St Vincent as her spiritual director and became one of his main helpers.[3] Together they founded the Confrérie de la

Charité, which was so successful that similar associations were set up in the provinces under the guidance of Louise Le Gras, who organised them to give care both in the community and in institutions. In Paris the Charité took on a new character, and, as with the Roman matrons and the twelfth-century nobility, nursing became fashionable and ladies of high rank became members. In order to assist them St Vincent recruited a few country girls whom he called 'Filles de Charité', and in 1633 Mlle Le Gras, realising that the Filles needed some preparation for their work took them into her own home and, devoting herself to this as her life's work, organised a system of training. The training consisted in lectures in ethics and in instruction in home nursing and such skills as using a lancet (*sic*) and a tourniquet and applying poultices and bandages.

In 1633 it was suggested that the Charity extend its work to the Hôtel Dieu, the city hospital of Paris, nominally in the charge of the Augustinian nuns of whom a contemporary wrote, 'some did nothing, others prayed and a few worked'. The sick were neglected, the hygiene appalling and, as was the custom of the time, there were several patients in one large bed, but often there were others on the floor waiting to scramble in when a corpse was removed.[4] However, St Vincent soon realised that the ladies of Paris were not suitable for hospital work and the need was eventually met by the Filles de Charité organised by Mlle Le Gras.

Although St Vincent had always impressed upon his 'Filles' that they were not nuns, in 1646 – as the Civil War in England was drawing to its close – their simple rule was approved by the Archbishop and the order became known to posterity as the Vincentian Sisters of Charity. By 1656 there were forty houses with the sisters extending their care to foundlings, lunatics, home nursing and the battlefield.

The Vincentian Institute marked two innovations: it was secular and it was of the people. Hitherto nursing nuns had taken vows; indeed, that was what the controversy over the Beguines had been about; they tried to give charitable care *without* taking vows; moreover, 'charity' had been considered the prerogative of wealth and of the Church. The Vincentian ideal sought to remedy the spiritual and social evils of its times, and although by no means the only movement of its kind, played an important part in the Catholic spiritual revival. From the point of view of nursing it was a milestone in the development of the Motherhouse system that was to dominate so much of European nursing for the next three hundred years, and was to be the standard by which, because of their failure to provide a nursing service, the Protestant countries were eventually to be compared.

While throughout Catholic Europe new nursing orders were developing within and without the cloister, often establishing daughter houses overseas, Protestant countries were relying on the parish system, the Poor Law and family responsibility. When the new-style charity hospitals were established in England in the eighteenth century (Chapter 5), there were no comparable nursing orders to staff them and they relied on civic resources. In both systems medicine was unscientific and nursing similarly so, but at least in Catholic countries there was an outlet for women of all classes who saw the giving of care as a vocation. In Protestant countries there was no such outlet and nurses for the new hospitals were hired and fired from the market place; some were good, some poor, no one pretended that nursing was a calling, for that somehow would have smacked of papacy.

However, while the Catholic reforms were producing new orders with nursing responsibilities, the Protestant countries, as they recovered from civil strife, and their intense concern with heresy and the salvation of souls, produced new groups with a social conscience. The Presbyterians, Baptists and the Quakers, who had known persecution, now, in a more tolerant society, settled down to a comparatively peaceful existence and often, because they were excluded from academic and political life, became practical men of business, and since they had austere lives and habits, often amassed wealth. Dissenters' wealth could not be expended on adornment, public or private, and for some even pictures were idolatory and portrait-painting a sin: wealth was therefore likely to be channelled into philanthropy and the relieving of what were seen to be the particular social evils of the day. In England by the middle of the eighteenth century there were movements on behalf of prisoners, lunatics, foundling children, law reform and on behalf of the abolition of slavery, although this later movement came mainly from the 'Clapham Sect' and the Church of England. But of all the reform movements of that century, probably none left a greater mark on posterity than John Howard, who apart from his great work on prison reform, left a detailed description of the life and care in most of the hospitals in Europe.

JOHN HOWARD (1726–90)

Although, a hundred years later, Howard felt, like St Vincent, that he had been 'called' to a special mission, he was a staunch Baptist and, as High Sheriff of Bedfordshire, he first met the social evils of his day when he visited the local prison and saw the corruption of the gaolers. The Bench refused his appeal for improvements, so Howard, an intensely practical man, in 1777 set off on a tour of the county gaols in England to see if he could discover a precedence for better conditions. What he saw he recorded in *A Winter's Journey*, which is one of the first attempts to give a factual survey of institutions. The conditions in the other county prisons were as bad as, and sometimes worse than, those in Bedford, and Howard now became interested in the whole subject of penal reform. He made journeys to the Continent, sometimes under appalling conditions, in order that he might compare conditions and particularly the incidence of gaol fever, with those in England. Back in England Howard made another tour and with the aid of Dr Arkin published *The State of Prisons and Bridewells in England*, which gives an account of his findings and deals with every aspect of prison life and the abuses he found; particular stress is laid on the consequences of contamination from typhus, not only to other prisoners but to those in charge and to the citizens around: prisons were focal points for community infection. Howard urged that the sick be separated from the well, that baths be made available, clothes baked as a means of destroying infection, and that sick persons, whether convicted or not, should have care from a physician or an apothecary.

The conditions in prisons stimulated Howard's interest in the way disease was spread and the cause of infection; having gained an international reputation on penal reform he now became an authority on hygiene. Howard then turned his attention to hospitals, visiting each in turn and using the same survey methods recorded the facts. The monumental *An Account of the Principal Lazarettos of Europe*[5] was published in 1789 and gives an account of the hospitals of the time, and shows how the new 'charity' hospitals were staffed and used in the first forty years of their life (Chapter 5). One thing seems clear, that in many cases they were used to deal with social problems rather than with the acutely sick, which of course accords with the reasons for their foundation; for example, the Middlesex Hospital opened its doors in 1745 to the 'sick and lame of Soho'. Howard frequently comments on the 'rules for patients' and the fact that when they were out of hospital they could visit the neighbouring gin shops, which suggests they were not acutely ill. For this reason it is hardly surprising that the so-called 'nurses' were really attendants and were regarded as such. Perhaps, like Miss Nightingale a century later, they used the 'term nurse for want of a better'. Howard would certainly have endeared himself to Miss Nightingale for his continual insistence on ventilation; he condemned the general standards of hygiene and the 'offensiveness' due to the fact that the floors were dry-rubbed – which meant the dirt was hidden by sand – and the heavy curtains round the beds. The diet in most hospitals comes in for his scorn, but praise is given where praise is due, and some hospitals, mainly outside London, are remarked upon as being clean and efficient; not all eighteenth-century management was bad. Howard's strictures on the lazarettos of Europe were no less pungent, for everywhere, both in Protestant and Catholic countries, there were too few staff to deal with the number of patients who wanted to be admitted; the waiting-list problem had begun.

In order to test his theories Howard took passage on a 'foul' ship bound from Smyrna to Venice, and had himself interned in the lazaretto at Venice under the quarantine regulations. The lazaretto was unfurnished, full of vermin, and the diet was bare subsistence; presumably, if the internees had not already got one of the rickettsial diseases before they arrived they had a good chance of being infected before they left. During this tour Howard visited the hospitals of the order of St John and was particularly outspoken about the lack of hygiene at Malta. The Knights had grown rich and effete and had fallen from their previous high standard; but Nemesis was at hand; within a few years, in 1798, they were ignominiously turned out by the Corsican corporal, Napoleon.

Howard continued his work reporting on conditions in European hospitals until he died of an infection in a military hospital in Kherson during the Turkish–Russian war. The infection was said to be typhus, but the signs and symptoms sound far from typical, a fact which illustrates the problem of studying morbidity rates before the bacteria and the germ theory of infection was understood. For over twenty years he had laboured and journeyed, collecting and recording social statistics, which he often put together without comment in order to let the facts speak for themselves and thus to lay the foundations for a new science in social study.

MRS ELIZABETH FRY (1780–1845)

In the pantheon of the early nineteenth-century reformers the one name associated with nursing before the advent of Miss Nightingale is Elizabeth Fry. Mrs Fry was of course best known for her work in prison reform, but in the pre-industrial era reformers and social workers seldom saw their work in separate compartments; physical, mental and moral health and welfare were all interrelated. In her youth in Norfolk Mrs Fry had been an ardent believer in vaccination, which she apparently performed successfully on the local villagers, a reminder of how quickly Jennerian Societies were formed and how often the 'parish' nurse or a lady from a charity performed this technique. The duties of the nurse were never static.

Mrs Fry's attitude to prison reform was strictly evangelical: as a devout Quaker she believed in a simple faith in which sinners, if they did not repent, would suffer eternal damnation. It was therefore the duty of every Christian to bring sinners to repentance, and while people lived in filth and degradation they had no hope of turning to a better life and being saved. For the same reason she opposed the death penalty; if you hang a man he has lost his chance of earning salvation. 'In history it is always earlier than you think,' and at the beginning of the nineteenth century there was a strong 'abolition of the death penalty' lobby.

When Mrs Fry first visited Newgate she was shocked by the squalor and depravity – it was as if the Howard reforms had never been; whatever she tried to do was hindered by the overcrowding and the lack of classification of prisoners. Being a practical woman she organised a committee of like-minded ladies who, in spite of opposition from the authorities, arranged a programme of visiting and drafted rules for the improvement of the female prisoners. The rules produced a measure of success and were recommended to reformers all over the world. Unfortunately, these reforms were never really consolidated in England because the government, impressed with the American system of large buildings with single cells, saw solitary confinement as the key to reform, and many of the present prisons were built at this time. Mrs Fry's work on prison reform brought her in contact with Pastor Fliedner, and she visited Kaiserswerth where she was impressed by the deaconesses and their many activities. On her return to England in 1840 she tried to establish a similar nursing system, but her work on penal reform and her international reputation made it impossible for her to give much time to the project. Eventually, with the help of her sister, Mrs Gurney, and her daughters, she founded the Institute of Nursing in Bishopsgate. The nurses, carefully selected, received some training at Guy's Hospital, but the training was unsupervised and the nurses were prepared to undertake other welfare work while others became attendants in private houses. Partly because of the lack of systematic training and probably because the time was not ripe, the impact on nursing was slight and in 1860 Pastor Fliedner confessed to Agnes Jones that he was disappointed in the results of the experiment.

THE DEACONESS MOVEMENT

As society became more industrialised and the population increased, the simple concept of the parish community accepting responsibility for its poor and sick no longer worked, and Protestant countries began to wonder how they could find women to give devoted nursing care without emulating the Catholics and having 'orders'. In 1822 a young Lutheran pastor, Theodor Fliedner (1800–64) found that his flock suffered hardship when the breadwinner was in prison, and even when the prisoner was discharged there was no aftercare and all too often no work; further economic hardship produced sickness and misery and a temptation to relapse into crime. On a fund-raising tour Fliedner came to England where he met Mrs Fry, and on his way back to Germany he was inspired by the work he had seen in Holland, where officers of the Church had appointed 'deaconesses' to help with charitable work in the parishes. Once back in Kaiserswerth he became interested in founding a similar institution, and met and married Frederike Munster who shared his inspiration. In his travels Fliedner had noted the wretched nursing in many hospitals and he was convinced if the right appeal were made to women with charitable instincts a new diaconate could be founded. With the money raised by subscription the Fliedners bought the largest house in Kaiserswerth, and in the face of local opposition opened a hospital. The first 'deaconesses' were chosen by Frederike, who undertook the work of organisation and became the first Superintendent. The sisters not only cared for the sick in the hospital they were also responsible for the housekeeping, the cooking, the laundry and the gardening and visited the sick in their own homes, often taking with them food from the motherhouse. Theoretical and practical instruction was given by a physician and an examination was taken in pharmacy, and, as the Institute became known it attracted more recruits and the motherhouse was asked to supply 'sisters' to other hospitals. The sisters received no monetary reward but they were maintained and supported in their old age in a House of Rest. As fund-raising occupied much of Pastor Fliedner's time, the main burden fell on Frederike, who not only worked as the Superintendent but bore nine children, four of whom died at birth. She died at the age of 42 years while giving birth to her last child, worn out by work and repeated pregnancies – a testimony to devotion, and also to the infant mortality rate of the times. Two years later Fliedner married Caroline Bertheau, a sister in charge of a department at the Hamburg Hospital, who became the second Superintendent of Kaiserswerth.

During the next forty years the Institute developed and attracted many visitors, one of whom was to be Miss Nightingale. In 1846 the organisation was granted a charter and the work was extended to include all forms of relief and social work. The motherhouse was responsible for supplying deaconesses to hospitals, schools, orphanages, almshouses and asylums, and like St Vincent's Daughters of Charity 200 years earlier, the deaconesses worked where the need was greatest; during war and its aftermath, among poverty and disaster, at home and abroad, and, by the time Pastor Fliedner died, there were thirty-two houses and 1,600 deaconesses. Now to some extent both Protestant and Catholic countries on the Continent were operating a motherhouse system.

Although the early founders recognised the importance of the woman superintendent, as time went by the control of nursing fell more into the hands of the pastors, who did not agree with the physicians about the function of the nurse and this led to schism. Even as late as 1950 when the deaconesses were being employed by the British authorities the pastors came to the conference and spoke on behalf of the nurses, and it was made clear that their first duty would be to the spiritual welfare of the patients. Nevertheless, the importance of Kaiserswerth lies in that it harnessed devotion and training at a critical time and, although the multifarious duties of the deaconesses went beyond anything the most ardent supporter of an 'all purpose visitor' would advocate, the experiment at least showed the later reformers what not to do.

THE CHURCH OF ENGLAND AND NURSING

The question was often raised, and repeated more frequently after the establishment of medical schools, why were there no nursing sisters in England and why had not the Church of England established an order? Whether the new 'teaching hospitals' with their multitudes of medical students really needed nurses is another matter. Apart from Mrs Fry's attempt there were in fact a number of organisations specialising in nursing care, the two most important being the Community of St John's House founded in 1848, where it was intended to maintain a community of suitable women of the Church of England who would undergo training to fit them to act as nurses and visitors to the sick and poor. This Community was associated with the King's College Hospital, and was the first society to offer its services to Miss Nightingale, whom six of its members did in fact accompany to the Crimea. The Community and others that sprang up in the mid-nineteenth century with the rise of the High Church movement continued to give service in nursing and teaching until the second half of the twentieth century.

The other society that was to act as a precursor to the Nightingale reforms was that founded by Miss Sellon in Devonport under the aegis of the Bishop of Exeter; the sisters who were active in the cholera outbreaks of 1848–9 that were so virulent in Devon, were known as the Sisters of Mercy, and again a number accompanied Miss Nightingale to the Crimea – referred to by her as 'Sellonites'.

By the middle of the nineteenth century, therefore, quite apart from the independent improvements that were being made by some hospitals, there was a considerable movement towards producing a different and more dedicated nurse. But by now the population was increasing fast, its health needs were changing and medical knowledge increasing at such a rate that the nursing needs of the community, and of hospitals, could not be met by devotion or religious orders alone. It was Miss Nightingale's strength that she saw this, and her good fortune that she launched her campaign when the time was ripe.

REFERENCES

1 Thucydides *The Peloponnesian War* Bk 3, ch. 5, 1962 edn, trans. Rex Warner, London: Penguin Classics, Penguin Books, pp. 208–12.
2 Trevor-Roper, H. R. (1969) *The European Witch Craze in the Sixteenth and Seventeenth Centuries*, London: Penguin Books (Pelican), ch. 1.
3 Janelle, P. (1971) *The Catholic Reformation*, Milwaukee: Bruce Publishing Co, pp. 234–5.
4 Baly, M. E. (1977) *Nursing Past-into-Present*, London: Batsford, p. 23.
5 Howard, J. (1789) *An Account of the Principal Lazarettos of Europe*, Warrington.

FURTHER READING

Chadwick, O. (1972) *The Reformation. The Pelican History of the Church*, London: Penguin Books.
History of Nursing Journal, Vol. 5, No. 1, RCN, 1994.
Purcell, M. (1963) *The World of Monsieur Vincent*, London: Harvill Press.
Trevor-Roper, H. R. (1969) *The European Witch Craze in the Sixteenth and Seventeenth Centuries*, London: Penguin Books (Pelican).

Chapter 5

The growth of hospitals in eighteenth-century England

Transition from one period to another is gradual, and no arbitrary date marks change, but because England in the eighteenth century was a meeting point between an agricultural age and industrial change it became an age of 'Challenge, Contrast and Compromise'.[1] Challenge came from all quarters. The seventeenth century had created new markets, the financial importance of England had increased, and for the first time the economies of Europe were influenced by extra-European trade. Now, instead of being a country that fed itself and used any surplus energy to produce wealth from industry, England became dependent on selling its manufactured goods abroad in order to import food for the home market. Money had a new meaning: it was no longer merely a means of exchange; more and more it was needed as capital.

The increasing emphasis on capital investment affected agriculture and hastened the changes begun in the sixteenth century. After 1740 the population began to increase rapidly (Figure 5.1) and, as trade and industry absorbed more people so the proportion of people producing food declined, a change that was to be intensified in the next century. By 1760, when George III came to the throne, England had ceased to export corn and was soon relying on imports. Land was more productive – in 1778, Lavoisier, the French scientist, estimated that the productivity of agriculture in England was 2.7 times that of France – and profits from the land and from trade were available for investment. At first this money was used for public utilities like the making of canals and better roads, but later it was invested in the mechanisation of industry. In this situation some people made money quickly, and the 'contrast' to which Marshall refers was the inevitable result. Although there was nothing new in social mobility and the creation of new wealth – the sixteenth century had seen plenty of this, there were now more opportunities than ever before for making money and the inequalities this produced were soon to be questioned by the new philosophies of the day which had profound results and produced what has been called the 'Age of Revolutions'.[2]

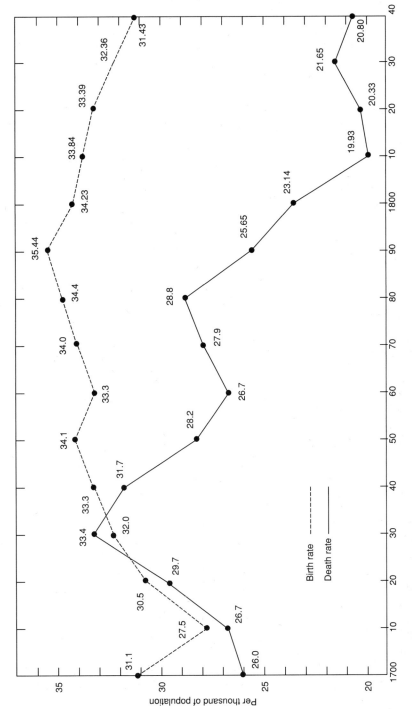

Figure 5.1 Comparison of birth and death rates between 1700 and 1840

Education through the grammar schools based on the humanist principles gave pupils a taste for the classics, and as Europe, except for its limited dynastic wars, became more peaceful, education was often completed by the 'Grand Tour'. This influence was reflected in the homecoming in new styles of architecture, sculpture, painting and literature; houses and public buildings were planned according to the laws and proportions of classical Greece and Rome, often using the design books of the much admired Andrea Palladio (1518–80), while the surrounding gardens were landscaped by men like Lancelot Brown, who worked out the 'capabilities' of the site. The wealthiest towns and families pulled down the old timbered Tudor buildings and replaced them with stone designed in the classical style.

THE EIGHTEENTH-CENTURY PHILOSOPHERS

The 'Enlightenment' is a label used to describe the general tenor of eighteenth-century thought. Fundamentally, it was a rejection of the old theocentric attitude, which was replaced by a new faith in reasoning and the ultimate perfectibility of man. Francis Bacon (1561–1626) had shown the value of inductive reasoning, while Descartes (1596–1650), by using mathematics, had demonstrated the importance of deduction, both of whom influenced the next generation in the importance of reasoning and logic. Then, in 1687, Newton published his *Principia*, which showed that the laws of terrestrial mechanics applied to the universe as a whole and, contrary to Aristotle, it was a vast interlocking system. Three years later John Locke (1632–1704), a physician, published his *Essay on Human Understanding* in which he argued that man was born without any innate ideas and his mind was a blank sheet, a *tabula rasa*, on which experience would write; all knowledge and wisdom came *through the senses*. Much of the subsequent philosophy, and indeed political thought, until well into the twentieth century comes from Newton and Locke; if natural laws governed the universe, then it was assumed, natural laws governed men and society and all that was necessary to achieve happiness was to discover the right laws. These conclusions led to a rejection of the idea of original sin, a secularisation of ethics and a new way of looking at society and the whole human condition. Later philosophers like Voltaire (1694–1778) and Hume (1711–76) produced variations on the theme, and Rousseau (1712–78) stood the argument on its head by stating that primitive man had been free and innately good – 'man is born free and everywhere he is in chains' – and it was civilisation that had produced vice, competitiveness and inequality. These ideas, especially those on inequality, had an influence on the French Revolution and the thinkers of the early nineteenth century. Now, instead of seeing suffering as inevitable, educated men and women were looking for causes.

Nevertheless, these ideas touched only the minority and for the majority life was still governed by a belief in portents, miracles and magical beliefs often older than Christianity itself, and witches were still burned in Europe in 1780.

RELIGIOUS THOUGHT IN THE EIGHTEENTH CENTURY

During the century there were several attempts at reconciliation between the Catholics and the rival Protestant sects, but ecumenical overtures were unsuccessful largely due to the pressures from outside. Orthodox religions were beginning to lose their dominance, and the greatest threat came from 'Natural Religion'; men of the Enlightenment, under the influence of Newton, agreed that the universe had been divinely constructed, nevertheless this 'Supreme Being' was not necessarily a Christian God. Deism, Latitudinarianism and Natural Religion were further stimulated by contact with other societies like Brahmins and Confucians, who had a different religion but who seemed to have a similar ethical code about duties to God and their neighbours. For the most part these ideas flourished where there was an educated middle class and a liberal-minded aristocracy, and where there was not there was a tendency to stay with the orthodox religion of the state.

Although these ideas were influential and affected the new science of sociology, for some, particularly those adhering to traditional religion, there was a positive reaction to the religion of 'Reason' and Deism. The most important of these reactions was the Methodist movement in England: John Wesley (1703–91), the founder, was hostile to the new 'liberalism' and distrustful of the physical sciences; his 'Method', which emphasised religion as an experience, used music as a way of arousing emotion, and placed great value on inspiration drawn from texts of the Bible. However, Wesley, following the example of St Francis de Sales (Chapter 4, p. 42) whom he admired, insisted that religion should be manifested by good works and in charity. Thus, the philanthropy which was the hallmark of the century united the Deists and the new Nonconformists; for the Enlightenment saw poverty, starvation and unnecessary suffering as an affront to reason and the natural law, while the Methodists saw it as an affront to God in whose eyes all men were equal.

NEW MEDICAL ADVANCES

New philosophy and popular religion coincided with a scientific revolution and advances in medicine, all of which interacted to make possible a new approach to illness. Until then, care in an institution was not only pointless, it was positively dangerous, but the situation was slowly changing.

An important advance had been made by William Harvey (1578–1657) who, challenging the theories of Galen, which were still held, researched the volume of blood in the body and in 1616 expounded his theory of the circulation, which he published in 1628. By the end of the century practical lessons from this theory were being put into practice; for example, it demonstrated the value of blood transfusion, though not of course its dangers. By this time Leeuwenhoek had discovered the microscope which enabled Marcello Malpighi to study tissue organs and to perceive that blood did not ooze 'into rivers of matter' as Vesuvalis had suggested, but returned by a hair-fine vascular system; thus the gap in Harvey's theory of the circulation was closed. Other anatomists made further discoveries: Sylvius (1614–1700) extended the knowledge of the brain and is still remembered by the aquaductus Sylvii. Then Sydenham (1624–89), taking the Hippocratic view that the doctor's duty was to help the sick organism in its natural fight, set about establishing a system of differential diagnosis, and, making a study of infectious diseases, was responsible for introducing iron for anaemia, mercury for syphilis and quinine for malaria, and of course for describing the chorea associated with his name.

There were also significant advances in physics: Robert Boyle (1627–91) realised the chemical nature of air and the possibility of a gaseous form of matter, and that 'in a given quantity of gas at a given temperature, the pressure is inversely proportional to the volume'. A century later Joseph Priestley (1733–1804), the philosopher, theologian and chemist, identified oxygen, recognising its indispensability to animals and its 'life force' in respiration and combustion. Towards the end of the century Lavoisier, who was guillotined in the French Revolution in 1791, conducted experiments showing that an organism takes in oxygen to maintain combustion by inhaling, and when it exhales carbon dioxide the waste products are eliminated. The foundations of modern chemistry were laid.

During the eighteenth century the Hunters transformed surgery from a craft into a branch of science, and John Hunter (1728–93) worked out important conclusions about inflammation, suppuration and regeneration. Meanwhile in Berkeley, in Gloucestershire, the village doctor, Edward Jenner (1749–1823) discovered that farm hands and milk maids who had cow pox were immune from smallpox, and from this he developed the idea that cow pox virus would provide a safer method of vaccination than the dangerous smallpox vaccination introduced by Lady Mary Wortley Montague from Turkey at the beginning of the century. Moreover there were now aids to diagnosis: Fahrenheit had invented the thermometer in 1736, and the idea of percussion had been introduced from Vienna. This 'scientific revolution' meant that doctors were now attaining a new prestige and were becoming far removed from the figures of fun they had been in the seventeenth century as depicted in Ben Jonson's *Alchemist* or Molière's *Le Misanthrope*.

NEW SOCIAL AND MEDICAL NEEDS

By the beginning of the century, in spite of the increased wealth, poverty was widespread. The growing towns were filled with insanitary warrens into which families were miserably herded. The state of the law was chaotic, crime went undetected and punishment was haphazard, those who did fall foul of the law finding themselves in Bridewells or prisons where typhus was rife. Cheap gin had replaced beer as the national drink, the horrors of which have been immortalised in Gay's *Beggar's Opera* (1728) and in Hogarth's panels of 'Gin Lane', 'Beer Street' and the Rake's Progress,[3] and by 1730 gin was certainly thought to be responsible for the high death rate. In 1715 a swingeing tax on gin persuaded the poor to revert to beer until a century or so later, when they took to the even more innocuous tea, usually a weak brew with plenty of sugar. As there was no reliable census until 1841 population estimates are hazardous, relying as they do on records of baptisms and burials; however, it seems likely that in the first years of the century the population was static, because every year or so an epidemic or a poor harvest checked the rise; certainly the death rate in the towns was twice that in the country because not only were the town dwellers exposed to the evils of gin and city violence but also to the greater likelihood of smallpox and typhus. Whatever the reasons, it seems the death rate between 1720 and 1740 overtook the birth rate (Figure 5.1) – this was true in the provinces as in London, for in Bath in 1710 there were 145 burials against 101 baptisms. The main victims of the high mortality rate were infants, at least one child in three died before the age of 6, and infanticide was by no means uncommon. In 1756, shortly after Captain Coram opened his Foundling Hospital in London, no fewer than 15,000 children were presented for admission. Since births and deaths were not registered until 1836 the reason for death is sometimes obscure, but studying the coroner's records at the beginning of the nineteenth century for Bath one cannot but fail to be struck by the high rate of accidents at work; workmen were continually being killed by accidents in building construction and in loading and unloading cargo, and surprisingly, from road traffic accidents where there was a real 'drink and driving' problem.[4]

MEETING NEW NEEDS – THE FOUNDATION OF THE CHARITY HOSPITALS

The initiative for founding the early charity hospitals came from philanthropic laymen who were either inspired by the new philosophy or motivated by an awareness of Christian duty. There were already in London the old 'Royal' hospitals, two of which, St Bartholomew's and St Thomas's, were hospitals for the sick and were now used for teaching purposes. To these were added the Five: Guy's, Westminster, St George's, the London and the Middlesex, all built between 1720 and 1745. These hospitals were intended as havens of care for the poor sick and they were often founded to deal with a specific problem; for example, Mr Guy, a governor of St Thomas's decided to set up a separate hospital for the incurables whom St Thomas's were now excluding. By 1789 there were about 30 similar charity hospitals for the poor sick in the provinces, but this only gave a ratio of about one hospital bed to every 5,000 of the population.

The charity hospitals were run by two groups of people, the paid and the unpaid. The governors who usually came from the upper echelons of society and often the treasurers gave their services free. The early foundations employed a doctor to visit once a week, probably a doctor personally known to the governors. However, as time went by it became customary for the doctors to become honorary; this was partly from charitable motives – it was, as it were, their contribution to the poor – and partly because the appointment gave status and therefore recommendations to private patients. Later, the doctors found independence important because they were then able to control which patients were to be admitted, and they chose those who were of significance for teaching purposes.

The paid staff were few and were employed by the governors rather like servants in a large house. The steward was responsible for the overall administration and the apothecary for the medicines, and over-spending on this item was the cause of more than one eighteenth-century boardroom row; the doctors would prescribe the more expensive new-fangled medicines instead of the old, well-tried herbs. The matron who was responsible for the female staff and the food and linen was also paid a salary, about £40 a year, usually about half that paid to the chaplain, a discrepancy that reflects as much the position of women as it does that of the matron or the relative valuation of spiritual and physical welfare. However, it should also be remembered that manual workers often only earned 8 shillings a week and average yearly wages were between £18 and £50,[5] so the matron was in fact quite well paid. The nurses and the sisters were relatively few in number and tended to stay on one ward; they took their orders from the doctors, the steward and the chaplain.

The patients were poor but they were not paupers, the stewards did not wish to incur the opprobrium or the expense of a pauper funeral and many hospitals insisted on 'caution' money. This was a sum the patient had to bring with him to defray the cost of his return journey or his funeral. The inaugural articles for the Bath Pauper Charity (see plates pp. 76–9) are typical, for they make quite clear that their new hospital, which in fact grew out of a Sick Dispensary and was at first in a doctor's house, was not for 'paupers' in the legal sense, but for the 'industrious labouring classes'.

Nursing in the charity hospitals

Although the matrons were recruited separately and were paid a salary, the nurses were rewarded in an infinite variety of cash and kind. As late as 1830 St Thomas's was paying its nurses 9/7d a week with beer, St George's £16 a year and 6 pounds of bread a week with 2 pints of beer daily. The quality of the bread and beer varied, and during the Napoleonic Wars when times were hard the quality of bread and beer went down and the Middlesex Hospital only averted a strike by distributing a small quantity of rice to the staff. In many cases the nurses lived out, but if they were resident they slept off the wards or in the basements or in the attics. Although the inducements to work in hospitals were not great, the nurses were probably as well off as the average factory worker where the wages in the post-Waterloo period varied between 11 shillings and 19 shillings a week, and at a time when the cost of bread was high due to the Corn Laws, the bread and the beer were quite a consideration.[6]

The best guide to the hospitals in the eighteenth century is that left by John Howard (Chapter 4). The mattresses were made of straw and often infested with bugs and the hygiene poor until the end of the century when those two great gifts to cleanliness came into universal use – iron, which was then used for bedsteads, and cotton, which was used for clothing and bed linen. Many patients were ambulant and helped with the work on the wards; they were, after all, receiving charity, and this of course helps to explain why the staff were so few. However, apart from the more conspicuous charity hospitals, philanthropic groups up and down the country were setting up sick dispensaries, or casualty hospitals to deal with the needs as they arose. Sometimes these were started by an enterprising doctor using his own house and taking on an apprentice or other assistance as the circumstances warranted.

But as medical knowledge increased the hospitals began to concentrate on the possibilities of cure, and, from the ever-growing hordes of out-patients, started to select patients for admission who were 'interesting'. Moreover, although the way infectious disease was transmitted was not known, fevers and skin diseases were excluded and most hospitals refused maternity cases and lying-in women for fear of infection. The Middlesex Hospital got over the problem of the admission of venereal diseases by charging such patients highly: the price of sin measured in hard cash.[7] Thus the real scourges of the day and the captains of death of the eighteenth century soon had no place in these havens of care. The intentions of the founders suffered a sea-change into something they would have found strange.

The development of medical schools

Until the end of the eighteenth century medical teaching was a combination of apprenticeship and some theoretical teaching conducted by private schools. The elite of the profession were, of course, the members of the Royal College of Physicians founded in 1518, who were university graduates, but they constituted a very small proportion. In 1800 the foundation of the Royal College of Surgeons led to a closer association between medical education and hospitals, and surgical practice became the prerequisite of training. At the same time the Society of Apothecaries began to require medical training for its members. This caused an influx of medical students and accelerated the change in the character of the hospitals. This change was interrelated with the growing middle class, a product of the changing industrial society, who no longer looked to estates and the land for a living but who were increasingly turning to the professions as a way of life compatible with the serious aspirations of the times. Law and divinity had been the leaders in this field, but now the scientific revolution, the new status of doctors with their more rigorous training made medicine a contender. The students paid well and most of the money went to the 'honoraries' in lecturers' fees. Now, more than ever, it was necessary for the doctors to control the admission of patients and divide the beds between them for teaching purposes. This changed the purpose of the charity hospital and the type of patient, but it must also have had an effect on the nursing staff.

As medicine became more scientific the hospitals might have looked for different nurses, since there was after all a precedent in Catholic countries. But with 200 students watching an operation and jostling for a place on the wards, what need of nurses? Medical students put on bandages, made poultices and made the beds, and in fact spent much of their time on nursing. No one had yet asked the question, 'What is the proper task of a nurse?' St Vincent's 'Filles' had wielded a lancet, medical students at St George's two centuries later were putting on poultices; jobs were done, as they had been done down the ages, by the person on hand to do them. In this situation it was hardly necessary to recruit, or indeed train, nurses.

Nevertheless, as more patients were admitted for treatment rather than custodial care, the doctors began to look for more trustworthy people to supervise nurses, and some hospitals recruited 'sisters' who were not promoted nurses but persons drawn from a higher status in society, perhaps widows in reduced circumstances or housekeepers from aristocratic families, and the records show instances of sisters teaching the medical students from their observation and experience. Before any firm conclusions are reached about the quality of the nursing, *within the light of its own time* a good deal more detailed research is needed, and this might well, to paraphrase Edward Thompson, rescue pre-Nightingale nursing 'from the enormous condescension of history'.

Teaching hospitals

Once the charity hospitals changed their character there was an impetus to found more hospitals, not this time as havens for the poor sick, but with the express purpose of teaching medical students, and to advance the art and science of medicine. In 1828, after the Catholic Emancipation Bill had failed to free Oxford and Cambridge from the Test Act, University College was founded in London in order to enable Roman Catholics, Dissenters and Jews, and those with no religious belief, to obtain a university education. The students were taught more and more on the lines of the Scottish and German universities, and this included medicine; University College Hospital was founded to give the medical students a background of practical experience, a foundation which prefigured the organisation of other new universities in the nineteenth century. At the same time other hospitals like St Mary's and Charing Cross, although not associated with a university, were founded on the initiative of doctors to provide a *teaching* situation and facilities for research. In 1850 there were 12 hospitals in London with medical schools controlling the greater proportion of the beds in London, the foundation of what was to be one of the greatest problems for the health service in the second half of the twentieth century. From the first these hospitals were designed to give demonstrations to large classes and to allow the students 'to walk the wards'. Unlike the charity hospitals of a century earlier, these hospitals started by grouping patients of the same diseases in wards or departments for teaching purposes. As more students applied for places and were willing to pay the increasing fees, so the honoraries seemed set for fame and fortune and the attraction of medicine increased.

The specialist hospitals

By the beginning of the nineteenth century being an honorary was a coveted position; the prizes for those who reached the top, as in law, were great and the profession attracted more ambitious young men than it could accommodate. The honoraries had their beds, but it was the juniors who organised them, and in many hospitals there grew up groups of men with specialised knowledge. Tired of waiting for promotion, they set out to found new hospitals where they could practise their expertise for greater reward. With the aid of grateful laymen the doctors set out to raise funds; at first there was a tendency to found hospitals for the groups excluded by the general hospitals, such as hospitals for children, but as time went by more hospitals were started for specialities already dealt with in the teaching hospitals such as ears, fistulas, hearts and chests. In a wordy piece of special pleading an eye hospital in the West Country appealed for funds because 'a special hospital was necessary because of the many nefarious practices by quacks who, with matchless imprudence, professing to cure the incurable, injure the tender organ and extract the last shilling out of the sufferer'. Often the founders did not move far from their parent hospital, and this led to a clustering of hospitals in certain districts and a concentration of beds out of all proportion to the needs of the population, a problem once started that was to have repercussions down to the present day.

The new hospitals often led to schism in the profession and acrimony in the medical press. 'An energetic surgeon makes up his mind to step to fame by means of bricks and mortar,' said the *British Medical Journal*, and, with heavy sarcasm, 'Stone cutting is a very limited occupation'. The battle raged and 'specialists' were often asked to leave the staff of the general voluntary hospitals. Undeterred, the specialists set to work to raise money, sometimes employing people to canvass and advertise, a practice not calculated to endear them to their colleagues. The specialists also operated in the provinces, where, as can be seen from their advertisements, there was clearly a spirit of competition. Some were no doubt motivated by a genuine spirit of research, but others merit the comment, 'Half the special hospitals were founded in the grossest self-seeking'.[8] Whatever the motivation, the legacy was the same, duplication and overlap and a gross disproportion of hospital beds in London unrelated to the needs of the population.

THE ORGANISATION OF THE VOLUNTARY SYSTEM OF HOSPITALS

The organisation of the early voluntary hospitals is important because it is the ancestor of the present hospital administration. The governing body consisted of a committee of distinguished, and often aristocratic personages, who decided on the hospital policy and were responsible for employing and discharging the senior officers. The lay administration was in the hands of the steward and to some extent the chaplain, while the matron remained subordinate. It was one of Miss Nightingale's triumphs that the matron eventually became supreme in matters pertaining to the nursing staff. As the number of honorary doctors increased, each with their own teaching commitment, they formed themselves into committees and divided the beds and the work between them, a division that was at times less than amicable. The overall smooth running of the hospital was in the hands of the steward, later called the hospital secretary, who was directly responsible to the governors.

Admission to the voluntary hospitals was usually by the ticket system, those who supported the hospital by donations were entitled to recommend patients and in some cases were like shareholders and entitled to attend the Annual General Meeting (see plates pp. 76–9) – the lady subscribers in this case having to vote by proxy. Sometimes an employer making a sufficient contribution could secure a ticket for his employees, rather like a sick club, and often the names of wards in voluntary hospitals bear witness to the donations from the traders around, a system that went on with modifications until well into the twentieth century.

The same system applied to the ever-growing volume of out-patients, and this became a source of controversy. Patients who attended an out-patient department when they were seen – and the waiting time was often considerable – were seen 'free', and thereby deprived the growing number of general practitioners of part of their income, and doctors in poor practices had many 'bad' debts. Not unnaturally, it was the doctors nearest London who were loudest in their complaints protesting that the out-patient system took the bread out of their mouths. At the same time as the emphasis on teaching continued the honoraries opposed the ticket system, preferring that their registrars should select the more interesting cases for teaching purposes. Furthermore, now hospital beds were at a premium with so many doctors in competition for them, the blocking of beds by long-term cases, who were not interesting, was to be discouraged. There was a further conflict of interest: the ticket system brought a predictable income to the hospital administration, while on the other hand, the number of patients treated and the dramatic nature of the work, especially sensational surgery, had more appeal when it came to attracting donations from wealthy benefactors. The in-patient turnover was already a sacred cow to both doctors and hospital administrators.

Within less than a century the charity hospitals of the middle of the eighteenth century had changed their character. From being the havens for the poor sick, the non-pauper class fallen on hard times and with some affliction, they became, together with the newer foundations of teaching hospitals, hospitals for the acute and esoteric. Advances in medicine and surgery led to a concentration on what could be done, a tendency that was accelerated once the use of anaesthesia became popular after 1840. The main needs of the population remained unmet and in the end had to find amelioration from different sources and in a different hospital system. For nursing the legacy was incalculable, for when they eventually had a training system it was based on the voluntary hospital and its values and it is not without significance that in 1973 the popular patient was the one who was 'clinically interesting'.[9]

REFERENCES

1 Marshall, D. (1962) *Eighteenth Century England*, London: Longman.
2 Godechot, J. (1971) *France and the Atlantic Revolution of the Eighteenth Century, 1770–1790*, London, New York: Collier Macmillan.
3 Hogarth Panels, now in Sir John Soane's Museum, Lincoln's Inn Fields.
4 Coroner's Records, City of Bath 1811–21, Bath Archives.

5 Eden, F. M. (1795) *The State Of the Poor*, A. G. Rogers (ed.), 1928, London: Routledge.
6 Cole, D. and Postgate, R. (1949 edn) *The Common People*, London: Methuen & Co., pp. 203–9.
7 Saunders, H. St George (1949) *The Middlesex Hospital 1745–1949*, London: Max Parrish.
8 *British Medical Journal* (1853) quoted by B. Abel-Smith, in *The Hospitals* (1964), London: Heinemann, p. 28.
9 Stockwell, F. (1973) *The Unpopular Patient*, RCN publication, London.

FURTHER READING

Abel Smith, B. (1964) *The Hospitals 1800–1948*, London: Heinemann Educational.
Graham, H. (1939) *Surgeons All*, London: Rich & Cowan.
Hobsbawm, E. (1973) *The Age of Revolution*, Cardinal edn, first published 1962, London: Weidenfeld and Nicholson.
Porter, R. and Porter, D. (1988) *In Sickness and in Health: the British Experience, 1650–1850*, London: Fourth Estate.

Chapter 6

The deserving and the undeserving poor

May never House, misnamed of Industry,
Make him captive.
'The Old Cumberland Beggar', William Wordsworth (1797)

In spite of the new philosophy, the scientific revolution and the new status of the doctors by the end of the eighteenth century there were only about 40 charity hospitals and their effect on the health of the population was minimal; most of the sick were still in their own homes or in poor houses and almshouses. In the late seventeenth century there had been an attempt to make the poor more profitable, and in 1696 the Bristol Corporation of the Poor, which other cities tried to copy, was founded with the intention of putting all the poor to work.[1] The 'workhouse' became the favoured weapon for the scheme, and Sir Edward Knatchbull's Act of 1722 allowed parishes who adopted the measure to withhold relief from any person refusing to enter a workhouse. However, towards the end of the century the new humanitarian attitudes prevailed and Gilbert's Act of 1782 encouraged adjourning parishes to co-operate and provide 'workhouses' or poor houses, not as a means of humiliating the indigent, but rather as a way of aiding the really destitute, what in the language of the day were called the 'perishing classes'.

Every parish interpreted the Poor Law in its own way and the coverage of the country by workhouses was uneven; Oxfordshire in 1777 had only one for every nine parishes, but in 1732 Bath, presumably encouraged by the Knatchbull Act, amalgamated the city parishes and bought a Poor House on the outskirts of the city. Because of the rivalry between parishes, the idea of setting the poor to work soon faded, as did that of putting all in need into a workhouse, and throughout the century the majority of Poor Houses or 'Houses of Industry' as they were sometimes misnamed, were seldom anything more than glorified almshouses, and even in that function they were not successful partly because they were prone to epidemic, but mainly because outdoor relief was cheaper, and if the records are studied, it will be seen that in most parishes about two-thirds of the applicants for relief were women and children.

THE INCREASE IN POVERTY AND THE AGRARIAN REVOLUTION

Towards the end of the seventeenth century there were a number of treatises on agriculture, and as the theory was put into practice there was a wave of agricultural reform. The potato, that was to save Ireland from starvation, was introduced in 1664, and by the beginning of the eighteenth century clover and turnips were being cultivated in Norfolk for winter feeding. Farmers like Robert Bakewell (1725–95) demonstrated how the quality of animal stock could be improved by selective breeding, while Viscount Townshend (1725–67) showed how the four-crop rotation could improve the productivity of the land. For the first time winter feeding was provided for livestock and fresh meat was available all the year round, and a direct consequence of this was that widespread diseases like scurvy began to disappear. The improved productivity and more vigorous trade with the colonies provided a better and more varied diet, which in turn fostered an increase in the population.

The other side of the coin meant there were more people for fewer jobs. Capital farming, greater use of mechanisation and the division of labour produced a sharp decline in the number of independent farmers and a rise in the number of labourers. It is the period of Goldsmith's *Deserted Village*, where 'Only one master grasps the whole domain'. Scattered holdings were consolidated and fenced, and between 1760 and 1800 something like 5 million acres of common land were enclosed. Although the enclosures undoubtedly improved the efficiency of agriculture and they were not the source of the dramatic hardship the Hammonds made out,[2] there is evidence that the loss of the plot of land, the grazing rights and the allotment were as bitterly resented as the new machines. The ordinary man had lost what the sociologists call 'defensible space', and he was the poorer, not only in produce, but also in dignity and spirit.[3]

THE GROWTH OF THE POPULATION

The remarkable growth of the population in Europe as a whole, and England in particular, after 1750 is an important factor in assessing the subsequent health needs of the community and one from which most lessons can be drawn. Why this spectacular growth occurred is complex and still the subject of debate. In the absence of reliable data the question arises: was the increase caused by a fall in the death rate or a rise in the birth rate, or both? And why did growth appear at this particular period *before* the Industrial Revolution? A very little disturbance in the balance of ecology can have a large cumulative effect, and McKeown and Brown assert that any fall in the mortality rate must have been due, not to the effect of medical science, which was minimal, but to the general improvement in the environment and especially the effect of better feeding.[4] Habakkuk and Krause have suggested that the rising birth rate was the key factor,

> that there was an excess of births over deaths in any year that was free from epidemic and war and in which the yield from the harvest was normal – any run of years that was fortunate in these respects was likely to enjoy an increase in the population. The second half of the eighteenth century seems to have been such a period.[5]

In this period women lived longer to have more children, some of whom were girls who had more children; the population increase was, as Thomas Malthus (1766–1834) was soon to point out, geometrical. There were, of course, a number of other factors currently being investigated by the Cambridge Institute on Population, such as the age of marriage – which varied widely – the use of birth control and the practice of abortion and infanticide, and even the variations in landholding and the need for labour; all these have a bearing and are difficult to assess. The fact remains that an agrarian revolution is usually a precursor to population growth, which in turn releases surplus labour for industry. There is then a situation where population pressure, technological invention and the resources available pursue one another and draw one another on in ever-widening circles. It is small wonder that the men of the late eighteenth century saw this growth as an alarming phenomenon and this alarm dictated much of their social and economic policy for the next half century. Malthus, in his *Essay on the Population* in 1798, argued that failing wars, plagues and famine, the increasing numbers would soon exhaust the nation's ability to feed itself and it would sink under famine and disaster. Although other economists, particularly the French *philosophes* believed that a rising population went hand in hand with prosperity, the depression and social unrest after the Napoleonic Wars ensured that the pessimists of the Malthusian school dominated policy.

THE INDUSTRIAL REVOLUTION

Mechanisation, which had begun on the land and in the mines as early as the seventeenth century, gathered momentum in the eighteenth. There have been many analyses of the 'causes' and much historical debate about a priori conditions. Historians like Ashton emphasised the economic factors, such as the lowering of interest rates, which quickened development; others have laid stress on the coming together of improvements in agriculture, better means of transport, increased availability of capital, a reorientated education and a 'growth mentality', while Rowstow, in his 'conditions for sustained growth', emphasised the importance of the growing markets. What is clear is that technological advances in one area soon brought pressure for innovation in another and that this process gathered momentum with such speed that the face of the country, and much of its life style, and therefore the health needs of many people, were changed in a lifetime.

The pace setter of this change was the woollen industry. In the early eighteenth century woollen cloth was produced in most counties by part-time workers, although there were a few areas where weavers and spinners had become specialists. In 1760, Kay (1733–64) speeded up the flying shuttle invented earlier, which allowed the weavers to work faster; this meant they were held up for shortage of yarn generally spun in the home by women and children whose wages eked out the meagre agricultural existence. In order to overcome the bottleneck there was pressure to speed up spinning, and in 1768 Hargreaves (1720–78) produced his jenny, and Arkwright (1732–92) invented a water frame which enabled more yarn to be spun by one person. But Arkwright's frame required power to work the rollers so spinning moved into the early factories which were often in the country, but many of the families of agricultural workers, unable to travel, lost their supplementary income. The poor became poorer.

Weaving as a semi-domestic occupation remained prosperous until the coming of the power loom. With the introduction of Compton's mule and Watt's steam engine patented in 1769, the factories tended to move to the towns, but it was not until after the Napoleonic Wars that there was a move to attach weaving sheds to the spinning factories. In the meantime, the number of factory workers was increasing and the number of hand-loom workers, and their wages, went down. As the skilled weavers were thrown on the scrap heap they became vocal, and some in their anger became 'Luddites' and initiated the sporadic outbursts of machine-breaking in Nottinghamshire and Yorkshire between 1811 and 1816. Their example was followed later by the agricultural workers who smashed the threshing machines in 1830.[6] A new interest has recently been taken in the Luddites, whose activities have been more thoroughly researched, and because the twentieth century, with its micro-electronics, is beginning to see the parallel with the power loom.

By the 1830s mechanisation had transformed the textile industry. Cotton consumption dramatically overtook wool, and by 1820 the industry employed two-thirds of all textile workers; as cotton became cheaper it replaced wool in importance in the home and overseas market. Mechanisation affected the iron industry, for which the demand was boosted by the coming of the railways in the 1840s, and the greater demand for pottery. As the new inventions widened their scope more and more women and children were employed in factories. There was nothing new in women and children working; Defoe (1661–1731) had said a child ought to be able to earn its keep by the time it was 5, but now they were regimented outside the home. In 1853, there were about 60,000 adult males, 65,000 females and 84,000 young persons, of whom over half were under the age of 14 years, working in the cotton mills. Unprotected by any legislation and under the economic philosophy of *laissez-faire*, the children were now exposed to evils that had not been present when they worked in rural cottages – at least not obviously so. There was a danger from industrial accident and crippling, and the effect of a brutalising life on their morals, and it was the latter, rather than the former, that stirred the early reformers. Since children were small and quick they were eminently employable, and this put a sickening premium on frequent pregnancies and a 'widow with a family of boys was considered a catch'. Thanks to the agitation of reformers like Oastler, Sadler and Ashley, and later the early medical officers of health (see Chapter 8), there were a number of investigations by various committees and commissions – the famous 'Blue Books' of the period, and the documentation is still there, like Howard's surveys, for the historian to read; much has been edited and published in an eminently readable form.[7]

Perhaps the saddest victims of this new industrial world were the children who worked as trappers in the mines, or in the early factories for upwards of 14 hours a day until their health broke. From what Arnold called the 'turbid ebb and flow of human misery', the commissioners often took verbatim reports, and the graphic and simple answers of these children still speak from the pages and remind us that much Victorian wealth was bought with these sad little lives.

> *Sarah Gooder* aged 8. 'I am a trapper in the Gawber Pit. It does not tire me but I have to trap without a light and I am scared. Sometimes I sing when I have a light, but not in the dark, I dare not sing then. . . . I have heard tell of Jesus, I don't know why he came on earth, but he had stones for his head to rest on. I would like to be at school far better than in a pit.'

> *Margaret Leveston* aged 6 – a coal bearer in East Scotland, described by the Sub-Commissioner as a 'most interesting child and perfectly beautiful'. She said, 'Been down at coal carrying six weeks, makes ten to fourteen rakes (journeys) a day, carries 56 lbs of coal in a backbit. The work is na guid; it is so vary sair. I work with sister Jesse and mother, dinna ken the time we gang, it is gai dark.'[8]

One fact that was brought home to the commissioners and other investigators was that, having denied the children any education and condemned them to work like mules, it was hardly surprising that the children did not even know the rudiments of the Christian doctrine.

Nor did those who reached adult stature fare much better; women were crippled with carrying heavy loads, particularly those who worked as 'drawers' in the narrow tunnels with belts round their waists and chains through their legs dragging the buckets. This crippling had an effect on the maternal mortality and the health of the next generation. Malnutrition and infection fanned the flames, and the death rate that had been falling since the middle of the eighteenth century now began to rise. The life expectancy of a labourer in Manchester was 17 years.

It was not only the working conditions that were detrimental to health; the living conditions were often not much better. As the unplanned towns grew up in the Midlands and the North around 'those dark satanic mills' land prices rose, and hastily built, cheap houses, often with little light and no drainage, were packed close to the factories into which were huddled the seekers for work. The social commentator, Alexis de Tocqueville, describing Manchester in 1835 wrote:

> From this foul drain the greatest stream of human industry flows out to fertilise the world. From this filthy sewer pure gold flows. Here humanity attains its most complete development and its most brutish; here civilisation makes its miracles, and civilised man is turned back into almost a savage.[9]

This is not to suggest that the living conditions of the rural labouring poor were much better. The rustic cottage idealised by the poets of the Romantic era was damp and unhygienic, the food often poor and unvaried and the general tenor of life what Marx called 'rural idiocy', but the rural poor had one advantage over their brethren in the town: they lived twice as long.

Now work had a new meaning. It was controlled by the machine and the hooter from 5 a.m. to 6 p.m.; the ebb and flow of the seasons, springtime and harvest, no longer had any relevance, and, as he grew old, the worker could no longer adopt a work rhythm to suit his physical and mental capacity. Man was now the slave of the machine and the machine favoured the young and nimble. The old concept of mutual responsibility between master and man had been replaced by the 'cash nexus':[10] the employer was there to hire and fire and to pay wages, but when the worker was old and sick the nexus was over and his only refuge was the support of his still working family or the local poor house.

THE PROBLEM OF PAUPERISM – THE OLD POOR LAW

Throughout the eighteenth century outdoor relief was the staple element of the Old Poor Law; the money was raised by a parish rate levied on holders of property and administered by two or more Overseers of the Poor. Outdoor relief was often intensely practical; it dealt with the insane, the crippled, the unemployed, provided pensions for the infirm, paid neighbours to look after children and took charge of orphans and bastards. The Bath Poor Law records[11] for the late eighteenth century show a wonderful miscellany of items, such as 'paid for mending Clarke's children's shoes'; 'a shift for Williams'; 'coals for a woman with smallpox'; 'for getting Mary Elacott's clothes out of pawn so that she could go to her situation'; and, poignantly, 'paid 3/- to Mary Southwell's daughter for laying out her mother and putting her in coffin'. The sick were attended by the parish doctor, paid for out of the rates, the lying in by the parish midwife, who seems to have been better paid than the nurse, but at least Nurse Philpots had her shoes mended periodically out of the rates. Nor were all poor houses the places of universal execration the reformers led us to believe. Between 1784 and 1800 the 40 or so paupers in the House at Bath complained to the Committee from time to time and caused at least three masters to be sacked and two doctors – the third only retained his post by signing in and out. The entries give some idea of the medicants in use and support Blaug's argument that the Old Poor Law did act as a safety net for the casualties of society,[12] and the poor house often sheltered the long-term sick who had no one to care for them. By no means everyone in the pre-industrial world lived in an 'extended family', and the records show, all too painfully and sadly, that there were many solitaries, men and women, often looking for work in a changing world.

For those who were not paupers but were tipped into poverty by poor harvests, harsh winters, floods, sickness and, above all, accidents at work, there were often a variety of charities which of course varied from parish to parish, but in a society imbued by Christian doctrines, charity was seen as an obligation and duty, and in a more leisured age it absorbed much of the time of the sober, well-intentioned upper middle classes. The recipients of this charity were usually the 'industrious labouring classes' or 'the deserving poor'. It is fair to say that in many towns as much money and food was handed out by charities as was given in Poor Law outdoor relief.

The system worked reasonably well in close-knit parishes when society was stable, but it was strained to breaking-point at the end of the century during the agrarian changes, the increases in the population and the violent fluctuations in prices during the Napoleonic Wars, so that in many rural areas the plight of the agricultural labourers reached a new nadir, some were starving.[13] In 1798 magistrates meeting at Speen in Berkshire to fix the agricultural wage, as they were bound to do under the '43rd of Elizabeth', yielded to a counter-suggestion whereby low wages were to be subsidised out of the poor rate with relief scaled to the price of bread (which acted as the cost of living index of the day). The system known as the Speenhamland Scale and commonly called the Allowance System was adopted for most counties in southern England and had far-reaching effects. It led to an outcry against the Old Poor Law and to the Poor Law Amendment Act of 1834, which in turn influenced the whole design of the health and welfare services in the twentieth century. The Allowance System meant that wages were kept low and high-priced bread subsidised out of the rates. It did, in a simple way, what sophisticated Family Income Supplements, differential taxes and things like school meals do today. Between 1800 and 1810 the price of corn trebled, and when the price fell after the war the Liverpool administration (1812–27), in order to protect the farming interest, introduced the Corn Laws, which forbade the import of wheat until the price reached 20 shillings a quarter. The price of bread rose and the Corn Laws joined the enclosures for pride of place in the popular anti-government slogans of the day. In 1775 the poor rate had totalled £1,500,000 a year; by 1818 it had risen to £8 million.[14]

Although industry was springing up in the Midlands and North, the agricultural workers found it difficult to migrate because of the Settlement Laws which made every pauper chargeable to his own parish; moreover, even if there had been the will to move there was little by way of transportation until the coming of the railways. The first factory workers were made up of two main groups to whom subsistence wages could be offered: the immigrant Irish, often refugees from famine, and apprentices from the poor houses in the South, a system that died out during the Napoleonic Wars when it was discovered that the supply of local children, for whom there was no contract, was cheaper.

The attitude to poverty in the post-Napoleonic War period was dominated by a number of factors. First, there was the Malthusian influence and the real fear of over-population. Second, and in line with rational philosophy (Chapter 5), Jeremy Bentham (1784–1832) had enunciated the doctrine of utilitarianism in his *Principles of Morals*. In this, Bentham set out the philosophy that 'the greatest happiness of the greatest number is the measure of right and wrong', and argued that it was the business of the law to make sanctions sufficiently strong so that men were induced to subordinate their own immediate happiness to that of the community. Third, and closely allied to utilitarianism, were the economic policies of the day. In 1776 Adam Smith (1723–90), reacting against the mass of restrictions surrounding mercantilism, produced *The Wealth of Nations*, in which he argued that the wealth of the country could only be increased by the unimpeded law of supply and demand – a doctrine that gave rise to 'laissez-faire' which was to dominate much nineteenth-century economic thought. The background against which these policies were argued was the fear of riot; most English intellectuals had lost their enthusiasm for the French Revolution with 'the Terror' and there was a tendency to see a Jacobin under every bed. Added to this there was the bitterness and rancour that surrounded the 40 years of debate on electoral reform which ended only after riots and the Reform Act of 1832.

The rise in able-bodied pauperism, or at least those having their wages subsidised, gave rise to much debate; some saw it as a blessing – unless men were driven by poverty who would do the most servile tasks?' – and a similar argument is used in the twentieth century with unemployment. On the other hand, there was a school of thought which argued that it was no business of the state to interfere and take away from people what was their Christian duty; the state did not differentiate between the 'deserving and the 'undeserving', and above all the pernicious Allowance System was interfering with the market mechanism.

THE POOR LAW AMENDMENT ACT, 1834

The reformed Parliament set up a Commission in 1832 to look into the workings of the Poor Law. The Commission was 'non-party' and included distinguished churchmen and lawyers, Nassau Senior, an Oxford economist in the Adam Smith tradition, and Edwin Chadwick (1800–90), a protégé of Bentham, as the secretary. The Commission was charged, not with looking into the causes of destitution, but of finding ways of dealing with pauperism. The Commissioners were diligent, but they were convinced 'utilitarians', they failed to look at any real statistical evidence and their conclusions were based on anecdotal stories and the false assumption that most pauperism was 'able-bodied'. The Report of 1834 was important not only for its content but because it set up a new form of government with a central department, the Poor Law Commission and its staff, exercising executive control, but not itself administering, a network of local authorities, a system that was to spread to other services like health and education. The Commission required the parish 'Unions' to elect Boards of Guardians who would be responsible for carrying out the new policy; it did not require them to build new workhouses – this would have added to the rates they were determined to cut – but in fact this is what energetic Boards did; but in spite of Chadwick's continual admonitions Boards interpreted the Act in different ways.

The main recommendation of the Poor Law Report was 'all relief whatever to able-bodied persons or their families, otherwise than in a well-regulated workhouse shall be declared unlawful'. In order to do this the Commission recommended that the Central Board appoint permanent officers to organise the parishes to form Work House Unions with each parish paying in proportion to the expense occurred. The main tenet of the Commission's philosophy was to 'cut off the disease of pauperism at its roots', and to do this it was proposed that able-bodied workers who applied for relief should be offered 'the House', where, since the purpose of the offer was to deter, 'their situation should be made not so eligible as that of the independent labourer of the lowest class'. This was the 'workhouse test' by the principle of 'Less Eligibility' that was to underlie most social policy for nearly another 100 years. As far as its primary task was concerned, the Poor Law Amendment was successful; agricultural wages rose, workers were no longer subsidised out of the poor rates and expenditure actually went down, but this was largely due to fortuitous circumstances, while grim stories of the new attitudes actually deterred those who needed help.

The Commission had assumed that able-bodied pauperism was the main burden, but it was not; any apprentice historian grubbing in the parish records can prove otherwise; nor had they taken into account the different circumstances in industrial areas where poor relief was not a subsidy but a form of unemployment benefit for workers periodically laid off by the vagaries of the system. To cut off outdoor relief and to bring them into the 'well-regulated House' was to make them the bane of the system with families constantly being uprooted and children separated from their parents. When looking at the old poor houses the Commissioners had been horrified at the agglomerations of the sick, the insane, the children and the adults in one 'mixed house', and they recommended that the new Unions should have four separate buildings, one for the aged and impotent, 'where the old might enjoy their indulgences', one for children where they could be educated, and the other two for the male and female able-bodied – strictly separate. It is the failure to carry out this policy that left so much bitterness, and the various attempts to implement it that account for the chequered policies on the Poor Law in the nineteenth century.

There were other initial problems. The Poor Law Commissioners themselves were sensitive to the outcry they had raised about the withdrawal of outdoor relief, and in this they were at odds with their secretary, who was a thoroughgoing utilitarian and who often overstepped his authority. A *cause célèbre* in Bath demonstrates the point: the new-style Chairman of the Guardians, a Benthamite almost straight down from Cambridge, who was determined to get a sick 80-year-old lady into the 'House', and was duly supported by voluminous correspondence from Chadwick himself, clashed with the old-style magistrates. The magistrates were equally adamant that the old lady should be 'relieved' in her lodgings and eventually threatened high court action; at this point even Chadwick saw the warning light. The old lady had her outdoor relief, and died.[15] Moreover, the first Boards of Guardians tended to be 'small aristocracies' and used to governing local affairs, and were often at odds with the peripatetic Assistant Commissioners who were seen as 'busy-bodies'. At the end of 1839 the number of paupers in the workhouses was 98,000, while 560,000 were receiving outdoor relief, a figure which suggests that only 3 per cent of the population were on relief, but this figure soon rose again during the 'hungry' forties and it gives no indication of the numbers who were refused relief or struggled outside the system. Probably between 30 to 40 per cent of the population was in poverty. By 1842 there were 1,427,499 on relief.

THE MOVEMENT FOR WORKHOUSE REFORM

It was never the intention of the Commissioners that large numbers of sick should be confined in workhouses, but they had not appreciated the extent to which sickness and poverty go hand in hand and that there had never been a large purely able-bodied problem. Although provision was made for the Poor Law doctor, often the old 'parish doctor', to visit those on outdoor relief, the cover to those in the House was variable. How many inmates were sick is not known, but it is likely that the aged infirm made up one-third of the workhouse population. In dealing with these the Guardians were to face the same conflict as when coping with children, if the paupers were given preferential treatment when they were sick the workhouse would cease to be a deterrent and the rates would rise.

With poor harvests and bad winters the rates did rise, and the Commission was the subject of a stinging attack in Parliament by Disraeli in 1841, the situation not being made easier by the constant attacks by Chadwick himself on his Commissioners' policy. In 1847 the Russell administration passed the Poor Law Board Act which transferred the power of the commissioners to a new Board with a President who was eligible to sit in Parliament. Under the new Board the inspectorate continued to investigate the categories in the workhouses for which the principles of the Act were not designed. Children constituted a quarter of the workhouse population; not to educate them was to render them likely to perpetuate pauperism; to educate was to offend the principle of less eligibility. A variety of experiments were tried, farm schools, 'scattered homes', 'cottage institutions' and boarding out, all of which came up against the problem of trying to reconcile two different objectives, and the bitter lesson that large conglomerations of under-fed children were easy prey to epidemic and often had a mortality rate twice that of the population outside. Another problem was persons of 'unsound mind'; policy was always confused on this subject and though there were generally about 5,000 idiots on relief, the Board took no steps to make provision for them. One explanation is the growth of a rival authority, the Lunacy Commission (Chapter 7), which had authority over all lunatics, and not being concerned with 'less eligibility' now put pressure on the Guardians to improve their facilities; but the Guardians could not off-load their imbecile and lunatic inmates into the asylums because they would have to pay out of the rates accordingly, so for a long time to come the inspectors' reports refer to children and the sick in the workhouses being in the care of feeble-minded inmates.[16]

Nevertheless, by the 1860s three strands were converging to stimulate reform. First, since Medical Registration in 1858, the status of doctors had improved and the more courageous of those employed by the Guardians began to protest, and some like Dr Joseph Rogers of the Strand Workhouse started an active reform movement. Dr Rogers' main complaint was that the sick were looked after by pauper nurses who were old and feeble, often illiterate and incapable of carrying out the instructions of the doctors. To these reports were added the disclosures by Sir John Simon (Chapter 8), now at the Privy Council, about the increase in infectious disease, especially diphtheria and cerebrospinal meningitis, and worst of all – guaranteed to send a shiver down the Victorian spine – cholera. Meanwhile, there were press reports of over-crowding in workhouses and the disgraceful neglect of the sick, who were a focus of infection for the community around. Even before the press scandals, reformers like Louisa Twining who in 1853 visited the Strand Workhouse 'to see a respectable old blind woman' were asking difficult questions. The indefatigable Miss Twining formed a Workhouse Visiting Society – rather as Mrs Fry had done for the prisons – which assembled and published information and pressed for debates in the House of Lords, where Miss Twining was not without influence. Miss Twining continued to press the cause of workhouse reform until the end of the century, with her ladies being particularly active in the cause of a reformed system of nursing.

However, before the reformer's case is accepted at their own valuation and pressed for the highest motives, it is as well to remember that the workhouses included many respectable women fallen on hard times. Indeed, they were often the majority of the applicants, and by no means all were drunk or feeble-minded; some, in a world that was particularly harsh to poor women, just could not get work. Here is Charles Dickens, to whom is owed that archetype of the untrained nurse, the caricature, Sairey Gamp, in a different mood, when he was not writing a money spinner:

> the morsel of a burnt child, lying in another room, so patiently, in bed, wrapped in lint, looking steadfastly at us with his bright quiet eyes when we spoke kindly to him, . . . as if he thought, with us, that there was a fellow-feeling in the pauper nurses which appeared to make them more kind to their charges than the race of common nurses in hospitals.[17]

There was obviously a community of suffering and mutual kindness, and the poor helped the poor not without intelligence and humanity.

The Brownlow Hill experiment

At the same time as Dickens was walking round that London workhouse on a Sunday morning, a wealthy philanthropist of Quaker origin in Liverpool shipbuilding, William Rathbone (1810–1902), was also interesting himself in the conditions of the workhouses. Because of his experiments in providing nurses in the community in Liverpool he was in touch with Miss Nightingale (Chapter 9), who had for some time been concerned with the state of the sick in the Poor Law institutions. The various workers for workhouse reform had all come to the same conclusion; that the sick must be separated from the well and proper nursing provided. Sometime earlier, in the 1850s, the Poor Law Board itself had suggested that suitable paupers might themselves be 'trained', for this they argued would relieve the rates and improve the standard of care, a plan on which Miss Nightingale, needless to say, poured scorn. Now in 1861 she had her own ideas for reform which, in alliance with Mr Rathbone, she put forward as her ABC plan in which she suggested that, first, 'the sick, the insane and the incurable and children must be dealt with in separate institutions and not mixed up in sick wards in the workhouses as at present'. This of course had been the intention of the Commissioners nearly 30 years earlier, but it had always proved too costly or too administratively difficult to put into practice. Second, 'there must be a single central administration. The entire medical relief of London should be under one central management which would know where vacant beds were to be found'. In this Miss Nightingale was looking forward to a London Health Service, the sort of thing that was eventually achieved by the London Council with its network of hospitals and institutions of all kinds. Lastly, for the purpose of providing suitable establishments for the care and treatment of the sick and the insane 'there should be Consolidation and a General Rate'.[18] The last point was of course *lèse majesté*, and would have undermined the sacred right of the parishes to deal with their poor in their own way out of their own rate, regardless of the fact it was a system in which the poorest and the unhealthiest were hardest hit. Miss Nightingale was right, for as long as the sick were paid for by the resented parish poor rate they would be penalised. That she could write, 'the first necessity is to change the mental attitude that made this hideous system possible', shows how radical her thinking was on this point compared with most of her contemporaries: she was saying then what the Webbs said in 1909, and even then they were considered *avant garde*.

Although reform of nursing in the workhouses came slowly there were improvements; one small beacon was the experiment at the Brownlow Hill Institution in Liverpool; working in conjunction with Miss Nightingale, Mr Rathbone promised to finance a scheme to provide proper nursing for the male part of the institution. At first the offer of a group of trained nurses from London was resisted by the Guardians; 'there has been as much diplomacy and as many treaties and as much of people working against each other as if we were going to occupy a kingdom instead of a workhouse', wrote Miss Nightingale,[19] but at last in 1865 her 'dearest and best pupil', Agnes Jones, and 12 nurses took possession of the male wards. It was a task to daunt the boldest but Miss Jones was an exceptional woman, beautiful and gifted, with a will of iron, and what was as important, the backing of Miss Nightingale. As a pilot nursing scheme it was a success, law and order was restored, the old pauper nurses dismissed, and better still, by good administration the costs fell; the medical men now began to ask for more such nurses and the local population sang their praises. But the work was overwhelming; just as victory was in sight and all the wards being placed under the administration of Miss Jones, an epidemic of typhus broke out and Agnes, aged only 35 years, fatigued and worn out, caught the infection and died; her last message to Miss Nightingale was, 'You have no idea how overworked I am'. The epidemic was a disaster and closed the scheme that was not likely to be repeated in a hurry; reform of workhouse nursing had to come from another quarter.

THE
PAUPER CHARITY,

HEREAFTER TO BE CALLED

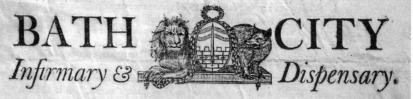

BATH CITY
Infirmary & *Dispensary.*

Mifs PULTENEY, PATRONESS.

Sir JOHN RIGGS MILLER, Bart. PRESIDENT.

Mr. CHARLES PHILLOTT, TREASURER.

CALEB HILLIER PARRY, M. D. ⎫
JOHN STARK ROBERTSON, M. D. ⎬ PHYSICIANS.
JOHN EWART, M. D. ⎭

Mr. FRANCIS MOLINY, APOTHECARY.

THE Subfcribers to the PAUPER CHARITY, having found it daily more difficult, fince the great extenfion of Bath, and the proportional increafe of its poor inhabitants, to adminifter, by their prefent plan, adequate relief to the numerous objects who apply to their Difpenfary; have determined to revife and new-model the form of their inftitution, fo as to enable them to confer the Benefits of their Charity, in urgent cafes, with better effect; to guard againft beftowing them on improper objects; and to rectify fome other abufes and mifapplications.

It is evident that the moft humane intentions of relieving our fellow-fufferers, who at the fame time labour under poverty and difeafe, muft often be entirely fruftrated, while they either live widely difperfed, or have no fixed place of abode. In acute and critical difeafes, medical advice, attendance, drugs, and other neceffaries, can only be adminiftered with certain advantage, when the patients are properly accommodated and collected together. The number of poor perfons, labouring under fuch difeafes in Bath, has grown too great to be vifited at their own houfes fo frequently as their cafes require; and many lives are loft by the want of a proper afylum to receive the fick-poor of this city and its neighbourhood.

While the benevolent contributions of the wealthy are chiefly conferred on an Hofpital, indubitably of extenfive ufefulnefs, which however excludes the inhabitants of Bath itfelf, there does not perhaps exift any other city of the fame opulence, in which the afflicted poor fuffer fuch mifery and want. It has come to the knowledge of the Managers of the Pauper Charity, that whole families have been lately fwept away by infectious diftempers, which probably would not have extended beyond the perfon firft feized, had there been an hofpital to receive him on his firft attack. Some have been found deferted in the laft extremity, whom the fear of catching infection deterred their neighbours from approaching. Others have wanted food, neceffary for the bare fuftenance of life, who in fuch circumftances could not be relieved from the anguifh of pain, or the oppreffion of

the

[2]

sickness, by any powers of medicine. Is it neceſſary to ſwell this catalogue of calamities, ſo ſhocking to humanity? The Subſcribers to the Pauper Charity are confident, that they require only to be mentioned, to render every good citizen, and every friend of mankind, zealous in providing a remedy.

Neither is it difficult to account for this ſtate of uncommon wretchedneſs, in which we find the Poor of BATH. Not to mention the many individuals, on whom unavoidable misfortunes entail diſtreſs, nor the ſlothful and the vicious, whoſe manner of life brings along with it the wages of miſery, there is a peculiar and local cauſe of poverty among the lower claſs in this city, which, being derived from their ſuperiors, demands from *them* commiſeration and relief. It is always obſerved, that the poor are multiplied by the numbers required in places of publick reſort for the more ſervile offices of life. Servants, being accuſtomed to rich and luxurious living in their maſters' houſes, find it difficult, when they marry and get houſes of their own, to ſubſiſt on humbler fare. They are tempted to live up to their laſt ſhilling, often beyond it; ſo that the viſitation of ſickneſs finds them totally unprovided.

The Subſcribers, in publiſhing the following ſketch of their New Plan, wiſh to prove the neceſſity of commencing an eſtabliſhment ſuited in ſome degree to remedy the foregoing evils; and are in hopes of procuring a more liberal ſubſcription to ſupport and to extend it.

They think it of importance to repreſent to the CORPORATION, as the Guardians of the City, to thoſe who compoſe Pariſh Veſtries, and to every inhabitant of BATH, that by affording early and effectual medical relief to the heads of families, and to other perſons by whoſe labour numbers are ſupported, not only diſeaſes are ſhortened and lives ſaved; butthat whole families may be prevented from becoming a burden on their reſpective pariſhes, and thus the pecuniary charges upon the occupiers of houſes in thoſe pariſhes would be eventually diminiſhed.

While the Subſcribers hope for the benevolent contributions of the Reſident Inhabitants, and of the Families who have property in the neighbourhood, to enable them to carry ſo uſeful a ſcheme into execution, they likewiſe flatter themſelves that the Company reſorting to BATH, who already ſee a well-endowed Hoſpital for the reception of Strangers from all parts of the kingdom, will, in return for the benefits ſolely appropriated to the poor of their reſpective diſtricts, contribute to relieve the Afflicted within BATH itſelf; who, without the aid of this inſtitution, have not even the means of employing the waters ſo bountifully beſtowed by Providence on their native city.

The Subſcribers, anxious to apply the benefits of their Charity to thoſe caſes, which moſt particularly preſs for relief, and in which they can be the moſt extenſively uſeful; and being ſatisfied that the Caſualty Hoſpital, by the preſent form of its conſtitution, is more eſpecially calculated to afford aſſiſtance to Surgical caſes, have thought it expedient to receive Medical caſes only. They are happy, however, to inform the public, that voluntary offers have been made by the moſt eminent Surgeons of Bath, to attend the patients in the Infirmary, whoſe caſes may happen to require their aſſiſtance and ſkill.

The Subſcribers truſt that they will be aſſiſted and ſeconded by the Community in general, in an attempt to reſcue BATH from the reproach of being the only city of its population and wealth in this country, which has neglected to provide an Aſylum for its own Sick Poor.

As they muſt unavoidably incur a conſiderable Preſent Expence over and above the Annual Expenditure, they have opened a particular Subſcription for Benefactions to defray the Firſt Coſt of providing and furniſhing a Houſe, &c.

N. B. Between Two and Three Thouſand Poor Perſons were relieved by this Charity in the courſe of the laſt year.

At

[3]

At a GENERAL MEETING of the SUBSCRIBERS to the PAUPER CHARITY, held the 3d Day of APRIL 1792.

THE Meeting having seriously considered the numbers and distresses of the SICK-POOR of BATH, and the impossibility of affording them Relief at their own Houses,

IT WAS RESOLVED,

1. THAT it appears necessary, not only to fulfil the duties of humanity, but to consult the interests of the public in general, that an Infirmary should be instituted to receive the diseased of this City and its Neighbourhood, who are incapable of supplying their wants in sickness; and that immediate steps should be taken to begin such an establishment, and every means used to enlarge it.

2. THAT a convenient House be immediately taken or bought, for the reception of In-Patients, containing commodious wards, a shop for medicines, apartments for a house-apothecary and female servant, a committee-room, an antichamber for out-patients to assemble in, &c.

3. THAT the same be fitted up with beds for at least six in-patients for the present, and with other necessary furniture.

4. THAT a proper assortment of medicines be purchased from Apothecary's Hall for the sole use of the Infirmary and Dispensary.

5. THAT an Apothecary be engaged at forty pounds a year, who is to live in the house, to prepare and dispense the medicines, to be accountable for the drugs committed to his care, to attend on the visiting hours of the physicians and surgeons, and to visit the out-patients under their direction, in cases which do not require the personal attendance of the physicians themselves.

6. THAT the Physicians shall examine the medicines of the Dispensary, to report occasionally the state and expenditure of the same; and that they be requested to draw out a *Pharmacopeia Pauperum* for the use of the institution.

7. THAT a proper Matron be hired.

8. THAT a Night-Nurse be occasionally hired, at the desire of the attending physician, when urgent cases require.

GENERAL REGULATIONS *for the* MANAGEMENT *of the* INSTITUTION.

9. That all New Regulations and Laws be determined at General Meetings of the Subscribers; at which every Subscriber of one guinea or upwards be entitled to vote; and that Lady Subscribers may vote by proxy.

10. THAT an Annual General Meeting be held in the beginning of January, to elect an annual President, Vice-President, and a managing Committee for the ensuing year, to audit accounts, and to transact such other business as may come before them.

11. THAT the direction of all ordinary business of the institution, and the providing for the maintenance of the in-patients, &c. be left to a Committee to be named annually as above, subject however to the revision of the general meetings.

12. THAT the said Committee consist of sixteen, including the physicians, who, by giving their assistance, are deemed subscribers; that they meet monthly; and that three shall constitute a quorum from the first of May to the first of October, and five from the first of October to the first of May.

13. THAT the members of the managing committee, who are not physicians, shall each in rotation visit the Infirmary weekly, to inspect the state of the same, and to enquire of the patients if they have any complaints to make; and if any gentleman cannot attend when it is his turn to inspect, he shall find a substitute from among his colleagues in the committee.

14. THAT any vacancy of a physician, or apothecary, be supplied, at the latest, one fortnight after such vacancy happens, by the nomination of the managing committee.

15. THAT the managing committee be empowered to call a general meeting of the subscribers, when any special business occurs to render such a meeting necessary.

Rules respecting the Admission of Patients.

16. THAT medical patients only be received on the foundation of this institution.

17. THAT patients living out of the city must attend at the Dispensary, or some friend for them, and cannot be visited at their own houses, on account of the distance.

18. THAT no persons can be admitted either as in or out-patients, who receive parish pay.

19. THAT no servants in place can be admitted on the fund of this institution; but the servants of subscribers may apply for advice to the physicians and may have their prescriptions prepared at the Dispensary, on paying a moderate price for the same on delivery.

20. THAT no person be admitted who does not bring a recommendatory ticket from a subscriber; which shall be likewise signed by an overseer of the parish to which the person belongs, before he presents himself at the Dispensary.

FORM

[4.]

FORM OF A RECOMMENDATORY TICKET.

I recommend the bearer to be a patient of the Bath City Infirmary and Dispensary, if his case is judged a proper one. Signed

A. B. *Subscriber.*

I certify that the bearer, is an inhabitant of the parish of and does not receive parish pay. Signed

C. D. *Overseer.*

To the Physicians of the Bath City Infirmary and Dispensary.

21. THAT each subscriber of a guinea shall receive six such printed tickets, or more in proportion to his subscription, to distribute to fit objects of this institution.

22. THAT recommendatory tickets be transferable from one subscriber to another.

23. THAT patients be admitted in rotation, according to the date of their recommendatory ticket; and that the apothecary be ordered to keep a register for that purpose.

24. THAT when a person is recommended, whose case is deemed improper by the physicians, the apothecary shall write to the subscriber who gave the recommendation, to explain why he is not admitted.

25. THAT the physicians are to select, out of the patients recommended by the subscribers at large, such cases as they shall deem most necessary to be received into the Infirmary; and in cases equally urgent they shall give a preference according to the date of the recommendatory tickets.

26. That each physician attend two days in the week to prescribe for, and to admit out-patients.

27. THAT all patients admitted be the peculiar patients of the physician by whom they are admitted.

DIRECTIONS *to* PATIENTS.

28. THAT all patients in person, or, if the case prevent personal attendance, that some friend for them, shall attend at the Dispensary on the days and hours of each their respective physician's attendance; on failure of which for three stated days following, the patients so neglecting shall be debarred from all future benefits of the Infirmary and Dispensary.

29. THAT all patients who are prescribed for at the Dispensary, be ordered to apply for what is prescribed before eight o'clock the same evening, otherwise they shall not be entitled to the benefit of their prescriptions; except in any particular case a physician shall have occasion to see a patient after that time; but such patient must apply immediately on receiving his prescription.

30. THAT if any patients be discovered to have wilfully neglected to take the medicine, or to have failed to follow the advice prescribed by the physicians; or if they have not used the medicine prescribed, from some unavoidable circumstance, and do not return it to the Dispensary; such patients shall be immediately discharged, and debarred from all future benefits of this institution.

31. THAT all patients behave themselves with propriety and according to order, otherwise they shall be dismissed and precluded as above.

32. THAT no patients under the same penalty go out of the Infirmary, or cease to attend the Dispensary, without a proper dismission from their respective physician; in order that the relief they have received, or the event of the case, whatever it may be, be registered for the satisfaction of the public.

33. THAT on the dismission of each patient from the Infirmary or Dispensary, a letter be sent by the apothecary to the subscriber who recommended him, to specify the event of his case, or the cause of his dismission.

34. THAT the apothecary shall keep a daily list of the admission and dismission of patients, of their diseases, and the event of their cases, to be signed by the attending physician, and afterwards to be copied into a register to be kept for that purpose.

The Three Physicians, together with the following Subscribers, are the Committee for conducting the Business of the Charity.

Sir JOHN RIGGS MILLER, Bart. *President.*

Rev. Mr. Leigh	Major Brooke	—— Monkland, esq;	Mr. Plura
John Waters, esq;	W. Baldwin, esq;	Henry Southby, esq;	Mr. Cruttwell
Mr. Charles Phillott	Granado Pigott esq;	Thomas Hicks, esq;	Mr. Hazard.
Rev. Mr. Dobson	Richard Milford, esq;	Major Velley	

☞ Subscriptions are received by Mr. PHILLOTT, *Banker*, Milsom-street; the Rev. Mr. LEIGH, Marlborough-Buildings; Major BROOKE, St. James's Parade; the Rev. Mr. DOBSON, Belvidere; by the Physicians to the Infirmary; and at the Libraries.

Back in London another blow had been struck for reform. In 1864 a pauper in the Holborn Workhouse had died 'from gross neglect and filth'. It is unlikely that Timothy Daly was the first so to die, but by this time the newspapers, which were becoming more widely read by the middle class, took up the case as a public scandal. Miss Nightingale had recently made a convert of Charles Villiers, the charming and handsome worker for the repeal of the Corn Laws and Free Trade, and she urged him to use the Daly case to press for radical reform. At the same time the editor of *The Lancet* sent out a commissioner to enquire into the state of the work-houses; now in 1865 with Charles Villiers as the President of the Poor Law Board, Delane, the editor of *The Times*, interested and John Stuart Mill and Chadwick as powerful allies, everything seemed set for radical reform on the lines of Miss Nightingale's plan. At that point Lord Palmerston died, and the Whigs fell from office after having had an almost unbroken run since the 1840s and the fall of Peel. The new Tory administration, with Disraeli becoming Prime Minister the following year, was cautious, and Gathorne-Hardy, a barrister and President of the Poor Law Board had no intention of dismantling 'less eligibility' or accepting his predecessor's Bill, and without consulting the reformers or the Association for the Reform of Workhouses in February 1867 produced his own Bill.

THE METROPOLITAN POOR LAW ACT: A NEW HOSPITAL SYSTEM

The Act, although disappointing to the Liberal reformers, remains a great landmark in Poor Law reform and marks the beginning of a new period of hospital-building. For students of the health services, however, its parti-cular significance lies in the fact that it set up a new hospital authority with different traditions, erecting hospitals for a different purpose, and all too often for a different class, thus creating a dichotomy that was later to create a problem for the health service. The main provisions of the Act were that separate institutions should be erected for the insane and for infectious fevers, and that small Poor Law Unions were to be encouraged to group together and large Unions should build separate infirmaries.

It will be noticed that 'groupings' are getting bigger and bigger, eventu-ally forming a basis for local authority boundaries. The weakness of the Act was that it only applied to London and it failed to provide overall administration and finance; because of this and the fact that Guardians were reluctant to incur higher rates and were often jealous of their own rights in 'amalgamation', reforms came slowly and unevenly. Even when new hospitals were erected there was difficulty in finding nurses, for in spite of the increase in the number of training schools the new matrons needed ever more nurses; moreover, even had there been nurses to spare it is unlikely that they would be attracted to the Poor Law system. Enlightened Boards of Guardians saw that the only answer was that they should train their own nurses. In 1873, prodded by Miss Twining and Miss Nightingale and other reformers, Section 29 of the Metropolitan Poor Law Act allowed Infirmaries to admit and train probationer nurses. In 1871, the new Local Government Board (Chapter 8) made .similar arrangements all over the country, but not all authorities responded, and until well into the twentieth century the poor sick were most often nursed by untrained nurses and not infrequently by pauper nurses. This was particularly true in the country districts, but as it was all too easy to slip into pauperism this is not to say that some were not kind and considerate to their charges.

One important outcome of the Act was a change in attitude towards the poor sick 'who were not proper objects of such a system'. According to the Webbs in their monumental work, the Poor Law Board now pressed the Guardians to form Sick Asylums *exclusively for the sick*, and the President of the Board asks 'how far it may be advisable to extend gratuitous Medical relief beyond the actual pauper class'. Here was a suggestion for a universal public medical service which, though not followed up, was always after 1870 considered a possibility. There was an interesting change in the attitude to the institution, long to leave its mark on the provision of services for the sick. Previously those on outdoor relief had fared better; now, in what the inspectors were calling 'state hospitals' with 'airy wards, improved dietary, resident doctors and trained nurses', the poor sick were being better cared for and they were certainly not 'less eligible', therefore it was logical that the outdoor sick be persuaded to come in *'where their medical needs could be adequately met'*.[20] There was now a positive encouragement for sick persons, whether destitute or not, to take advantage of these new institutions. Gradually the less eligibility principle was being eroded. In 1885 The Medical Relief (Disqualifications Removal) Act decreed that Poor Law medical treatment did not pauperise, and the recipients of such relief were not disenfranchised.

However, while the poor sick were getting a better deal, if they happened to be nursed in a new 'infirmary' little headway was made where workhouses merely set aside part of the building as the sick wards. As well as having a depressing atmosphere they were managed in a different way. Workhouses were run by 'masters and matrons' many of whom had worked for years in the old system and had little understanding of the sick. Nurses who had worked under trained nurses and doctors did not easily accept this interference with their work, but infirmaries run this way remained until the National Health Service of 1948 finally swept away the last remnants of the Poor Law. Many of the buildings remain – sometimes 'listed' with their high windows and airing courts – to remind us how the poor sick were dealt with in the nineteenth century and the first half of the twentieth.

REFERENCES

1 Butcher, E. E. (ed.) (1932) *Bristol Corporation for the Poor 1696–1834*, Bristol Record Society, 1932, III.
2 Hammond, J. L. and Hammond, B. (1910) *The Village Labourer*, reprinted 1966, London: Longman.
3 Thompson, E., 'Time and Work Disciplines', *Past and Present* (Dec. 1967), pp. 93–4.
4 McKeown, T. and Brown, R. G. (1969) 'Interpretation of the rise of the population in England and Wales', *Central African Journal of Medicine*, also quoted in McKeown in Preface to the *Role of Medicine* (1976), Rock Carling Fellowship, Nuffield Provincial Hospitals Trust.
5 Habakkuk, H. S. (1958) *Population, Commerce and Economic Ideas*, New Cambridge Modern History, ch. 8, London and Cambridge: Cambridge University Press, pp. 25–7.
6 Rudé, G. (1964), *The Crowd in History*, London: Wiley & Son.
7 Pike, R. (1966) *Human Documents of the Industrial Revolution in Britain*, London: Allen & Unwin.
8 *Parliamentary Report 1482*, 17, p. 513.
9 de Tocqueville, A. (reprinted 1958) *Journeys in England and Ireland*, trans. G. Lawrence and Mayer (eds) pp. 105–6.
10 Carlyle, T. (1843) *Past and Present*, III, also quoted in Karl Marx, *Das Kapital*.
11 Overseers Account Books, Poor House Committee Records; Rate Books Parishes of St James, St Michael, St Peter and St Paul and Walcot: Bath City Archives. County Record Department, Taunton; unpublished thesis, M. E. Baly.
12 Blaug, M. (1964) 'The Old Poor Law re-examined', *Journal of Economic History*, XXIV.
13 Cole, D. and Postgate, R. (1961 edn) *The Common People*, London: Methuen and Co, pp. 121–3.
14 Webb, S. and Webb, B. (1910) *The English Poor Law History*, Part I, (reprinted 1963), London: Cass.
15 Spencer, T. *The Failure of the New Poor Law in 1836*, Poor Law Tracts, Bath, 5, p. 15.
16 Webb, S. and Webb, B. (1911) *English Poor Law History*, Part II, vol. 1, London: Cass.
17 Dickens, C. (1860) 'A walk in the workhouse', from *Household Words*, reprinted in *The Uncommercial Traveller*.
18 Nightingale, F. (1865) taken from a memorandum to Mr Charles Villiers quoted in Cecil Woodham Smith, *Florence Nightingale*, London: Constable, p. 467.
19 Nightingale, F. (1864) Letter to the Rev. Mother Bermondsey.
20 Webb, S. and Webb, B. *English Poor Law History*, Part II, vol. 1.

FURTHER READING

Ashton, T. S. (1968) *The Industrial Revolution 1760–1830*, London and Oxford: Oxford University Press.
Frazer, D. (1973) *The Evolution of the Welfare State*, London: Macmillan.
Laslett, P. (1979) *The World We have Lost*, London: Methuen.
Thompson, E. (1968) *The Making of the English Working Class*, London: Penguin Books.
Webb, S. and Webb, B., *English Poor Law History*, Part I, reprinted 1963, London: Cass.

Chapter 7

Those of unsound mind

The cultural and social background and restrictions on human behaviour have a far-reaching effect on mental health, and attitudes to those whose behaviour deviates from normal vary from society to society and from age to age. In the world of classical Greece the physicians of the Hippocratic tradition recognised the various forms of insanity and prescribed different regimes for the separate categories. Treatment included a good diet, exercise, music and occupational therapy, and, of course, the Aristotelian adjustment of the four humours by purging, emetics and blood-letting. As far as treatment was concerned there was little advance on this until the nineteenth century and, even then, Bethlem Hospital was still purging and blood-letting, having unfortunately forgotten the music, the exercise and the occupational therapy. However, in the intervening centuries the attitude to mental illness, as it was dominated by the different cultures and religious practices, went through many vicissitudes. Sometimes it was confused with sin, at other times it was regarded as proof of demonic possession, and there was a very narrow margin between what was considered to be the vision and ecstasy of a saint and what was thought to be contact with the devil.

In most primitive societies so-called insanity can be absorbed in the community, but as society becomes more complex the mentally handicapped are increasingly disadvantaged and for this reason it is impossible to make a comparison of insanity from age to age or between different cultures. It would appear that in periods of comparative stability, as in the Middle Ages, it was easier to absorb the mentally aberrant and there was more tolerance to deviation; on the other hand, in periods of rapid social change there is more general anxiety and a decreased tolerance to any abnormal behaviour. One such example has already been seen in the witch craze of the sixteenth and seventeenth centuries; another period is the early nineteenth century, when there was an apparent increase in mental ill health and the incidence of suicide accompanying the disturbances and the changed values brought about by the French and the Industrial revolutions. Today there is an apparent, though not measurable, increase in anxiety and neurosis that seems to be concomitant to increasing competitiveness and secularisation and the fact that we are unable to fit the more simple-minded into the pattern and the working methods of a sophisticated society.

TREATMENT OF THE INSANE BEFORE THE NINETEENTH CENTURY

Evidence is scanty, but it seems that in the medieval period the mentally and the physically sick were frequently accommodated together, although St Mary's of Bethlehem in London, which originally cared for vagrants, concentrated on lunatics as early as the fourteenth century. From the legal point of view, and in order to protect estates, a distinction was made between idiots and lunatics, which was set out in a statute of Edward II in 1324. The Elizabethan Poor Law tended to focus attention on the unemployed, and made no separate provision for the insane who were left at liberty so long as they were not a nuisance, if they were, they were apprehended under the vagrancy laws. Interestingly enough, the 'fools' depicted in so many Renaissance plays, particularly Shakespeare, were thought to have special 'insights', and there is a splendid example of this sixteenth-century juxtaposition of 'wisdom in the Fool and folly in the Wise' in *King Lear*.

The seventeenth century saw a change in attitudes throughout Europe and the beginning of the 'Great Confinement';[1] increasing use was made of houses of correction erected under the Poor Law, and in the reign of Queen Anne an Act of Parliament for the first time distinguished between 'poor lunatics' and 'rogues, vagabonds, sturdy beggars and vagrants', and authorised Justices of the Peace to apprehend dangerous lunatics, who could be locked up in a safe place. The cost of dealing with such lunatics fell on the parish, and one way of disposing of the parish lunatics was to board them out in private houses. From the evidence given to the Select Committee at the beginning of the nineteenth century it is clear that this practice had been widespread at the beginning of the eighteenth century and was one of the origins of the private madhouse system. The affluent insane were placed in the more genteel custody of medical men or clergy 'experienced in dealing with distempered persons' who found their disordered charges a useful supplement to their income.[2]

By the end of the eighteenth century the mentally ill were to be found in a variety of places. Many, of course, were cared for in the community, especially in rural areas, where the village idiot was an accepted part of village life.[3] Because, until 1800, insanity was no defence at law, others were to be found languishing in prisons under the conditions described by John Howard. Still others were in houses of correction or in workhouses, while many were boarded out and, for the more prosperous, there were a growing number of private madhouses run for profit; nearly 200 are known and listed, and there were presumably others.[4] Besides these there were 'single lunatics' confined alone, sometimes kept like animals in attics or cellars, sometimes, like the wife of Mr Rochester in Charlotte Bronte's novel, *Jane Eyre*, in special apartments with a private keeper. It is interesting that Charlotte, intelligent and compassionate as she was, implied something evil and sinister about Mrs Rochester's mental state.

The one public institution for lunatics was 'Bethlem', a contraction of Bethlehem, and colloquially known as Bedlam, which had been incorporated by royal charter in Tudor times for the reception of the insane but had deteriorated and become a byword for inhumane treatment where visitors were charged for the privilege of baiting the inmates. The abuses of Bedlam were exposed in 1735 by the famous Hogarth panels on the 'Rake's Progress' and the literary comments of men like Defoe and Jonathan Swift who wrote of the 'hundreds of spectators making sport of the miserable inhabitants of Bedlam provoking them to furies of rage',[5] and this publicity helped towards a new concern for the mentally ill.

NEW ATTITUDES TO MENTAL ILLNESS

At the end of the eighteenth century a number of factors combined to produce a new attitude to the treatment of the insane. First, there was the philosophy of the Enlightenment as propounded by men like Locke (1632–1704), and particularly the epistemiology of David Hume (1711–76) with his 'association of ideas' and his psychological explanations for our false beliefs and fictions; this new type of 'psychological philosophy' exerted considerable influence on psychiatric thought and formed a new basis for the classification of the insane. Second, there were the advances in general medicine and the example of the new charity hospitals which by the end of the century were tending to become 'teaching hospitals'. Inspired by these new hospitals, similar institutions for the insane were founded by public subscription; Guy's Hospital started to provide accommodation for lunatics in 1728, and St Luke's at Muswell Hill was founded in 1751 with the idea of providing treatment early for the less severe cases. The teaching of Dr William Battie of St Luke's illustrates the new approach, for he maintained that 'madness was as manageable as many other distempers and that purging, restraint and incarceration in loathsome prisons was the worst way of dealing with a disordered mind'.

However, the greatest spur to improvement was not so much the miserable fate of the poor lunatics but the legal position; cases had been brought before the courts on writs of habeas corpus and a number of people detained in madhouses were found to be sane. In 1774 a Madhouse Act was passed which made provision for the inspection of the madhouses around London by five Commissioners appointed by the College of

Physicians, and significantly it was only non-pauper patients who had to have a certificate confirming insanity before confinement – paupers, of course, had no legal rights – but apart from this defect there were other difficulties and the Act was largely unenforceable.

In 1785 attention was focused on the problem for a different reason. George III (1738–1820) the first Hanoverian king to identify himself with England, became the victim of an intermittent mental disturbance, now thought to have been caused by porphyria, and had he had the benefit of modern treatment his life and the political situation could have been different. As the attitude to royalty was only just removed from regarding the king as unimpeachable, it was difficult to hold to the theory his afflic- tion was due to sin. To complicate matters the question of the Regency was at stake, and although George III had been obstinate and a trial to his ministers, interfering, and favouring the Tories, the Prince of Wales and his association with Fox and the 'left' Whigs was by no means universally popular, so there were a number of people in high places with a vested interest in George's sanity. Moreover, those like Dr Francis Willis, a clergyman turned physician, who treated George III – not in the modern manner – claimed that insanity was curable, which all added respectability and optimism to the profession of doctors for the mentally ill. When George III died in 1820, he was not referred to as 'mad' or 'insane' but as 'this honest man who passed the last years of his long reign in darkness, mental and bodily'.[6]

The new attitude was reflected in an appraisal of methods of treatment and more enlightened experimentation. On the Continent Phillipe Pinel (1745–1826) the director of the Bicêtre Hospital in Paris, had taken the chains off patients and had written a number of treatises on the manage- ment of the insane. Pinel, who visited England in 1793, approved of the new principles of moral treatment being practised in some hospitals, though he commented, with Gallic pride, that the English physicians had no exclusive claim 'for great superiority of skill' for he had been using such methods for 15 years.

One place that called forth Pinel's approval was the Retreat at York. In 1791 William Tuke (1732–1822), a tea merchant and the head of a well- known Quaker family connected with the Frys, became interested in the York County Asylum where a young woman committed to the care of the Quakers had died in suspicious circumstances. When the governors refused an enquiry Tuke persuaded the Society of Friends (Quakers) to raise money to found a hospital where he could demonstrate that a compas- sionate regime for the insane was both possible and desirable. The name 'Retreat' was chosen by the Society, and was indicative of the spirit of the founders. The advisory physician, Dr Rush, was a man with humane ideas who was interested in the efficacy of occupational therapy; the governors were intelligent and wealthy and held liberal views, but above all the staff were carefully selected and beyond reproach. The Tuke family established a dynasty in the reform movement for the care of the insane, and four generations laboured in the cause, with Daniel Hack Tuke (1827–94) becoming a mental illness specialist, a governor of Hanwell Asylum and the author of the *History of the Insane* (1882).

This attitude and changed philosophy inspired the foundation of the Reform Movement for Lunacy, which in 1807 persuaded Charles Williams-Wynne, the Under-secretary to the Home Office, to set up a Select Committee to enquire into 'the state of the criminal and pauper lunatics in England and Wales and the laws relating thereto'. The Report, which revealed the wretched state of pauper lunatics, led to the County Asylums Act 1808, which laid down specifications for the construction and mainte-nance of county asylums, and although by 1821 only nine such hospitals were completed, the Wynne hospitals, some of which can still be seen, are the forerunners of the present county hospitals. The Act is important because, by providing special legislation for the control of mental hospitals, the way was prepared for a separate hospital system for the mentally ill unconnected with the development of general hospitals for the physically sick and outside the Poor Law (see Chapter 8, Figure 8.1).

THE LUNACY REFORM MOVEMENT

The concept of county asylums was not new, for a number had been built in the eighteenth century by public subscription, but because of the new competing demands for public money for such projects as turnpike roads, bridges, canals and houses of correction, progress on the Wynne Act was slow. But now there was a new alarm; many medical practitioners thought that they detected an increase in mental illness although, needless to say, there was no firm statistical evidence on this point. In 1815 another Select Committee heard further evidence of the exploitation of patients and their relatives by proprietors of private madhouses and the abuses in some asylums. It was to this committee that Godfrey Higgins, a friend of William Tuke, gave evidence about the barbaric cruelties that had been discovered in the York Asylum and of the convenient fire that had destroyed the evidence, and there was further evidence about the degradation and ill-treatment of the patients in Bethlem.

Following the report of the Committee attempts were made by the reformers to bring Bills to deal with the worst abuses, but like all other attempts at reform in other fields, they met with opposition. Lord Eldon, the Lord Chancellor, an extreme Tory, believed that all 'reform movement and philanthropy smacked of dangerous liberalism and could only lead to social unrest and Jacobism', and it was not until after another Select Committee in 1827 that effective legislation reached the statute book. The Madhouse Act of 1828 embodied some of the principles of 1774, did nothing for the single lunatics and left the county asylums uninspected, but the Act did set up a Commission of 15 members with more power over private madhouses and one of the commissioners was Lord Ashley (1801–84), who became the Earl of Shaftesbury in 1851. Ashley perhaps more than anyone else represents the new social conscience of the mid-nineteenth century; he laboured continuously for the cause of children employed in factories and mines and for Ragged Schools, but no cause occupied him so deeply as the care of the insane. It is largely due to Ashley's efforts that an Act in 1842 gave the Commissioners more powers, which in due course led to the Lunatics Act of 1845; this Act set up a Board of Commissioners in Lunacy as a permanent body with powers to inspect all asylums and private licensed houses with the exception of Bethlem, which was not brought under the control of the Commission until 1853. It was now compulsory for all counties and boroughs to make provision for the insane and a large number did so within the next two decades, many of which are still in use, a testimony to solid Victorian building and the fact that land was cheap.

The Commissioners were stringent in their requirements insisting on accurate records of admissions, discharges, deaths, escapes and the use of restraint and solitary confinement. However, in spite of the building programme, the demand for admission soon exceeded the places – an early example of a better service creating its own demand, although of course some of this demand was due to the rising population. The Act, however, had a number of unlooked-for effects. First, it changed the character of the private madhouses, which, having lost their 'inferior' patients, concentrated on the wealthy, who, but for a few private beds in the old voluntary asylums, were excluded from the county hospitals. Meanwhile, the disuse of restraint meant the need to employ more, and a better type of, staff, and this increased the running costs which in its turn had further repercussions. The Poor Law Amendment Act of 1834 had forbidden the admission of 'dangerous lunatics' to Union workhouses, but this was rarely adhered to because transfer to an asylum might cost the poor rate twice as much; in other words, the bed cost in the asylums was rising and the poor could not afford to use them. The Annual Reports of the Poor Law Commission show that they were aware of the problem but they were suspicious of the powers of the magistrates in asylums and feared an extension of this control to *their* paupers.[7] Therefore, instead of using the asylums, there was an increasing tendency for workhouses to set aside 'Lunatic Wards' and in 1853 the Poor Law Board admitted that out of 126,000 inmates, 7,000 were known to be insane, and while the Lunacy Commissioners were convinced that many of these patients were ill-treated and under-fed, there was little they could do. The situation did not improve until the Irremovable Poor Act of 1861, which allowed the cost of maintenance for pauper patients in asylums and registered houses to be transferred from the parish funds to a

Common Fund. However, while this relieved the workhouses of most of their mentally ill, it overburdened the county asylums with chronic cases, and the high hopes of 'moral management' and therapy for comparatively small groups of patients were dashed as asylums became larger and able to concentrate on no more than custodial care.

Nevertheless, the change that had come over the more enlightened hospitals within half a century was remarkable and can only be compared with the changes in the last twenty years. Although psychiatry was yet to become a discipline of medicine there was a great interest in the 'moral management of the insane' and a new specialism evolved; visits were exchanged, papers read, and professional journals published the results of experiments in treatment without coercion or restraint. Dr Conolly (1794–1866) of Hanwell, a pioneer in new methods, realising the implications of the new outlook, encouraged the use of occupation and education as a means of rehabilitating patients and established a rudimentary system of aftercare. Conolly knew, however, that the programme needed a new type of nurse who would be able to co-operate intelligently in the management of the patients, and he requested the governors to introduce a training scheme. At first this was rejected on the grounds of cost, a reason for not introducing or improving nurse training to be repeated for many years to come, but as the idea spread, a number of asylums provided lectures for nurses. Later, when the Medico-Psychological Association was founded in 1841, the campaign for better nursing gathered momentum and by 1891 examinations were organised on a national scale.

WAVES OF SUSPICION AND EXCITEMENT

Unfortunately, what had happened in the past was to happen again – the sudden flowering withered. In 1882 Daniel Tuke wrote, 'waves of suspicion and doubt occasionally pass over the public mind in regard to the custody of the insane',[8] and this was such an occasion. While Ashley and the reformers were working for better conditions, urging specialisation for doctors and better pay for nurses, public attention was again focused on the evils of the private madhouses, the worst abuses of which were now checked by inspection. Pressure groups were formed to prevent illegal detention, and backed by lawyers, a campaign was mounted to secure more rigid control of entry into institutions for the insane. It was suggested that the private system be abolished altogether, which led to a debate that has echoes in our own day with such arguments being raised that 'abolition of the "registered houses" would lead to a clandestine private network', and 'a healthy, but supervised, private sector was a spur to public hospitals' and, above all, 'was it right to let the public hospitals have a monopoly?'. The so-called 'Reform' movement was opposed by Ashley and most of the medical profession, who were against the piling on of safeguards that would detract from early treatment. But one or two sensational legal cases added grist to the campaign's mill and, for good measure, the subject of illegal detention became the theme of melodramatic novels, in which sympathy was directed not at the fate of the mentally sick, but as in Wilkie Collins' *The Woman in White* (1860), at those who assisted the escape of patients who were detained for nefarious reasons: stories as gripping to the Victorians as the 'spy' genre in our own day.

The result of this wave of excitement and pressure from the Lord Chancellor was a complicated set of regulations concerning safeguards and 'certification'. Although the Bill was bitterly resented by the Earl of Shaftesbury, who died before it was introduced, and men like Henry Maudsley (1800), the son-in-law of the great John Conolly, the battle was lost. The Lunacy Act of 1890 was long, complicated and legalistic; it covered every contingency and put restraint not only on admission to asylums but on the further development of the mental health services.

The main provisions of the Act which governed the mental health services for the next 40 years was that the ultimate control was with the Lord Chancellor who appointed the Lunacy Commissioners, but the local control was now with the local authorities set up by the Local Government Act two years earlier (Chapter 8). There were four methods of admission, and the Act introduced the 'reception order'. In the case of a private patient, this was obtained on the petition of relatives or friends, and in the case of a pauper, the petition required two medical certificates, the case to be heard by a magistrate and the order signed by a Justice of the Peace. For short periods admission could be obtained for a private patient through an 'urgency order', and for a pauper on the initiative of the relieving officer or a police constable.

It is doubtful if the safeguards protected anyone, but the rigidity of the process prevented people from seeking treatment, and 'certifiable' became a pejorative word setting mental illness apart. The other disadvantage was that the Act operated through the Poor Law so that mental illness bore the double stigma of being associated with pauperism and the process of the law. It is ironical to recall that as the Act was being forced through by the lawyers, Freud (1856–1939) was just starting to write his seminal works on psychology.

CARE IN THE TWENTIETH CENTURY

By 1900 the main county hospitals were averaging 1,000 patients each and the era of overcrowding had begun. In spite of this and the fact that 'being put away' as a fear of the day ranked with the old outcasting of lepers, advances were made under the inspiration of men like Maudsley, and with better and more organised instruction the nursing improved. Unfortunately, the demands of the First World War robbed the hospitals of doctors and nurses alike, and the more liberal ideas of the better hospitals received a setback. This setback probably more than offset the advances that were made in the treatment of shell shock and the greater understanding of neurosis. It took a Royal Commission sitting from 1924 to 1926 before the Mental Treatment Act of 1930 was introduced, which did what might have been done nearly half a century earlier; it offered admission for voluntary patients and set up out-patient clinics for psychiatric patients, and, by no means least, it was the Mental *Treatment* Act, not. the Lunatics Act.

The decade following the Act saw the introduction of controlled physical treatment for mental illness by such measures as electroconvulsant therapy, insulin treatment and developments in neurosurgery such as prefrontal leucotomy (1935); this gave not only a more optimistic outlook, it also raised the status of the mental hospital and its doctors and nurses. The right thing was done for the wrong reason.

THE CARE OF MENTAL DEFECTIVES

The statute of Edward II made a distinction between idiots and lunatics; and the Lunatics Act of 1845 between 'mental defectives and those of unsound mind'. During the nineteenth century a number of applications were made to license houses for idiot children, like the small school opened in Bath in 1846; this was a variation on the private madhouse theme. During the next few decades a number of idiot asylums were established as charitable institutions, some, like Starcross in Devon, maintaining that they were outside the lunacy laws because their object was *training* and the age limit 15. In 1886 the Idiots Act permitted local authorities to build and maintain special institutes for idiots and imbeciles, but before the challenge could be taken up the Law Lords had stated with conviction in the Lunacy Act, 'Lunatic means idiot or person of unsound mind'. Local authorities reluctant to spend money on the unspectacular task of caring for mental defectives now had the blessing of the law. The case for the feeble-minded was then taken up by voluntary organisations, and the powerful Charity Organisation Society founded in 1868 to prevent the overlap of philanthropic endeavour took up the cause. The Society, which had distinguished and influential members, including Miss Octavia Hill (1838–1912), who was then working on housing reform, turned its attention to mental deficiency, conducting special surveys and organising classes. The Society believed that many such children could be improved, their lives made less burdensome and their usefulness increased by special training. In the debate on relative effects of nature and nurture, the Society was definitely on the side of nurture.

But as the Society was urging optimism a new note was struck by Francis Galton (1822–1911), a cousin of Charles Darwin, who held that Mendel's law not only applied to physical characteristics but also to human intelligence; these views, often misunderstood and sometimes wilfully misinterpreted, underlay much of the argument about Social Darwinism and the philosophy of Nietzche, which in turn were exploited by Hitler to support his pure Aryan policy. Meanwhile the issue was inflamed by the publication of sensational and exaggerated case studies which purported to show a high correlation between feeble-mindedness, delinquency, alcoholism and – still more depressing – fecundity. It was another example of public suspicion and excitement whipped up by the press. On the positive side in France in 1905 the Simon-Binet tests were published, and although their implications were not properly understood the way was open to testing the mental age of a child and to classify defectives according to intelligence.

In 1904 the Balfour administration set up a Royal Commission to 'investigate the existing methods of dealing with idiots and epileptics, and with imbeciles, feeble-minded or defective persons not certified under the lunacy laws'. The Commission sat for four years, and finally recommended a course which steered between the optimism of those who thought defect was susceptible to treatment, and the alarm of the more extreme exponents of eugenics. The outcome was the Mental Deficiency Act of 1913 which replaced the Lunacy Commission with a Board of Control responsible for making better, and further, provision for the feeble-minded and moral defectives. Mental deficiency was defined as 'a condition of arrested or incomplete development of mind existing before the age of eighteen years, whether arising from inherent causes or injury'.

Under the terms of the Act defectives could be sent to special institutions or placed under guardianship. Unfortunately, legal machinery for 'certification' of mental defectives was introduced and the new mental health authorities were soon divorced from the general work of the public health departments. These barriers hampered a social approach to the problem, and the mental defective, like the mentally ill, was set apart. However, new colonies were built, with many of the existing ones dating from this Act, and authorities began to undertake not only institutional care but responsibility for guardianship, supervision and home visiting and teaching. At the same time the voluntary movement stressed the need for community care, and the Central Association for Mental Welfare, co-ordinating a number of agencies, organised training courses for voluntary workers. Some of these social workers were used by local authorities to do assessment and case work and to augment the community services; there was a growing awareness that institutions alone could not cope with the problem and that community care was not only cheaper, but was also better for the handicapped person. Unfortunately, the war and its aftermath of economic depression meant that little real advance could be made in this direction and the mental health services in the community remained poorly developed.

Nevertheless, between the wars there was more fruitful research in genetics, and this with the now more widely accepted teachings of Freud and his disciples, together with the new understanding of psychopathology, changed the attitude to, and the interest in, the mentally sick; a new bridge was being built between the mind and the body. The wheel was coming full circle to the teachings of the Greek physicians.

REFERENCES

1 Foucault, M. (1967) *Madness and Civilization*, London: Tavistock, p. 38.
2 Parry-Jones, W. Ll. (1972) *The Trade in Lunacy*, quoting A. Fessler (1956) *The Management of Lunacy in Seventeenth-century England*, London: Routledge & Kegan Paul.
3 Wordsworth, W. (1798) 'The Idiot Boy', in *The Poetry of Wordsworth*, Crehan, T. (ed.) (1965), London: Hodder & Stoughton.
4 Parry-Jones, *Trade in Lunacy*.
5 Swift, J. (1710) *Letters to Stella*, G. A. Aitken (ed.) 1901.
6 *Gentleman's Magazine*, 1820.
7 Select Committee on the Poor Law Amendment Act *Fifth Report*, 1838.
8 Tuke, D. H. (1882) *History of the Insane,* quoted in K. Jones, *Lunacy Law and Conscience* (1953), London: Routledge & Kegan Paul.

FURTHER READING

Foucault, M. (1967) *Madness and Civilization*, London: Tavistock.
Jones, K. (1953) *Lunacy Law and Conscience*, London: Routledge & Kegan Paul.
Parry-Jones, W. Ll. (1972) *The Trade in Lunacy*, London: Routledge & Kegan Paul.

Chapter 8

Local government and sanitary reform

> I wander through thro' each charter'd street,
> Near where the charter'd Thames does flow,
> And mark in every face I meet
> Marks of weakness, marks of woe.
>
> 'London', William Blake (*c.* 1794)

One of the main difficulties in implementing social reform to meet the changed needs of the nineteenth century was the lack of effective local administration. British local government had evolved from the Saxon parish system where freemen were grouped in hundreds and formed subdivisions of the shires and counties. Over the years the counties had become uneven in size and, although the 'Hundreds' were still often used as a basic division of a parish, they were no longer indicative of a density of population. After the introduction of parliamentary representation in 1265, towns and cities obtained privileges, some had the 'charters' referred to by Blake, which freed them from the surveillance of the County Sheriff and enabled them to send their own representatives to Parliament. By the end of the eighteenth century many of these privileges were no longer justified and in some places, the so-called 'Rotten Boroughs', the candidate was returned by a handful of electors; others were 'Pocket Boroughs', where patrons could secure their own nominees. As the population increased and moved to new areas, the privileges of the old boroughs seemed more anachronistic, for the new towns often had no civic organisation and London itself was in the hands of the parish vestries and the county Justices. It was discontent with these anomalies that led to the 'Reform Movement', which, after terrible bitterness and rancour, recalled by Miss Nightingale as a childhood memory, led to the Reform Act of 1832 which redistributed parliamentary seats and granted a limited increase to the male franchise.

After the setting up of constitutional monarchy under William of Orange (1689–1702), it became an accepted principle that there should be no interference in local affairs by the central government; the structure set up by the Elizabethan statutes continued to operate: local government was largely self-government. In order to provide some of the services needed, tentative attempts were made by Acts of Parliament to introduce local Improvement Acts, and semi-private concerns grew up with local commissions dealing with matters like street lighting, sewers and the relief of the poor. In spite of the haphazard nature of the system and the corruption of much local government, improvements were made, and by the end of the eighteenth century roads, street lighting and sanitation were much better than the descriptions given of England in the 1720s by writers like Defoe (1660–1731). But as the population and urbanisation grew there was an urgent need for more stringent control of the municipal services.

Early reform came from central commissions which required local 'Unions' of parishes to undertake specific tasks of which the requirement to set up Boards of Guardians (Chapter 6) is a good example. However, after the Reform Act 1832 the Municipal Corporations Act of 1835 allowed boroughs to apply for a separate court of the Quarter sessions, and some appointed stipendary magistrates who were paid and who were now invariably trained judicial officers, a good example of the nineteenth century change from the gentleman amateur to the professional. By the terms of the Act, 184 corporations were suppressed and replaced by elected councils chosen by the ratepayers; the council chose a mayor who held office for a year and aldermen who made up half the council who held office for six years. According to the Webbs, the expansion of middle-class power in the nineteenth century is to be found in the towns and not in Parliament, which remained distinctly aristocratic.[1] Needless to say, the magistrates and the Guardians came into conflict from time to time, and as the issue of public health began to impinge on the question of pauperism and the legal problems surrounding drainage and water supply, so the battle for sanitary reform became inseparable from the campaign for a strong, all-purpose local government.

EARLY ATTEMPTS AT DEVELOPING PUBLIC HEALTH SERVICES

In 1720 Richard Mead (1673–1754), a protégé of John Radcliffe, published a treatise on the plague, in which he argued the case for a Central Board of Control. In 1798, Edward Jenner (1749–1823), having discovered a means of vaccination, had been instrumental in setting up a Vaccination Board, and although it did not make vaccination compulsory until 1853, when, ironically, smallpox had ceased to be a major killer, it and the quarantine regulations of 1743 were the only public health measures in existence.

In 1804 yellow fever crossed from the West Indies to the Mediterranean where, because in Gibraltar it killed a third of the population, it was known as 'Gibraltar sickness'. Fear of its spread created alarm and the Privy

Council consulted the College of Physicians – the general advisory body on all health matters, which advised the establishment of a Central Board of Health. The recommendations included the setting up of an epidemiological centre, the establishment of isolation hospitals, the rigid separation of the sick, the employment of nurses at public expense, regulations about fumigation and the handling of infected material with forceps. Towns where fever was reported were required to set up a Local Board and the Justices were to regulate relief, grant certificates and make arrangements for the transfer of infected persons. Perhaps the most interesting recommendation was that yellow fever should be dealt with at its source in the West Indies. Had yellow fever reached England in 1805 it, and not cholera, would have been the driving force behind health legislation. Compared with later events this enlightened attitude is yet another proof, if one were needed, that health care and attitudes to it are not continuously progressive.

In the 1820s there was news of another sickness crossing from Asia, the acute epidemic disease cholera, that is spread by contaminated water. As earlier, the Privy Council got in touch with the College of Physicians about setting up a Board of Health; as before, the College responded offering the names of distinguished physicians and a Board was established. Like its predecessor, it lasted only two years. The regulations were rigorous, requiring the setting up of Local Board of Health consisting of Justices, clergymen and doctors, and the sub-division of towns into district committees which were given the wide powers of removal and fumigation; it was even suggested that a reward be offered to the first person to detect a case of cholera morbus and that those found guilty of concealment be fined. It was hardly surprising that the regulations were unpopular and no one reaped the reward; nevertheless, 1,200 local boards were formed, and the machinery was there when the need came.

In October 1831 the first death from cholera was reported, then as the disease spread the Physicians' Board was replaced by a General Board of Health and in 1832 the Cholera Act was hurried through; by the middle of the year 5,000 people had died. Local boards were built up, but once they began to extend their activities into prevention they overlapped with other local boards and groups and there were disputes about who did what, and who paid for what. As the epidemic abated so did the enthusiasm; the Cholera Act was allowed to lapse and at the end of the parliamentary session the Board of Health was dissolved.

NINETEENTH-CENTURY PUBLIC HEALTH PROBLEMS

In spite of epidemics of the plague in the Middle Ages and the outbreak in London in 1665, England never suffered epidemics to the same extent as other countries, partly owing to the absence of widespread famine and malnutrition on the scale often found on the Continent, and to the limited advances in hygiene, but the main reason was probably that the cool climate was not favourable to the animal vectors of disease. Therefore the outbreaks of cholera and the marginal rise in the death rate at a time when the population was becoming more prosperous was surprising and challenging.

There were three main reasons for the rise in cases of infection. First, there was the rise in the population numbers and rapid urbanisation (Figure 8.1). The population of Great Britain rose from 12.4 million in 1810 to 16.5 million in 1830, a rise of 30 per cent in 20 years; in 1800 no city had a population of over 100,000, by 1837 there were five and by 1891 the number was 23. In 1841 only 17.27 per cent of the population lived in cities of this size, by 1891 the proportion was 31.2 per cent.[2] More people were living in close proximity, and although the new artisan houses were solid by present-day standards they lacked the basic amenities of drainage and sewerage and this was the great health hazard. But not only was there the threat of infection in the home, life at work was fraught with health problems in a way that agricultural work was not. Apart from industrial accidents there were new dangers from work processes. In 1832 Dr James Kay* (1804–77) wrote a report on the cotton operatives of Manchester, where he says that workers not only lived in a polluted atmosphere and pestilential streets, but they also toiled in workshops for 12 hours a day, breathing dust and filaments of cotton, where they were totally exhausted by unremitting toil.

> These artisans are frequently the subject of a disease in which the sensibility of the stomach is morbidly excited and the alvine secretions deranged and the appetite impaired, . . . as the disease worsens the victim becomes depressed and falls into despair, a mental state we can only conclude associated with infection or some toxic state.[3]

The second reason was that, however medical knowledge may have progressed in other ways, it was no nearer the light as far as the spread of infection was concerned than Galen had been, although there were a number of people, Dr Kay among them, who recognised the predisposing causes. But the mass of infections from which people suffered were neither differentiated nor clearly understood. Finally, there was the attitude to poverty outlined in Chapter 6. The theories of Malthus about the population overwhelming resources; the economic obsession with *laissez-faire* and the non-interference with the labour market, and the social policies of the utilitarians who believed that poverty could be abolished if poor relief were made sufficiently unpleasant and the poor (in their own interests) stopped breeding, all combined to produce a harsh, though

---

* Changed his name to Kay-Shuttleworth, created 1st Baronet 1849.

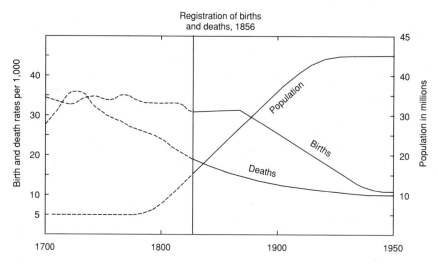

Figure 8.1 Population growth in England and Wales, 1700–1950 (Crown copyright)

well-intentioned, attitude to the poor and the casualties of the industrial system. However, by setting up the New Poor Law as a deterrent to pauperism, the government had unwittingly opened up the whole question of the causes of pauperism and the ill health with which it was intrinsically bound.

EDWIN CHADWICK AND MID-CENTURY PUBLIC HEALTH

Edwin Chadwick (1800–90), one of the architects of the New Poor Law and secretary to the Commission, during his work began to see preventable ill health as having a strong, and causal, link with pauperism. In 1838, at the behest of the Home Secretary, the Poor Law Commission investigated a complaint into the cost of the removal of nuisances, and this led to the so-called 'Fever Report' by the three doctors who did the survey, James Kay, Neil Arnott and Southwood Smith, and this gave Chadwick a chance to press for a full enquiry. Chadwick, who was notoriously contumacious and unpopular with the Commission, was readily, and one suspects thankfully, given leave to conduct the survey. In spite of the difficulties put in his way Chadwick, with indefatigable energy visited the worst towns and slums for himself, and in a manner that recalls John Howard, quarried a mine of information, and his *Report on the Sanitary Conditions of the Labouring Population of Great Britain* (1842) remains one of the most informative Blue Books of the nineteenth century. In his report Chadwick showed that there was a strong link between environment and disease and there was wide variation between the average life expectancy in different parts of the country. A professional man in Kensington could expect to live until he was 44 years old, but in Bolton his expectancy was 34; at the same time a labourer in Manchester had an expectancy of a mere 17 years but in Rutland he might live twice as long.[4] Chadwick argued that much of this death was preventable and was a waste of manpower, and in terms of dependants was an added burden on the Poor Rate.

> That of the 43,000 cases of widowhood, and 112,000 cases of destitute orphanage relieved from the poor's rates in England and Wales alone, it appears that the greatest proportion of deaths of heads of families occurred from the above specified and other removable causes; that their ages were under 45 years; that is to say, 13 years below the natural probabilities of life as shown by the whole population of Sweden.[5]

Chadwick was now admitting that the main demand on the Poor Rate was not the able-bodied but widows and children. He now believed that in order to prevent disease it would be necessary to have a more powerful local administration, which he saw as being accountable to a central authority – not a popular idea. However, the most practical part of the Report concerned 'the means by which the sanitary conditions of the labouring classes may be improved'; these consisted of proper drainage, the removal of refuse, and above all, the improvement in the supplies of water. Health depended on sanitation and sanitation was largely a matter of engineering. Chadwick was the first to advocate the modern method of sewerage disposal by glazed round pipes flushed through with water; this, of course, implied a great increase in water supplies, and water was controlled by private companies for profit. The control of the water supply was therefore ultimately the key to the problem. Among Chadwick's other recommendations was the employment of salaried Medical Officers of Health. The first of these was Dr W. Duncan, who was appointed to Liverpool in 1847, which had then the distinction of having the highest death rate in the country and a life expectancy rate of 24 years as an average for all classes; Dr Duncan's heroic efforts in tackling this problem is rightly one of the legends of public health.[6]

Apart from the fact that Chadwick had stumbled on the way to break the causal chain of water-borne infection without any scientific proof about the mode of transmission, it is interesting to note the change in his philosophy, which was typical of much of the utilitarian movement. Chadwick, like other 'liberals', was moving away from the doctrinaire *laissez-faire* to the idea of collectivist intervention to secure, by direct legislation if necessary, the 'greatest good for the greatest number', the control of water supplies being the classic example. Later, John Stuart Mill expounded this doctrine more elegantly and is one of the economists with whom Miss Nightingale corresponded and with whose views she was largely in accord.

Chadwick's Report had a wide circulation and its findings were backed by the Health of Towns Commission set up by the Peel administration in 1844, a report which incidentally led to the setting up of such associations in a number of towns and whose reports are still available. Both Chadwick and the Commission knew that reform could not come without a long and bitter struggle, and freedom from cholera, a spell of good harvests and the inevitable conflict with those who had a vested interest in selling water led to procrastination; then, in 1847, a bad harvest and the renewed threat of cholera succeeded where reports and public debate had failed, and the Public Health Act of 1848 was passed. The Act, cautious and vague, established a General Board of Health with three Health Commissioners, Kay, Arnott and Southwood-Smith, for a period of five years. Unfortunately the Board began its life during an outbreak of cholera, and as there was no effective local machinery to carry out its recommendations, what it could achieve was limited. Above all, the whole ideology of central interference was unpopular and subject to a bad press, although, ironically enough, 'interference' and control to deal with paupers had been accepted quickly. Chadwick, who had always been tetchy and difficult to work with, was dismissed in 1854, and from then on, although it remained in existence for another four years, the Board ceased to be effective.

However, although the Board was disbanded advances were made. In spite of rivalries and chicanery in local affairs and accusations of corruption and patronage when contracts for water and sewerage works were handed out, many towns started their own sanitary schemes and some appointed Medical Officers of Health. The City of London accepted with reluctance the appointment of Dr John Simon, who already had a distinguished career in pathology; the City intended Simon to be a mere figurehead but they were soon to learn otherwise. In the much-vaunted square mile Simon showed that the infant mortality rate was higher than in almost any other city, while the housing density was up to 291 persons to an acre with three families in a room and perhaps nine in a bed. Sewers were open and unconnected, water was supplied to dark, crowded alleys through a stand-cock operating for half an hour a day and never on Sunday. Burial grounds reeked with a stench, and the blood from slaughterhouses ran down Aldgate. Simon asked for accurate information, prompt notification of deaths, reports of sickness in workhouses and prisons, and from the Poor Law Officers a co-ordination of effort. By a triumph of tact and persuasion he built up a new concept of a Medical Officer of Health with his first annual report, a model of factual information which set the standard for many years to come. Unlike the pioneers in the industrial North, Simon was reporting on conditions within a few miles of Parliament, and *The Times*, hitherto a bitter critic of Chadwick and the Board of Health, hailed the City report as 'a great milestone in the cause of public sanitation'.

Meanwhile in 1854, when Miss Nightingale was helping with the nursing of the cholera cases at the Middlesex Hospital, a mile or so to the south in Soho, young Dr John Snow was confronted with an outbreak in an area that had hitherto been free. By careful observation and logic he tracked down the cholera cases to the people who had been supplied with water from the Broad Street pump. The pump handle was removed and the epidemic abated. Dr Snow wrote up his findings in what he called 'a slender pamphlet', which clenched the argument that cholera was spread by faecal contamination of water.[7] Professor Fraser Brockington comments laconically, 'now that the world is drowned in words it does good to contemplate so much benefit to mankind from so few'. In Somerset, William Budd had made similar observations about typhoid. Now, although the causal organisms remained elusive, incontrovertible evidence was building up about the mode of transmission, and men like Chadwick and the early Medical Officers of Health, and women like Miss Nightingale, could advocate the right thing even if they did not know the right reason for it.

As the great cholera epidemic of 'the long, hot summer' of 1854 subsided, so did support for public health measures and what were called 'the clean party' in the cities; the General Health Board was dissolved and its functions transferred to the Privy Council – another Victorian maid-of-all-administrative work – with Dr John Simon as the medical officer. It was a period of consolidation; Simon gathered around him a team of distinguished doctors, who, unlike their successors in the twentieth century, moved easily from careers in medicine to studies of health and disease in the environment. Between 1860 and 1862 Edward Greenhow made a comparative study of deaths in the different parts of England and analysed the morbidity rates from pulmonary disease according to occupation, showing the wide variation for the different parts of the country and for different occupations. Thomas Spencer Wells (1818–97) studied the results of quarantine, and Sir Thomas Clifford Allbutt, a Cambridge professor, investigated the prevention of disease by better housing. It was now clear to Simon and his team that although the Factory Act of 1833 had limited the hours worked by women and children and the further Acts of 1844 and 1850 pioneered by Lord Ashley had made some improvement in working conditions, manufacturing processes were themselves creating new hazards; phosphorous poisoning, arsenite of copper producing arsenic poisoning, chimney-sweep's cancer, fork-grinder's lung and other new occupational diseases, often with colourful demotic names were described at this time. At the same time, although improved sanitation was beginning to reduce the incidence of the water-borne diseases, and vaccination had apparently lowered the rate of smallpox and tuberculosis was declining, their places as killers had been taken by virulent outbreaks of diphtheria, scarlet fever and whooping cough.

The result of the exposure of the more glaring public health evils was a welter of confused legislation. There were Public Health Acts which permitted the setting up of local health boards and the appointing of salaried officials; then there were the confusing, and sometimes conflicting, Acts dealing with nuisances, the control of burial grounds, slaughterhouses, common lodging houses, smoke, noisome trades and the like. Besides these there were new 'Sewer Authorities' created by an Act of 1865, and finally, the Disease Prevention Acts and a wide range of private and confusing local Acts. In 1865 Simon wrote in his report that the time had come for unifying action, the result of which was the Sanitation Act of 1866, which made available to all authorities the powers of the 1848 Act, enlarged the field of nuisances and made it a duty for authorities to fulfil sanitary functions. Unfortunately, the Act, badly drafted, carried little conviction and less action and the inevitable Royal Commission was set up to sort out the muddle. Reporting in 1871, the Commission was loud in its condemnation of the casual and experimental public health system and recommended speedy action 'to consolidate the present fragmentary and confused legislation'. The need for speed was reinforced by the threat of cholera, a possible epidemic of smallpox and the distant rumblings of the approaching 'Great Depression' of the 1870s. The Commission had stressed the need for separate machinery to deal with public health and stated that it should not be confused with the functions of the Poor Law, which of course had been the point made by the Workhouse Reform Movement in 1867: the deterrent attitude of the Poor Law was inimical to good public health. Unfortunately, both the public and Parliament had been long educated in the principles of less eligibility, and the idea of deterrence was so ingrained that the message of public health and the 'sanitary ideal' failed to find reflection in satisfactory legislation. However, in order to implement some of the Commission's recommendations, the Gladstone administration compromised and passed the Local Government Board Act in 1871. The Local Government Board was in fact a continuation of the old Poor Law Board which it replaced, and it took under its wing the Registrar General's Department and the Medical Department of the Privy Council, with John Simon as a subordinate – a situation which had a subsequent effect on the status of preventive medicine. Moreover, the shadow of the Poor Law was cast forward to rest on local government itself, a fact that was later to effect the attitude of the medical profession to the health services run by local authorities. The Local Government Board remained in being until the Ministry of Health came into existence in 1919, and when the National Health Service was set up, it found itself in possession of property marked 'LGB'.

In order to implement the provisions of the Local Government Board Act at local level the Public Health Act of 1872 was passed. This mapped out the country into sanitary authorities, each of which was to have a Medical

Officer of Health; then in 1875 the great Public Health Act consolidated many of the previous sanitary Acts and this continued to control most public health legislation until 1936, and some until 1948. To the 1875 Act was added the important Artisan's Dwelling Act of the same year, which allowed authorities to replace insanitary housing and was the forerunner of municipal housing schemes – in fact, the 'council houses'.

LOCAL GOVERNMENT AT THE END OF THE NINETEENTH CENTURY

Since in 1867 the Second Reform Act had extended the franchise, the various strands of the Labour Party were beginning to come into being, and by 1883 there were 11 Labour members in Parliament; there was an increasing tendency, in all groups, to promote greater democracy. In local government this was still confused, and in 1888 the Conservatives removed some of the anomalies by the Local Government Act (not to be confused with the LGB), which set up elected County Councils to replace the nominated justices in the administration of county affairs, and created County Boroughs from the larger towns which were also to set up popularly elected councils to control local policy and administration. In 1894 a further Local Government Act established urban and rural councils as health authorities. Now the health and Poor Law functions were combined centrally under the Local Government Board, whose chief functionary was the President of the Poor Law Board, but locally the Poor Law functions were administered by the Boards of Guardians, and the health functions by the Health Committee of the new authorities, whose chief officer was usually the Medical Officer of Health. As time went by the new local authorities, in a variety of different ways, took under their aegis other services; for example, the county asylums for which they were responsible to the Lunacy Commission, and eventually the new education services, soon to require health services themselves (Figure 8.2).

Local government in London

In the middle of the century there were no fewer than '250 local Acts of Parliament relating to particular districts and there were 10,000 commissioners exercising varying functions and degrees of authority'.[8] The result was muddle and confusion that led to the London depicted by Dickens (1812–70) with its seamy, uncleansed alleys and courts around the polluted Thames, that dark underside of the city that attracted and repelled so many writers, the London of Mayhew's *London Labour and London Poor* of 1851, where the 'masses' had their being.

The main problem was that the population ebbed and flowed like the tide; Londoners moved out to the sprawling suburbs and immigrants

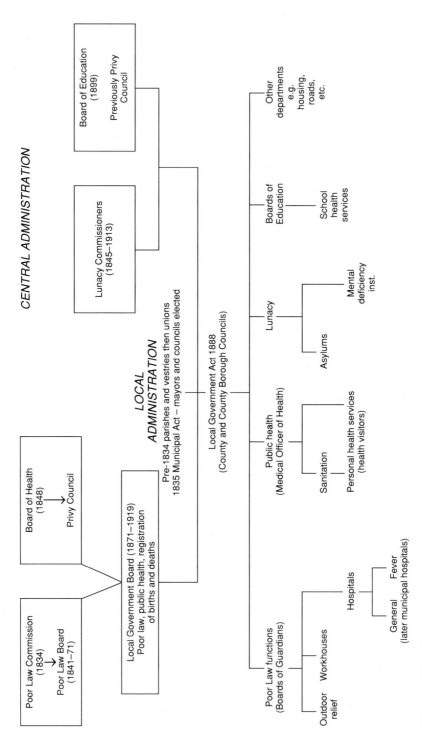

Figure 8.2 Health services in the nineteenth century

moved into the centre. Partly because of this Chadwick wanted to see London's sanitary administration in the hands of a small, powerful commission, but the idea was not popular with the many groups favouring democracy and in 1854 a Royal Commission pronounced against one authority, and instead the Metropolis Local Management Act was passed; for a number of purposes London was administered by the Metropolitan Board of Works, whose hallmarks are still to be seen and which was responsible, among other things, for acquiring a number of London's parks and gardens. The Board itself consisted of delegates chosen by the parish vestries, but it in no way reflected pressure from below, merely trying to implement the various Acts from above. By the 1880s there was new radicalism about the concept of civic needs and duties, with the Socialists and the new Liberals urging greater action. However, it was the Conservatives who eventually introduced the London County Council Act of 1888 which allowed for the direct election of 118 councillors. The greater range of civic functions, the possibilities of such services as public libraries encouraged initiative and debate, and now that the struggle between the different interests took a political form, there was at last the possibility of London leading the way with good civic government. Then in 1899 Balfour, reacting against centralisation, passed the Metropolitan Boroughs Act which created 28 metropolitan boroughs each with its own mayor and council, the move being opposed by the Liberals as creating, 'instead of one London, 29 little Birminghams'. London was again sub-divided, but not in a way that reflected any particular civic loyalty and people began to ask, where does London begin and end? The Act left an important legacy for the health services in London because every borough had its own medical officer and its own peculiar employment arrangements about school nurses and health visitors, which was yet another problem to be dealt with by the National Health Service and the post-war reorganisation of local government.

Education

The French Revolution had paved the way for a new educational system in France with the Ecole Polytechnique enabling France to take the lead in science. Then, in the second half of the century, Germany under the leadership of Bismarck (1815–98) rapidly developed its universities and a highly organised system of technical and general education. England lagged behind. In spite of the efforts of Dr Kay-Shuttleworth, now secretary to a committee of the Privy Council on teacher training, and the founding of his Training College at Battersea, little headway was made because on the one hand there were the claims of the different religious denominations that education must remain in their hands, and on the other the fear of the *ultras* who thought if people were educated above their station there would be social unrest and revolution. Nevertheless the new technical advances of the day required workers who understood them, and in 1869, W. E. Forster (1818–86) as Vice-President of Education in the Gladstone administration conducted a survey in which he found that in four major towns only 10 per cent of the population had any schooling. The result was the Education Act of 1870, known as the 'Forster Act', which, although it did not provide universal education, did allow School Boards to be established and elementary education to be provided from the rates and a government grant. In 1899 a Board of Education was set up and in 1902 the Balfour Education Act made the new local authorities 'Local Education Authorities' (LEAs) and placed a statutory duty on them to provide elementary education for all children up to 14 years and allowed for the provision of secondary education, and last, and controversially, to make grants to former religious schools provided certain conditions were met.

After 1870 for the first time the poor health of children was brought to the notice of the authorities. At the same time the physical deterioration of children, due to poverty and ignorance, was revealed not only to the school teacher but also to the recruiting sergeant, for between 40 and 60 per cent of the recruits for the Boer War (1899–1902) were rejected on grounds of physical defect. This led to the formation of the Interdepartmental Committee on Physical Deterioration, whose report in 1904 must be regarded as a seminal document in the history of the health services. Its recommendations were far-seeing, and included the training of mothers, referring to the Salford Ladies; the need for health societies all over the country; for the feeding of schoolchildren; for games and physical exercises for girls as well as boys; it urged that schools should provide cookery classes for the older girls; and, striking a modern note, it pointed out the dangers of juvenile smoking. It was all a strange mixture of forward-looking health and educational policy and Edwardian paternalism, some of which called forth outraged letters to *The Times*.[9] Letters to *The Times* or no, it was this Report that underlay much of the social legislation brought in by the new Liberals after their landslide victory in 1906 and which in many ways became the foundation stone of the modern welfare state.[10]

In 1906 the needs of destitute children were partly met by the Education (Provision of Meals) Act, which allowed educational authorities to supply meals for children in deprived areas; and the Education (Administrative Provisions) Act of 1907 marked the beginning of school medical inspection and enabled the local authorities to provide schoolchildren with medical care. One suggestion of the Interdepartmental Committee had been that there should be a unified state health service for children organised on a local basis; or alternatively, that doctors in private practice should give care to schoolchildren and be reimbursed from public funds. Had either of these suggestions been adopted, curative and preventive medicine would not have suffered the divorce that was to bedevil it for years to come. As it was, the British Medical Association protested, and in the end the preventive services and the 'School medical inspection' was given to the local authority and the Medical Officer of Health, but curative services remained with the private doctor, whose services the parents of under-fed children could not afford, a disability that was to remain until 1948.

In 1907 the Notification of Births Act required all births to be notified to the Medical Officer of Health, and this gave a statutory basis for the health visitor, and the Children's Act of the following year codified earlier legislation, with some of the provisions remaining until 1968; it was the 'Children's Charter' for the best part of 40 years and provided juvenile courts and the Child Life Protection regulations.

POVERTY AND HEALTH AT THE BEGINNING OF THE TWENTIETH CENTURY

In spite of the fact that many towns had tackled the problem of sanitation with vigour, and because of the water closet – perhaps the greatest boon to public health in all time – and better water supplies, and diseases like cholera had ceased as epidemics, the death rate was still 22 per 1,000 in the last decade of the century and the infant mortality rate 163 per 1,000. In 1886 Charles Booth (1840–1916), a wealthy Liverpool shipowner, organised an elaborate survey of the East End of London. His original study carried out in Tower Hamlets showed that about one-third of the population were living below a line that he himself had worked out, called 'the poverty line'. The poor were not the trade unionists or skilled workers but the unorganised men and women in sweated industries, the casual workers, women, and the unemployed and unemployable – the same groups that were on parish relief in the eighteenth-century – not the wilful able-bodied so often referred to by opinion but never found in the statistics. Like Mrs Fry and other philanthropists, Booth asked the question, how under these conditions the poor could be expected to lead moral lives. This led to the monumental work, *Life and Labour of the People of London*, which appeared in 17 volumes between 1889 and 1902. Booth, who can be classed among the pioneer social scientists, showed, among other things, that there was a cycle of poverty for low paid workers – when the young family were growing up, then again in old age – and that the problem of poverty was far beyond the scope of private charity or exhortations to thrift. What was needed was government intervention, a finding which gave weight to the argument already going on about the possibility of state pensions for the elderly poor. In York, Seebohm Rowntree (1871–1954), a Quaker and a member of the great chocolate family, became interested in Booth's work and conducted his own survey. *Poverty – a Study in Town Life* showed that 28 per cent of the people of York lived below the poverty line, but Rowntree distinguished between 'primary' poverty, where there was not enough money for subsistence, and secondary poverty, where earnings were sufficient but waste and ignorance reduced the family to poverty. Rowntree continued his labours until well into the twentieth century, and in 1937 in *The Human Needs of Labour* showed the extent of poverty in the inter-war years.

These and other surveys 60 years after Chadwick's revelations showed that the doctrines of the utilitarians had not reduced unemployment; the poor, suitably deterred, had not died away. The reasons for Victorian poverty are complex; industrialisation had led to a pattern of booms and slumps which economists did not know how to manipulate and control, and of course many thought should *not* be controlled. Second, in the early years social policy was determined by the notion that intervention did more harm than good. As the century wore on men became converted to the need for some collectivist intervention, and Radicals, Liberals, Socialists and even the Conservatives accepted the idea of state control in varying degrees, but in the gap between the acceptance of the idea and legislation lay Booth's 'submerged third'.

NURSING AND THE SANITARY IDEAL

There was a tendency among reformers to concentrate on the living conditions of the poor and the effect on their morals rather than on the working conditions and low wages that made them poor. Societies for sanitary improvement grew up, and in Manchester a Statistical Society conducted an enquiry into the living conditions of the poor. Then in 1851 a Sanitary Association was formed 'to teach the laws of health', followed ten years later by the Ladies' Sanitary Association which was formed to teach health to mothers. However, the ladies were not particularly successful and their leaflets made little impression, so they employed a 'respectable woman' to go from door to door giving advice and help as the opportunity offered. At first the 'health missioners' were employed by the Association, an example of a voluntary service pioneering the way for a statutory service; then the Association changed its name to the Ladies' Health Society, and the missioners were called Health Visitors. As the work developed and the importance of lowering the infant mortality rate became recognised, an arrangement was made with the Manchester City Council for the work of the health visitors to be brought under the direction of the Medical Officer of Health and a proportion of their salary to be paid by the local authority.

In 1892, when Miss Nightingale was staying with her brother-in-law, Sir Harry Verney (see Chapter 9), she had a chance to promote her idea that the work of the district nurses should be backed by *trained* health visitors. The Local Government Act had given the County Councils the power to spend money on technical education, and Miss Nightingale's nephew, Frederick Verney, was, fortuitously, the chairman for education in North Buckinghamshire, and with his aid she managed to get a training for 'lady health visitors' classed as technical education. Sixteen lectures were given, followed by discussion, and the students did practical work with the Medical Officer of Health and the general practitioners; the pass rate was only 50 per cent, so it was obvious that Miss Nightingale's contention that 'health visitors required a different, but not lower, training was being endorsed.

At first health visiting was seen as a separate profession from nursing, requiring different skills. Indeed Frederick Verney wrote, 'the health visitor is not a nurse and does not pretend to be one'. The work of the early visitors was primarily educative and persuasive; the visitor came as a friend and counsellor to the *whole family*, and it was always emphasised that she was not an inspector. However, by the end of the century there was increasing concern about the health of children and the infant mortality rate, and this and the maternal death rate were the reasons for the Midwives Act of 1902, which required midwives to undergo a training and to register with the new Central Midwives Board; then the Notification of Births Act gave the opportunity for a statutory basis for health visiting which fitted the same pattern – the health visitor would take over from the new-style midwife. In the same year the Health Visitors (London) Order required all health visitors to have either a medical degree, which a number did in fact have, or the full training of a nurse, or the certificate of the CMB, and some training as a nurse and the certificate of an 'approved society'. The Sanitary Institute, founded by Chadwick in 1876, later the Royal Sanitary Institute, was already holding examinations for inspectors of nuisances, and now prepared a course suitable for teachers or trained nurses and continued to be the certificate-granting body until 1962.

The idea of a 'health missioner' came into being as the result of the sanitary campaign started in the middle of the nineteenth century by men like Chadwick, who instinctively equated disease with poor hygiene. Sanitary reform eventually brought to an end the great water-borne epidemics, and the identification of bacteria paved the way for the control of infectious diseases. By this time health visiting had become established as a branch of nursing, but the situation that called her into being was to change. Like so many situations in medicine the wheel comes full circle, and once again it is the whole family that needs her guidance, but over problems that are more difficult to ameliorate than was cholera by the removal of the handle of the Broad Street pump.

REFERENCES

1 Webb, S. and Webb, B. (1910) *English Local Government*, vol. I, Private edn, reprinted 1963, London: Cass, p. 222.

2 Briggs, A. (1963) *Victorian Cities*, London: Penguin Books (Pelican), p. 59.
3 Kay, J. P. (1832) 'The moral and physical conduct of the working classes employed in cotton manufacture in Manchester', reprinted (1970) in *Industrialisation and Culture*, London: Macmillan, pp. 9–12.
4 Chadwick, E. (1842) 'The sanitary condition of the labouring population of Gt Britain', reprinted as Introduction by M. W. Flinn, 1965, London: Longman.
5 Chadwick, Ibid.
6 Frazer, W. P. (1947) *Duncan of Liverpool*, London.
7 Snow, J. (1855) *On the Mode and Communication of Cholera*, quoted C. Fraser Brockington (1958), *World Health*, London: Penguin, p. 203.
8 Briggs, A. (1963) *Victorian Cities*, London: Penguin Books (Pelican), p. 321.
9 Read, D. (1973) *Documents of Edwardian England*, London: Harrap, pp. 211–26.
10 Fraser, D. (1973) *The Evolution of the British Welfare State*, London: Macmillan, pp. 144 ff.

FURTHER READING

Briggs, A. (1963) *Victorian Cities*, London: Penguin Books (Pelican).
Brockington, Fraser (1965) *Public Health in the Nineteenth Century*, London: Churchill.
Finer, S. E. (1952) *The Life and Times of Edwin Chadwick*, London: Methuen.
Lambert, R. (1963) *Sir John Simon 1816–1904*, London: MacGibbon & Kee.
Lewis, R. A. (1952) *Edwin Chadwick and the Public Health Movement 1832–1954*, London: Longman.
Longmate, N. (1966) *King Cholera*, London: Hamish Hamilton.

Chapter 9

The influence of Florence Nightingale

Florence Nightingale was literally a legend in her own day. Neither the miasma of sentimentality, nor the exegesis of psychologists nor modern scholarship can destroy her achievements. For the best part of 50 years she laboured unremittingly for the 'sake of the work'. She is rightly remembered for her work in the Crimean War, but work for nursing is but a small part of her reforming zeal. The Army Medical Service possibly owes more to her than does nursing. She probably made a greater impact on Poor Law nursing than on general nursing, and her designs for hospitals and barracks have stood the test of time for a longer period than probably her present-day successors can expect for theirs. It is not for nothing that Cecil Woodham-Smith, her biographer, described her as 'The Greatest Victorian of them all'.[1]

EARLY LIFE

Florence Nightingale was born in Italy in 1820 while her family was on the 'Grand Tour'. Her parents were wealthy, and her mother, Fanny, was a great beauty and a successful hostess, W.E.N., her father, was a cultivated man with liberal views. As his estate was entailed the fact that there was no son was a disaster, but he took great pains with the education of his two daughters, Parthe and Florence, which he largely supervised himself. Neither girl inherited Fanny's striking beauty, but Florence was graceful, quick and an apt pupil. However, she was not a comfortable child and did not fit into the restless round of the Nightingale homes. This was partly because she resented the unhealthy life of idleness, which resulted in depressive brooding. She tried to fill the emptiness by excessive devotion to favourite members of the large Nightingale family, to good works in the neighbourhood, and at one time she felt that she had a vocation for mathematics. There is no doubt but that her brooding and imagination led her to over-dramatise the situation, a tendency that remained with her for life, but which sometimes produced that telling aphorism. Then at the age of 17 years she received a 'call from God'. Unhappy and taut she was in fact living in a dream world, but she was always adamant that the voice was clear, and although she did not then know what the voice called her to do it affected her subsequent decisions. In spite of this she went to Italy where she was a social success and where she became imbued with the idea of Italian freedom and liberation, in the cause of which she declared herself prepared 'to go to the barricades'.[2]

SPIRITUAL EXPERIENCE

It is important to see Florence Nightingale in the context of the social change of her day. A century earlier, middle-class women would have found plenty to do because, before the benefits of the Industrial Revolution arrived, the actual business of living took longer. Those who lived in the eighteenth century accepted poverty, and, if morally motivated, they dispensed charity. Now, as the result of the French Revolution and the Enlightenment, the intelligent were concerned with the causes of poverty and unemployment. Florence Nightingale appeared on the scene when the middle classes were benefiting from the conveniences of industrialisation but their social mores belonged to the last part of the eighteenth century. Fifty years later the growing middle classes had accepted the idea of professions for educated men, if not for women, and by the end of the century in earnest Victorian families a useful occupation for anyone was considered 'worthy' – and more worthy if it was unpaid.

In looking at the span of Florence Nightingale's life it is only necessary to compare the outspoken young ladies in Shaw's *You Never Can Tell* (1897) with Jane Austen's *Emma* (1816). For this advance we have to thank the battles fought by women like George Eliot, Harriet Martineau and Elizabeth Browning, and Florence Nightingale herself, who achieved freedom from conventional restrictions at the cost of personal sacrifice, inner conflict and mental stress. This conflict sometimes looked for metaphysical answers. Much has been made of Florence Nightingale's 'voices', but in an age revolting against 'reason' there was a turning to the development of the inner vision. Blake was inspired by aural and perceptual visions, Wordsworth and the Romantic poets tried to achieve the contemplative state which gave them a blessed vision of unity with nature. There was an interest in the works of mystics, and Florence Nightingale herself, while in Rome in 1848, was given instruction by Madre Santa Columba who helped her to submit to the will of God.

However, before the visit to Rome there had been much soul-searching. Florence was much affected by the famine of 1842, and she knew by then that her destiny was with the poor and the miserable, and in 1845 she decided that she wanted to be a nurse. She suggested to her family that she should go to Salisbury, near her home, and learn about nursing. The result at home was predictable; Fanny and her sister, Parthe, were terrified and her father retreated to the Athenaeum.

VISITS TO KAISERSWERTH

In spite of Florence's resentments, the social round had its compensations. Fanny had aspirations as a political hostess in the grand Whig manner, and Florence became friendly with her neighbours, the Herberts, Lord Palmerston (1784–1865), later to be Prime Minister, and Lord Ashley (1801–85), and it was at the suggestion of the latter that she began to read the 'Blue Books' on health matters. At night, when everyone else was abed she studied the reports of Kay, Southwood Smith, Arnott and Chadwick (see Chapter 8), and had started on the path that was eventually to make her one of the first experts on public health in Europe.

Among this circle of Nightingale friends were a Mr and Mr and Mrs Bracebridge, who now persuaded Mrs Nightingale to allow Florence to accompany them abroad. Mr Bracebridge had a positively Byronic enthusiasm for Greek freedom, and it was during this tour that Florence contrived to make her first visit to Kaiserswerth and at last met Pastor Fliedner (see Chapter 4). The 1849 visit was merely one of observation, but it revived her interest in nursing and she dashed off a pamphlet of 32 pages on the subject, duly corrected by the scholarly Mr Bracebridge and printed as 'The Institute of Kaiserswerth on the Rhine for the practical training of Deaconesses under the direction of the Reverend Pastor Fliedner'.

On return to Embley, the old resentments broke out again, with the family determined that Flo should stay at home and do her duty, but Sidney Herbert, who recognised Florence's potential, persuaded the family to let her return to Kaiserswerth in 1849. In later years Florence Nightingale denied that she had been trained at Kaiserswerth; she said that 'the nursing was nil and the hygiene horrible' but that she was impressed by the atmosphere of devotion and the fact that many deaconesses were peasant women.[3] But what she did learn was that good nursing cannot be achieved by devotion alone. She was now filled with a desire to nurse in a large hospital and she again asked her family to be released; they refused.

THE INSTITUTE IN HARLEY STREET

The following year the family physician, Sir James Clark, who was also Queen Victoria's physician,[4] with more than usual perspicacity suggested that for the sake of Parthe's health the sisters should be parted and that Florence should leave home. The Herberts seized the opportunity and arranged that Florence be appointed the superintendent for the 'Institution for the Care of Sick Gentlewomen in Distressed Circumstances', in Harley Street. While waiting to take up her appointment Florence contrived to visit Paris, where she worked with the Sisters of Mercy, nursing and helping, watching the doctors and making her own tabulations. At the same time she circulated all the hospitals in Germany, France and England with a questionnaire which she assembled and collated.

Eventually, in 1853, she took up residence in Upper Harley Street. Her requirements were revolutionary: there were schemes for lifts, piped hot water and all manner of labour-saving devices. She was her own work-study expert and did not believe in nurses doing non-nursing tasks: 'to scour was a waste of power', she wrote. By efficiency she put up the standard of care and reduced the expenditure, and the patients were loath to be discharged. Apart from organising the Institute, she continued visiting hospitals and collecting information on the subject on which she was making herself an expert, and now she began urging her friend, Sidney Herbert, on the need for nursing reform. It was during this period in Harley Street that Florence Nightingale made friends with a number of medical men, like William Bowman (later Sir William) and Bence Jones, who were later to help her with the foundation of the Nightingale Schools.[5]

THE CRIMEAN WAR, 1854–56

In the spring of the following year an event happened that made all that had gone before a mere prologue. The Turks refused to accept a Russian demand to protect the Christians in the Turkish Empire; England, fearing Russian expansion, and anxious to uphold the Turkish Empire as a barrier, had an alliance with France and declared war on Russia. Forty years had passed since the Napoleonic Wars, and their horrors were forgotten, while in the meantime the army had been run down and was riddled with corruption; nepotism was so rife that the brothers-in-law, Lord Cardigan and Lord Brudenell, who had ill-defined commands, spent most of the campaign playing off a personal family vendetta.[6] The army's tactics were based on Wellington's campaigns, and the main climate they knew, or were equipped for, was India. To make matters worse, the politics of the war were confused and carried little conviction. At home there was a strong anti-war lobby headed by Cobden and Bright, and abroad it was a campaign of unmitigated disaster, mismanagement and incompetence, with an appalling disregard for life.

This was not the first time that the army had sustained losses, but this time there was a difference: the British public knew what was happening. This was the heyday of *The Times* under the editorship of Delane, who sent to the Crimea the war correspondent William Howard Russell, an Irishman with literary talent whose dispatches hit the public like a bolt from the blue.[7] He spared no one, but his greatest acerbity was reserved for the lack of hospital provision. Much of the public indignation that followed fell on the head of Sidney Herbert, Minister at War, who was responsible for the financial provision of the war and who was suspected of dragging his feet because his mother was a Russian. Herbert wrote to Miss Nightingale on 15 October 1854, when she was nursing at the Middlesex Hospital and invited her to take a party of nurses to Scutari at the government's expense. Miss Nightingale had already offered her services and had begun to look for nurses. The expedition actually left on 21 October, so although much had been made of the fact that '40 nurses were not to be found', what seems more remarkable is that 38 *were* found at such short notice and were prepared to leave England for they knew not what in a matter of two or three days.

Miss Nightingale had no illusions about the difficulties, and that this could be an experiment that could prove the value of good nursing to the world. Therefore, discipline must be strict and, above all, if she were to gain her main point, the party must be non-sectarian. In the end 14 professional nurses were engaged with experience in hospital work, and 24 others – including five nuns from Norwood and the five Bermondsey nuns, whose Superior became one of Miss Nightingale's greatest friends – and finally, there were eight from the Anglican Sellonites.

On 3 November in atrocious weather the party reached the Bosphorus. To the south on the Asian side at Scutari, the army had taken over the Turkish barracks. This was their destination; the party disembarked and climbed the slopes to the gateway over which Miss Nightingale said should have been Dante's inscription, 'Abandon hope all ye that enter here'. The barracks themselves were built round a vast courtyard and everything was filthy and dilapidated; the courtyard was a refuse dump, equipment and sanitation were non-existent and the building was over a dammed-up cesspool, from which came a frightful stench. In the cellars below lived 200 prostitutes and around the walls lodged a filthy rabble. Across the Bosphorus, in great splendour, lived the British Ambassador who had orders to equip the hospital but had never even visited it until compelled to so by Miss Nightingale.

The arrival of the Nightingale party was greeted with sullen opposition; the doctors received the news with disgust, but because of government backing and the power of the press they dared not show open hostility. They simply refused the help offered by Miss Nightingale and her nurses. Of all the tests this was the sternest; years of self-discipline had trained her for this moment and she refused to let the nurses nurse until the doctors requested it. Meanwhile Miss Nightingale had charge of the money raised by public subscription and the party employed their time buying equipment, stuffing mattresses, making bandages and cleaning the place.

On 9 November the situation changed. The battle of Balaclava over in the Crimea was a disaster, the harbour heaved with dead bodies, and in the chaos and confusion the sick and the wounded began to pour across the Bosphorus to Scutari. The hospital filled, the doctors were overwhelmed and they turned to Miss Nightingale. Out came the mattresses and the bandages, and although the doctors 'worked like lions' it might be two weeks before they could see a patient. At one stage there were 4 miles of patients on mattresses on the floor and there were more than 1,000 cases of diarrhoea. In the confusion it was realised that someone had the power to spend money. Miss Nightingale had at her disposal £30,000. A visiting Member of Parliament and the administrator of *The Times* Fund were pressed into service as quartermasters, and the main requirements were bought in Constantinople. Now opposition collapsed and Dr McGrigor, an energetic man, became Miss Nightingale's principal ally.

By the spring of 1855 she was exhausted; she would be on her feet for 24 hours and was known to spend eight hours on her knees dressing wounds. Her influence was extraordinary; the men described her as 'full of fun' and kissed her shadow, but perhaps her greatest contribution was that she was one of the first people who regarded the British soldier as having a dignity of his own and not as 'the scum of the earth enlisted for drink'.[8]

Troubles with administrators, purveyors, doctors and the Gift Fund were nothing compared with the troubles with nurses. Mrs Roberts from St Thomas's and Mrs Drake were excellent; so too were the old friends, the Bermondsey nuns, but some of the hospital nurses she pronounced as 'not fit to look after themselves'. One of the Sellonites became overwrought and had to be sent home, then, to pile Pelion on Ossa, other well-intentioned ladies wanted to join the party; to refuse help seemed churlish, but help in the form of Mary Stanley's 'Lady Ecclesiastics' could endanger the whole enterprise. Mary Stanley was of the High Church Party and on the verge of conversion to Rome. Firmness was essential, and at all costs Miss Nightingale had to keep control herself and keep the party non-sectarian.

Having established some order at the Barrack hospital, Miss Nightingale was now free to visit the hospitals in the Crimea itself, and here the flaw in her instructions showed, for she had been sent to 'the military hospitals in Turkey' and now the struggle began all over again. In the Crimea, the army were smarting under defeat and criticism and were determined to teach meddling civilians a lesson. While she was battling with these odds Miss Nightingale contracted 'Crimean fever' and her life was despaired of, but by now she was a legend and it was said that Balaclava seemed a place of mourning and at Scutari soldiers 'turned their faces to the wall and cried. All their trust was in her.'[9] However, she recovered and returned to Scutari. During the next year, until the Peace of Paris in 1856, she struggled to improve the standard of care, hygiene and the general facilities for the troops. During this time 'a mystical devotion grew up between her and the British Army' and she now set herself a new task: to improve the lot of the private soldier.

Now the nation longed to honour her; ironically, she was all they could honour for the war had ended ingloriously and the casualties had been enormous. Of the 98,000 British soldiers who took to the field 22,000 had died, and of these *17,000 had died from disease.* Nevertheless, that was better than the casualty rate for the allies, and for Russia the total death rate was 50 per cent. Refusing the offer of a man-of-war, Miss Nightingale, emaciated and her hair cropped short, crept back incognito to Embley knowing that her battle had only just begun. Every day she delayed soldiers would die unnecessarily through lack of sanitation, patients in hospitals would die because nursing at its worst was poor and unsupervised and at its best, devoted and unscientific. Exhausted and ill, she set about asking for a Royal Commission.

THE ROYAL SANITARY COMMISSION

In September 1856 Miss Nightingale paid an informal visit to Balmoral; Queen Victoria became, and remained, an admirer. By sheer personality and a little push from Victoria and Albert she won over Lord Panmure, Secretary for War, and drew up a list of names for the Commissioners, who included Sir James Clark, Dr Sutherland, who had been sent to the Crimea on the Sanitary Commission, and Dr Alexander, who had been fearless in his criticism of his medical superiors. Sidney Herbert was to be chairman but the war had broken him; he was already sick and he refused. Miss Nightingale moved into Burlington House to be on hand, then when all was set, Panmure capitulated, a disturbing report had been published and he wanted to prevent further disclosure. Miss Nightingale had one weapon left: she would publish her own report. Moreover, the nation was angry and wanted the truth, so in May 1857 the Commission began to sit with Sidney Herbert as the chairman. Miss Nightingale's evidence can be found in *Notes on Matters Affecting Health, Efficiency and Hospital Administration of the British Army*, 1,000 pages of closely printed tables and statistics. The strain was enormous, she worked night and day immolating herself for 'the sake of the work', scarcely eating or sleeping. Her position was incredible, she alone had the statistical facts and she alone knew how to use them. 'She had to teach her helpers', said Dr Sutherland; 'nobody who has not worked for her daily could know or have any idea of her clearness of mind, her extraordinary powers combined with her benevolence of spirit.'

The report dealt with a number of subjects, including the need for a statistical department, army medical departments and an Army Medical School. A month after the report was ready Miss Nightingale collapsed. Until now, although she did not appear in public, she rushed around; now her life was despaired of and her family talked of its 'hanging on a thread'. There is no doubt but that at the time she was acutely ill, possibly with a relapse of the Crimean fever, or a heart condition, but she did not die and was splendidly nursed by her favourite Aunt Mai. She was now 37 years old. Once she recovered, she used her illness to free herself from her family, who were now mercifully diverted. Sir Harry Verney, head of the distinguished Verney family and the owner of Claydon in Buckingham-shire, who had previously proposed to Florence, now turned his attention to Parthe, who gladly accepted him. Later, Sir Harry was to become the greatly valued chairman of the Nightingale Fund Committee.

Thanks to the skilful chairmanship of Sidney Herbert, the reformers gained most of their points and four sub-committees were set up that were to have far-reaching effects on the army and especially the army medical service. Now there was a new task; when the Indian Mutiny broke out in 1857 Miss Nightingale asked for a second commission to deal with the conditions of the army in India. Once again the work was tremendous; she was now on her bed or couch continuously, but her family ceased to talk about her life ebbing away. Fortunately for the work she was yet to under-take there was, it seems, an unending stream of friends and relatives to take charge of the household that was run with military precision. Such was her personality and the regard in which she was held that even the most eminent did not mind taking their turn in the appointment list at South Street. Claiming herself to be a semi-invalid Miss Nightingale was about to embark on another 40 years of labour in a variety of causes of which nursing was but a small part.

THE FOUNDATION OF THE NIGHTINGALE SCHOOLS

In 1855, while Miss Nightingale was still in the Crimea, Sidney Herbert set up a committee to collect from a grateful nation a Nightingale Fund. At the time Miss Nightingale insisted that she did not want the Fund and she had no plans for its use. Almost fanatical about the high mortality rate in the army and the conditions for soldiers, the last thing she wanted to bother about was starting a nursing school or a 'Fund'. When she did return she had more pressing matters with which to concern herself, such as the reform of the army medical services, and, if necessary, the army itself, the collection of medical statistics, the redesign of hospitals, and, of course, the great sanitarian movement.

For over two years the Nightingale Fund was quietly forgotten. Tentative approaches were made to various London hospitals with the idea of attaching a school of nursing to them, but no one wanted *that* cuckoo in the nest. Then Miss Nightingale's attention was directed to St Thomas's which was selling its site to the South-eastern Railway and were about to rebuild. There was a faction led by Richard Whitfield, the Resident Medical Officer, who advocated rebuilding outside London in the healthy suburbs, a view to which Miss Nightingale ascribed, and who wrote enthu-siastic articles in *The Builder* using statistics that Mr Whitfield had purloined. Most of the doctors headed by John Simon were against such a move, and there followed a Machiavellian intrigue with both sides bombarding each other with statistics in the press. During the course of the correspondence there is a letter from Richard Whitfield to Miss Nightingale suggesting that the governors might be persuaded to accept a school of nursing in her name.[10]

It looks as if Miss Nightingale now clutched at a straw. There is correspondence to show that she envisaged a school of nursing like a medical school, but Mr Whitfield turned that down and put up a counter-plan; they would accept 15 probationers as assistant nurses, but he insisted that they must be under the surveillance of the present matron, Mrs Wardroper, and not under an independent superintendent, as Miss Nightingale had suggested. Miss Nightingale put the Whitfield plan to the Nightingale Council, who were unhappy about the power to be given to the matron and the contract that was being proposed. But the public, the donors to the Fund, were beginning to get restive and they eventually agreed to the plan, *faute de mieux*. Contrary to myth, Miss Nightingale did not go to St Thomas's because she thought it was well run – it was, in fact, run down, but because she thought it would be a new hospital out at Blackheath and she would have a say in the design.

The contract was drawn up by Sidney Herbert, now Secretary of State for War, and Miss Nightingale's poet cousin, Arthur Clough, both of whom were mortally ill, and who were no match for the treasurer of St Thomas's. The Fund paid for the board and lodging of 15 probationers who would work on the wards under the instruction of the present sisters, and a fee to both Mrs Wardroper and Mr Whitfield. No one asked if the sisters were capable of being teachers. The probationers had to sign a contract 'which bound them to enter into service as hospital nurses in such situations as may be offered them for a further four years'.[11] It was a contract for a servant. Miss Nightingale protested, but to no avail. She then drew up her famous Character Sheet with its 14 heads and retired to nurse her griefs over the deaths of Lord Herbert and Arthur Clough and to reform the sanitary services in India.

The first ten years of the school were disastrous. Mrs Wardroper selected working class girls who came and went with amazing rapidity; there was no rush of candidates in spite of the advertisements. Analysis of the register shows that comparatively few probationers were nursing at the end of their four years. During the first ten years, 196 nurses were entered on the register but fewer than 60 were still nursing, 64 had been dismissed, 4 had died in their training, and, with the exception of Agnes Jones, few had made any mark on nursing. The fact that so many were dismissed for glaring defects like drug addiction, phthisis, syphilis and insobriety suggest that either Mrs Wardroper's judgement was at fault or that there was no choice. Nevertheless the Fund's publicity continued to be good and members of the Council wrote authoritative articles on 'reformed nursing', but by the 1870s most of London teaching hospitals had a training school, often with a less restrictive contract. The new antiseptic surgery was needing a different type of nurse and the publicity brought a few better recruits to the Nightingale school, but they were critical of what they found.

For a variety of reasons after 1867 Miss Nightingale had more time to give to the school. She was furious that the governors had decided to build, not in the suburbs but on the banks of the dirty Thames 'on the worst site in London'. With the Council now headed by Sir Harry Verney there was talk of moving the school elsewhere. Now, a little late, she realised 'our school is not a training school, it is taking on half the hospital's work'.

But the Council was in a cleft stick. There was no expectation that any other hospital would drive a less hard bargain – and where else could you train nurses other than in hospital? Meanwhile, it was discovered that Mrs Wardroper was not keeping the register and did not know one probationer from another and that Mr Whitfield did not give lectures and 'had been in habits of intoxication for years'.[12]

How the Council dealt with this crisis is important, because it largely set the pattern of nurse training for years to come. First, having failed to get a separate superintendent, the Fund Council instituted the idea of a Home Sister who was to be responsible for helping the nurses to revive their lectures and for their general care and moral behaviour in the Nurses' Home. It was not until 1913 that St Thomas's had a separate Sister Tutor. Second, Henry Bonham Garter, secretary to the Fund Council and Miss Nightingale's cousin, obtained Mr Whitfield's resignation and instead instituted a series of lectures to be given by medical men to the nurses. The medical model had begun. Third, nurses were to visit Miss Nightingale in her home – and from her notes, their letters and their diaries we know what they were doing, mainly it seems, non-nursing tasks: 'these are horaries, not of probationers, but of ward assistants'. Fourth, at the same time it was agreed that the Fund should take on 'Special' probationers who would be groomed for superintendence. These were to be better-educated candidates who would pay for their training; the Fund now needed the money. This idea was not popular with Mrs Wardroper who saw the Specials as a threat to her authority. The Specials have gone down in history as 'paying probationers' or 'lady probationers', in fact, they did not all pay and some were, alas, not ladies. Miss Nightingale herself was ambivalent about the scheme, insisting that 'the lady be educated with her cook'.

The idea of grooming was fine but it was never put into practice, Mrs Wardroper insisted that the Specials laboured on the wards as hard as anyone else, Miss Nightingale was to moan to Henry Bonham Carter: 'I have said this scores of times, you must be weary of hearing, we do not to those we expressly hold out a career of superintendence offer any special training.' The fact that St Thomas's, along with other London hospitals, turned out a few leaders is not, as nurse historians would have it, because they were 'trained to train' but because a few were educated Victorian women anxious to carve out a niche for themselves in a world where opportunities were few.

Now the Fund started to diversify and try to influence nursing elsewhere. In 1872 the Fund sent a team of nurses under Miss Barclay to Edinburgh. Later the Superintendent was Miss Angelique Pringle, the 'Pearl' who, Miss Nightingale thought, with some justification, would produce a better school than Mrs Wardroper. When the opportunity came Miss Pringle's deputy, Miss Williams, was sent to St Mary's, Paddington, as Superintendent, but after a series of clashes with the administration was forced to leave. Not all the Specials were successful.

Perhaps the most successful of the diversifications was the extension of the Nightingale system into Poor Law hospitals, of which the most notable was Miss Vincent at St Marylebone (later St Charles). Miss Nightingale always insisted that she was the Head of the Nightingale Schools, whether voluntary or public hospitals. Apart from sending teams to other hospitals and abroad, the Fund Council undertook to assist with the combined training for district nurses for the Metropolitan and National Nursing Association, which became the foundation training for the Queen's Institute of District Nursing (see Chapter 10).

The Fund's contribution to nursing was that it enabled the concept of secular nurse training based on a general hospital to have started earlier than would otherwise have been the case. Whether this was a good thing is a moot point. The so-called Nightingale system tended to eclipse other systems because it was claimed to be so successful. Some other systems had merit in that they trained nurses for the community as well as the hospital. For better, for worse, nurse training was based on the acute general hospital for years to come.

Was 1860 too early to base a reform of nursing on a general hospital? A few years later with the Education Act of 1870 and with universities opening up for women there would be more women with higher education who could have been trained as tutors with a better understanding of the health needs of the population and the new possibilities of medicine, and there might have been a chance to develop a separate philosophy for nursing, what it was and what it was not.

For all its vaunted publicity the Nightingale system was not a break with the past. The personnel used to train probationers were products of the past and without a new controlling hand there could not be a new profession. We do nursing, and particularly nursing education, a great disservice by pretending that nursing suddenly became homogeneous and educated. Believing the myth, we have clung like a drowning man to a raft. Those who came after Miss Nightingale for the most part lacked her willingness to experiment and they emphasised obedience and discipline long after hospitals had ceased to be the lawless places complained of by the early pioneers. Obedience breeds conformity, and an unquestioning profession was bred that was resistent to change.

If nurses themselves clung to the system that made them fashionable, so did hospital administrators to a system that kept down their costs. As hospitals changed and hospitals opened their doors to the middle classes, so there was a demand for more and better nurses. Hospitals wishing to fulfil this need seized on the humble experiment of 1860 and turned it into the orthodoxy of the 1900s. Hospitals, both voluntary and public, were poor, and probationers were cheap. As far as the hospital was concerned, the longer the training the better. It was even better if some probationers paid for the privilege. Hospitals budgets were costed accordingly. This is another legacy of the system. This is not what Miss Nightingale intended. She saw what was happening and was powerless to do anything about it and turned her attention to the metaphysical world and, now that nurses were becoming doctors' assistants, to the idea of training a separate corps of women as sanitary educators. Towards the end of her life she was disillusioned about nurse training and the way it had developed.

Under the Nightingale system undoubtedly nursing and hygiene improved. There developed a career structure for nurses, and the strong position of the matron was secured though, interestingly enough, by the 1890s Miss Nightingale had doubts about giving the matron so much power. But the arrangements for analysing the central purpose of the workforce and designing a training to fit were neglected. 'What the nurse was taught and who taught and examined her are questions which are left unanswered.'[13] Miss Nightingale did not answer them and, over 100 years later, they are only just beginning to be answered.

REFERENCES

1 Woodham Smith, C. (1956) 'Founders' Day Lecture', The Royal College of Nursing.
2 Keele, M. (ed.) (1981) *Florence Nightingale in Rome: letters written by Florence Nightingale in Rome in the Winter of 1847–1848*, Philadelphia: American Philosophical Society.
3 Nightingale, F. (1897) *Recollections of Kaiserswerth*, London: British Library.
4 Longford, E. (1966) *Victoria RI*, London: Pan Books, p. 200.
5 Baly, M. E. (1986) *Florence Nightingale and the Nursing Legacy*, London: Routledge, p. 7.
6 Woodham Smith, C. (1953) *The Reason Why*, London: Constable.
7 *The Times*, Dispatches, 9, 12 and 13 Oct. 1854.
8 Longford, E. (1969) *The Years of the Sword*, London: Weidenfeld & Nicolson, p. 321.
9 Woodham Smith, C. (1950) *Florence Nightingale*, London: Constable.
10 Baly, *Florence Nightingale*, p. 30
11 Baly, ibid, p. 36.
12 Ibid, p. 156.

13 Abel-Smith, B. (1960) *A History of the Nursing Profession*, London: Heinemann.

FURTHER READING

Cook, Sir E. (1913) *The Life of Florence Nightingale*, London: Macmillan.

Baly, M. E. (1986) *Florence Nightingale and the Nursing Legacy*. London: Routledge

——(1991) *As Miss Nightingale Said . . .*, London: Scutari Press.

Pickering, Sir George (1974) *The Creative Malady*, London: Allen & Unwin.

Skretkowicz, V. (ed.) (1992) *Florence Nightingale's Notes on Nursing*, revised, with additions, London: Scutari Press.

Smith, Barry (1982) *Florence Nightingale – Reputation and Power*, London and Canberra: Croom Helm.

Woodham Smith, C. (1950) *Florence Nightingale*, London: Constable.

Chapter 10

Nursing reforms extended

Although the nineteenth-century nursing reforms are associated with Miss Nightingale, the circumstances produced the leader and the time was ripe. Towards the end of the century a number of factors came together to give the concept of 'trained nursing' an impetus undreamt of by the mid-century reformers. First, there were the medical advances stemming from the work of men like Joseph Lister (1827–1912) and Louis Pasteur (1822–1895); antiseptic surgery required a more intelligent and conscientious type-of nurse, whilst the introduction of anaesthesia in the 1840s by James Simpson (1811–70) called for a more observant one; but above all there were the effects of the identification of the pathological bacteria which followed hard on Koch's discovery of the tubercle bacillus in 1882. Within a matter of 40 years there was a new public expectation of what medicine could do – and what it would do in the future. For the first time in history people began to see medicine as scientific, and therefore the new image of the hospital nurse was associated with doctors, science and cure. From now on nursing was to become eclectic, often taking over duties and techniques, and sometimes acquiring the knowledge and skill once considered the prerogative of other professions and callings.

These new requirements for nurses coincided with the change in the population profile. Late marriage, a falling birth rate after the 1870s, the high emigration rate of sons to the growing Empire, together with the economic depression of the 1870s produced a large pool of middle-class spinsters, who for the most part were condemned by social sanctions to idleness in the home. Good works were praiseworthy, but delicacy – that hallmark of refined Victorian womanhood – had in the past precluded nursing; but once nursing was made 'respectable' it represented an escape from Mama and boredom in a way no other occupation could. Nursing did not involve vulgar competition with men, as did those pioneer women in medicine like Elizabeth Blackwell and Elizabeth Garrett, and no one could accuse nurses of being inspired by pecuniary motives; above all it was the fulfilment of a Christian duty, and for the most part the men approved. Although more upper-class women were attending university extension courses, and some, like Beatrice Potter (later Mrs Webb, 1858–1943), embarked on sociological studies, these were a minority and were generally considered rather 'advanced' and not quite *comme il faut*. Therefore, until well into the twentieth century nursing as an occupation for a middle-class girl had no serious competitor other than teaching, and later, and to a lesser extent, the civil service. However, it must be remembered that it was only the 'reformed schools' that exercised this pull and 40 years after the foundation of the Nightingale School, by the time of the 1901 census, of the 67,000 'nurses' and midwives recorded, Burdett estimated that only 25,000 to 30,000 were trained.[1] Even this figure is suspect; the actual number was probably much lower, and from all accounts it is clear that most nursing was still being done by the untrained and often quite elderly nurses who had received little instruction or supervision. In 1901, 45 per cent of all nurses were married or widowed, but in 1931 the figure was 12 per cent,[2] a figure which indicates how in the next decades the 'reformed' system took over and the old and the married were ousted by the young and the single.

THE NEW DEMAND FOR NURSES

The success of the Nightingale reforms led to a rapid expansion of nurse training schools, first to the London voluntary hospitals, then to the larger provincial voluntary hospitals, and finally to the new hospitals being built under the auspices of the Local Government Board and the Poor Law authorities. As the new nurses were appreciated so the demand increased, and within 40 years of Mr South's famous *obiter dictum*, hospitals were bidding to become training schools, and as more offered training so the standard and length began to vary and the whole system showed signs of being caught in the web of its own success. By the twentieth century voluntary hospitals with hoardings outside saying 'Half a Million Pounds Required – Give Generously', were not slow to see the advantages of offering a nurse training school; lady probationers added prestige, they were biddable, but above all they were cheap. Consciously or unconsciously, all connected with hospital administration now had a vested interest in nurse training – the longer the better. Miss Nightingale's consideration had been 'how quickly can a reasonably intelligent girl acquire the necessary skills and then pass them on?'; now it was how long could a hospital enforce the 'probationer contract' without noticeable defections? Ironically, the hospitals best able to select pupils with the most suitable attributes now required the longest training, and the length of training became the hallmark of prestige. Furthermore, the heirs to the first Nightingales, lacking the prescience of their founders, worked on the principle that reform had improved status, therefore more reform along the same lines would make status even better; but from Lot's wife to Orpheus, history and legend are littered with the dangers of looking back, and the price, as Lot's wife found, was petrification. Now praised as 'ministering angels' and sickled o'er with the pale cast of sentimentality, the matrons of the twentieth century too often clung to the traditions that had raised them to their new pinnacle and particularly the tradition of discipline. In so doing criticism was stifled, orthodoxy and conformity bred and, in spite of Miss Nightingale's acid remarks about obedience being 'suitable praise for a horse',[3] obedience was seen as a cardinal virtue.

Two other legacies of the Nightingale experiment soon became a travesty; the nurses' home and the method of payment. The Nightingale nurses' home was intended to be a real 'home', with a small 'h', to provide a cultural and educational background for young women who had left an educated middle-class home, and to raise the sights of those who had not. Only a few favoured teaching hospitals continued to emulate the pattern of poetry readings and musical soirées, and as time went by, and the probationers became the main workforce, the nurses' home, now a Home, all too often became an adjacent barracks built because it was the cheapest way of housing the labour force that was required to work round the clock and for seven days a week. Now, instead of sights being raised, probationers often felt severed from the educational and cultural interests they had formed at school.

The method of rewarding the first Nightingale nurses was quite logical in 1860 at a time when the only women earning a living were working as domestics, in shops or factories; and although they helped on the wards the first pupils were supernumerary to the hospital labour force. Moreover, once she was trained, the nurse's salary was three or four times her training allowance – a differential never to be seen again. Forty pounds a year for a ward sister may not sound princely, but at that time the average agricultural worker only earned about £30 a year, and in the Edwardian period a woman secretary in the civil service was paid £79 per year, so the ward sister with everything found was clearly much better off.[4] Compared with other women workers nurses have not always been at the bottom. However, this method of paying probationers continued after they had ceased to be supernumerary and when they had become the main labour force of the wards; now 'low pay' for probationers was seen to have some intrinsic merit of its own in 'getting the right type of girl'. With this casuistry the great debate had begun; was the probationer a pupil or a worker? Nevertheless, it is only fair to add that this method of training was not unusual, and that pupil teachers were miserably exploited, as were apprentices in shops; as there were more applicants than jobs for women, all women were badly paid.

DISTRICT NURSING

The idea of the sick being cared for in large institutions is, except in cases of extreme indigence, a comparatively modern one. From the diaconate of

St Paul to St Vincent's Sisters of Mercy and the Deaconesses of Kaiserswerth, emphasis has always been placed on the importance of providing care in the home. The move to care in hospitals came when medical techniques became, or in some cases doctors liked to think that they had become, too sophisticated for domesticity, and doctors found it easier to have research and teaching material under one roof, and the nineteenth-century administrators decided that 'bigger is cheaper'. But in spite of the voluntary hospitals, large and small, and the Poor Law institutions, by the second half of the nineteenth century most of the sick were where they are today, in their own homes.

In 1859 Mr William Rathbone (see Chapter 6), the senior member of a firm of wealthy shipowners whose father had been an associate of Robert Owen, decided to keep the nurse he had had for his wife who had just died of tuberculosis, and get her to nurse the poor in a district of Liverpool. Mrs Robinson was a good nurse but it was soon obvious that one person was quite inadequate, and in 1861 Mr Rathbone wrote to Miss Nightingale to seek her advice about supplying 'trained nurses' to care for the sick poor in their own homes. Miss Nightingale was sympathetic to the idea but she could not spare her first 'nurse missioners', and she replied with a counter suggestion that Liverpool Infirmary train its own nurses for this purpose. Mr Rathbone responded by donating a new building as a 'school of nursing' which in 1862 began to train nurses in a comprehensive course for work both at home and in the hospital. Once the nurses were trained, Liverpool was divided into 18 'districts', each with a ladies' voluntary committee responsible for the dispensation of medical comforts and a trained nurse was attached to each district.

In 1874, while Miss Nightingale was immersed in the family problems at Embley, Mr Rathbone, now a Member of Parliament, asked her help in organising a district nursing scheme for London. She gave what help she could and wrote several pamphlets[5] and a letter to *The Times*. At last the Metropolitan Nursing Association was founded, with Miss Florence Lees, one of the ablest of the first Nightingale nurses and who had since served with distinction in the Franco-Prussian War of 1870, as the Superintendent. The Association had strict conditions of entry because 'district nurses would be placed in positions of greater responsibility than hospital nurses'. The training was integrated: the successful candidate spent the first month in the Central Home learning about district nursing, then did a year's course in a hospital operating the 'reformed system' of nurse training, and finally she returned to the Central Home to do six months' special training in home nursing. Like her counterpart in hospital, the new district nurse had to be almost perfect: it was another experiment that could raise the status of nurses in the eyes of the public. Careful selection and supervision paid off, and in 1887, Queen Victoria, always interested in Miss Nightingale and nursing, gave the greater part of the Women's Jubilee offering of

£70,000 for the extension of district nursing schemes; William Rathbone was one of the advisers to the trustees, and the following year the Queen Victoria Jubilee Institute for Nurses came into being. The principles of training remained the same as those advised for the Metropolitan Nursing Association, and they continued until state registration was introduced in 1919, when registration with the General Nursing Council became the prerequisite for district nurse training as registration with the Central Midwives' Board had been for district midwives. Mr Rathbone continued to be associated with the scheme until his death in 1902 and, together with Miss Nightingale with whom he worked in harness – another 'Member for Miss Nightingale' – he must be seen as the founding spirit. Like so many of the health services district nursing started as a voluntary service, run by voluntary committees with the money being collected from the recipients, if they could afford it, and the remainder from charitable efforts and donations. As time went by and the value of the service was seen, legislation required local authorities to accept more responsibility for the sick in the community, which many chose to do through what in 1928 was to become the Queen's Institute for District Nursing.

PRIVATE NURSING

The first Nightingale nurses were exhorted not to undertake private nursing. The object of the training was to produce nurses capable of training others and to go forth and found new training schools. Nevertheless, as the improved standard of nursing became obvious there was a demand for trained nurses in private houses. Doctors with large and lucrative practices encouraged patients to employ trained nurses; obviously, it made their task easier and added to their prestige. Commercial agencies were not slow to see the opportunities in supplying this need, but in the absence of registration or any sound criteria by which the patient could judge whether a nurse were trained or not, agencies were not particularly scrupulous about being sure that the nurses were actually trained; this became a scandal and therefore grist to the mill for those who sought to control nursing by registration. It is impossible to say how many nurses worked privately because, apart from those supplied by the agencies, there were still a host of women who hired themselves out for a few shillings a week to watch the sick in their own homes, and indeed the poor could not have managed without such people especially in terminal illness.

NURSING IN INDUSTRY (see also Chapter 21)

As early as the beginning of the eighteenth century Bernardino Ramazzini, an Italian professor of medicine, had recognised the significance of a man's occupation as a contribution to his expectation of health and that certain occupations carried special risks. In England, a century later, men like Edward Greenhow (see Chapter 8) were studying the effects of industrialisation and the fact that a wide range of occupations appeared to cause pulmonary disease. However, it must be emphasised that medical opinion in the nineteenth century with its middle-class orientation, the work ethic and the self-help philosophy of that class, tended to stress the failure in physical or moral personal hygiene rather than look for illness as an effect of work, and for this reason occupational medicine was poorly developed.

The struggles with the various Factory Acts highlight the dilemma; on the one hand there was the Benthamite belief in the freedom of the individual combined with the economic theories of Adam Smith and his followers, who held that any state interference upset the market forces and made matters worse for capital and labour alike. On the other hand there was an uncomfortable awareness that industrialisation was producing social injustices and, in the case of child labour, conditions that affronted Christian consciences, and for women, conditions that produced moral depravity. In these cases, it was argued, the community had a duty to step in; the political differences towards the end of the century were therefore mainly about the extent of intervention with the socialists and the new Liberals calling for more radical reform. The Factory Act of 1874 forbade the employment of children under the age of 10 and those between 10 and 14 were only to work half time, and of course by now the new 'Board' schools were coming into being. Some firms, like Colmans, began to see the labour force as a valuable asset, and in 1872 Colmans actually employed a nurse to look after the health of their employees. Because there was not a medical inspector of factories until 1898 it is not known how many firms followed Colmans' lead, but if they did, the duties of the nurses would have been mainly welfare. It was not until the First World War with the increase of young women working in the munitions factories that the importance of preventive health in industry was appreciated, and it was not until the inter-war period that nursing in industry was regarded as a speciality needing a distinctive training.

HEALTH VISITING

Early health visiting has already been mentioned in Chapter 8; legislation at the beginning of the twentieth century increased the demand for health visitors and to some extent changed their purpose and function. The rising concern over the infant mortality rate and the health of mothers led the new Medical Officers of Health who were becoming more concerned with personal health than with sanitation, to direct the health visitors, who might be women doctors, to visit all the homes of newborn babies and advise the mother and follow up the visit at intervals. Thus maternity and child welfare became the most important aspect of the scheme, which of course suggested that the health visitor ought also to be a midwife. But other duties were added, for the early health visitors were nothing if not adaptable; they became increasingly concerned with child life protection after the Children's Act of 1908, and had the duty of supervising children under 9 living apart from their parents, and apart from this many of them had duties as school health nurses, although some boroughs employed the school nurse as a separate category. After 1913 there was an increasing tendency to make the health visitor responsible for visiting mentally deficient children in their own homes; inevitably the health visitor was becoming not only a health educator but also a medico-social community worker, which produced confusion in the minds of the public, medical colleagues and sometimes her own as to what was her true function and role.

THE ARMED SERVICES OF THE CROWN

After the Crimean War the first female 'trained' nurses were attached to the new Army Hospital at Netley, then later at the Herbert Hospital at Woolwich, which had been built on Miss Nightingale's 'pavilion' style and where an Army Medical School was opened as a memorial to the work of Sidney Herbert. What was to be the Army Nursing Service was officially recognised in the Boer War and graced by the patronage of Queen Alexandra, the wife of Edward VII, to become the Queen Alexandra Imperial Nursing Service with a similar service founded as the Royal Naval Nursing Service. Both services were small and highly competitive, promotion was by examination conducted by a Nursing Board, and the sisters in the service were required to take a course in administration. The army nursing service was backed up by the Territorial Force Nursing Service, generally known as the 'TANS', which, said a significant advertisement in 1910, 'would be mobilised in the event of the invasion of the country'. The war, when it did come in 1914, proved the value of these two nursing services to the full, but during that war the Royal Flying Corps came into being and after the war, in 1920 the Air Force developed its own medical service to which was then attached the Princess Mary Royal Air Force Nursing Service.

Apart from the armed services another opportunity was offered to trained nurses, that of manning the various nursing services of the Empire. By the beginning of the century the Colonial Nursing Service was recruiting carefully selected trained nurses to send abroad. Cassell's *Textbook for Nurses* of 1910 explains why the selection was so rigid and the possible hazards ahead, but it is good to know that the passage out to the selected station would be first class. Nurses continued to man this service, many with distinction until the sun finally set on the British Empire in the Second World War. By then the Nightingale system, with modifications, was covering perhaps half the world; its only rivals were the various religious houses still training nurses, the Red Cross and the American system, and even that, although it developed along different lines, in its early stages owed much to the idea of the professional nurse fostered in England.

REFERENCES

1 Burdett, H. (1905) *Evidence to the Commission on Registration*, London: HMSO.
2 Registrar General, Census Returns 1901 and 1931, London: HMS0.
3 Nightingale, F. (1859) *Notes on Nursing* (ed. 1952), London: Duckworth, p. 130.
4 Burnett, J. (1969) *A History of the Cost of Living*, London: Penguin Books.
5 Nightingale, F. (1874) *Suggestions for Improving the Nursing Service for the Sick Poor*, Metropolitan and National Association for providing nurses for the Sick Poor, *On Trained Nursing for the Sick Poor*.

FURTHER READING

Baly, M. (1987) *A History of the Queen's Nursing Institute*, London: Croom Helm.
Stocks, M. (1960) *A Hundred Years of District Nursing*, London: George Allen & Unwin.
Summers, A. (1988) *Angels and Citizens: British Women as Military Nurses, 1854–1914*, London: Routledge.

Chapter 11

Towards a health service

By the end of the nineteenth century the hospital services were developing along three main paths (Fig. 11.1). The charity hospitals with their origins in the philanthropy of the eighteenth century – originally havens for the non-pauper infirm – were now transformed into voluntary hospitals often associated with the teaching of medicine and sometimes with schools of nursing. These hospitals were financed by public donations; they treated selected cases usually for whom there was hope of cure or who were interesting to medical teaching; treatment and accommodation were free except when a token fee was asked.

The second path was provided by the Metropolitan Poor Law Act (Chapter 6), which allowed Poor Law Unions to introduce a hospital system, and by 1891 16 per cent of the Poor Law hospital beds were in specially designed hospitals – the hospitals that became the municipal system. Here the first Poor Law Medical Inspector, Dr Edward Smith, noted that the 'inmates are better fed, better clad, better housed and better cared for than they were before admission and better than the great mass of the working class who earn their own living',[1] and now few people regarded this as an offence against less eligibility. However, this path had another branch: many Unions had either merely set aside a workhouse ward as the sick infirmary, or in some cases had 'upgraded' one complete workhouse in the Union; these were often referred to by the new nurses as 'the unreformed infirmaries', and they were warned that working in them would mean being under the control of the workhouse master and matron.[2] There was yet another path within the Poor Law system: in 1881 a Royal Commission recommended the general accessibility of the Poor Law hospitals and by 1891 the citizens of London had the right to hospital treatment for infectious disease. This, together with the Notification of Infectious Diseases Act of 1889, led to a spate of building isolation hospitals, and by 1911 there were 32,000 beds for infectious diseases under the control of the Metropolitan Asylums Board – the authority set up by the 1867 Poor Law Act – and many other cities followed this example producing a network of isolation hospitals where non-pauper patients were treated free.

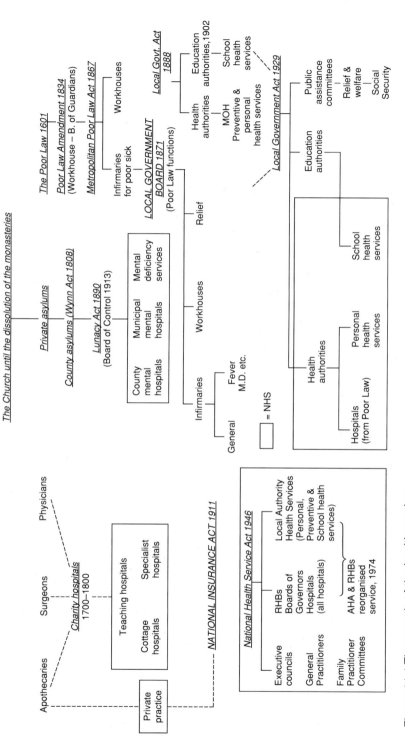

Figure 11.1 The growth of the health services
Note: See also Figure 8.2

The third main path had grown up because of public concern about madhouses, and with a few exceptions, the county asylum system for the mentally sick had developed outside the Poor Law and the voluntary system. After the Lunatics Act of 1845 (see Chapter 7), the asylums were controlled by the Lunacy Commission and after 1913 by the Board of Control.

CARE IN THE COMMUNITY

The intention of the Poor Law Act of 1834 had been to minimise relief given in the community and subject all applicants to the workhouse test, but each Union interpreted the Act in its own way and the objective was only partly achieved mainly because Guardians soon found that outdoor relief was cheaper. The Workhouse Reform Movement advocated not only a hospital system for the pauper sick but also Sick Dispensaries where the poor who were not in need of hospital care could get advice and medicine. Many towns did in fact have such dispensaries, but they had usually been founded by charitable effort – Bath, for example, had four such dispensaries serving the different areas – and although George Goschen, who was the President of the Poor Law Board in the Liberal administration of 1868 tried to persuade Boards of Guardians to fill the gaps, most were disinclined to take on this form of relief. One reason for this reluctance was that, now they were building hospitals or upgrading wards, these seemed to offer the poor more satisfactory treatment. As the Webbs point out, there was now a new drive against outdoor relief and the sick were now pushed into infirmaries for their own good.[3]

For the non-paupers there were two possible sources of help in the community in times of trouble: the friendly societies and the various charities.

Friendly societies

Friendly societies were a working-class response to Samuel Smiles's (1812–1904) dictum about the value of work and 'saving for a rainy day'. After the failure of the Grand National Consolidated Trade Union in 1833 and the collapse of the Chartist movement in 1848, the trade union movement had settled down, much to the chagrin of Marx and Engels, not to overthrow the system, but to get the best they could for their members in a capitalist world. The aristocracy of labour, the skilled unions organised along Smiles's precepts, they developed Institutes for Mechanics and working men's adult education schemes so that through education their members might rise in the industrial system, and at the same time they encouraged members to save in good times that they might be tided over hard times. Since only people earning above the subsistence level could hope to belong, membership of a friendly society gave not only working-class solidarity but also a sense of status. As the friendly societies multiplied, the government, anxious to encourage this form of self-help, intervened to prevent fraudulent practice, and in 1855 appointed a Registrar of Friendly Societies and under the Friendly Societies Act gave him the power to inspect rules, accounts and financial transactions. The lack of outdoor relief, occupational sickness schemes and the dread of the workhouse all acted as a spur to membership, and by 1875 there were 32,000 societies covering 8 million members and dependants. As banking facilities increased and capitalism expanded, the small friendly society gave way to commercial undertakings run for profit, and the man from the Prudential became a familiar figure to working class homes. Thus the employed, and the skilled, were able to survive a rainy day – if it did not rain too hard.

Trade unions, first developed in the eighteenth century, had been rendered ineffective by the Combination Acts of 1800, but after they were made legal in 1825 the membership increased. After the frustration of early and revolutionary hopes, they settled down into performing functions that were often indistinguishable from those of the friendly societies, but with memories of the Chartists, this form of self-help was looked on with less favour by the government and an attempt was made to deprive them of their status. Eventually after a decade of legislation and counter-legislation, in 1875 the unions gained a number of advantages at law and membership began to spread to the unskilled workers. There were a number of strikes, including the 1889 dock strike and the miners' strike in 1893, but it was many years before organised labour was able to affect the level of wages or protect the poor on a rainy day.

Charities

The other source of help for the deserving poor, and sometimes the undeserving, was charity. In an age of strong religious feeling many charities were sectarian and aimed at proselytising; the rise of Methodism was a spur to other sects competing for converts, and, as Major Barbara pointed out, 'you can't save a man's soul when he is hungry'.[4] Equally, many societies stemmed from a concern about law and order; the cities were infested with gangs, mugging was rife and the streets were unsafe at night. A number of reports showed a correlation between pauperism and crime, but probably more telling were the fashionable novels of Charles Dickens. Besides those who were motivated by religious principles there were a number of people who were genuinely uneasy about the effects of industrialisation and were conscience-stricken when they saw so much poverty. Finally, in a socially volatile society, association with charitable work could be a way of climbing the slippery rungs of the social ladder.

Apart from the fact that charity was merely a panacea, much of it was haphazard and societies overlapped, and many saw this indiscriminate almsgiving as undermining the incentive to thrift and the less eligibility principle. Moreover there were now some critics who were looking at the more fundamental problems. The Social Science Association was founded in 1857, and this discussed the problem of the unemployed and led to the concept of a Charity Organisation to co-ordinate effort. After many initial struggles because societies were loath to give up independence, eventually the great social prestige of the Central Committee persuaded many of the value of amalgamation. In 1875 Charles Stewart Loch, a deeply religious man, was appointed general secretary and he influenced the society for the next 38 years. Laudable and humane though its aims were, the Charity Organisation Society (COS) soon moved away from radical ideas and became a pillar of the establishment and the *status quo*. The Society, however, was immensely important because its committee was aristocratic and powerful and it gave evidence to the various commissions dealing with social problems, not least of which was its evidence to the Royal Commission on the Poor Law. Its reactionary attitude must be considered a delaying factor in the cause of social reform. The Society under-estimated the extent of poverty and disagreed with the Booth findings. It was wedded to the policy of non-state intervention – Loch was firmly against the old age pension scheme; it preserved the myth that the 'deserving' and the 'undeserving poor' could be differentiated; finally, it completely under-estimated the effect poverty had on health and the vicious circle of poverty, ill health, unemployment and more poverty.

MOVES TOWARDS A FREE HEALTH SERVICE

Throughout the nineteenth century there had been limited attempts at providing a free health service for certain categories; these categories changed as public anxiety changed. Free treatment for the insane was inspired by the fear of people being wrongly put in madhouses. Free treatment for both in- and out-patients in the voluntary hospitals was now mainly motivated by medical teaching needs; free treatment for infectious diseases became a popular idea once it was appreciated how these diseases were spread; and free treatment for paupers was the logical outcome of separating the sick from the well. Those interested in the health of the community wanted to extend these services to a universal service; those like the Charity Organisation who saw these services as a blow to the incentive to save, and to whom the less eligibility principle was the Ark of the Covenant, wanted these 'abuses' curtailed.

Now a new problem had arisen in the community: because the country was alarmed about the fitness of the recruits to the army and what this could mean in the event of war, attention had been turned to the health of school children who were having free medical examinations and in some cases free treatment. 'Where', asked *The Times*, 'would it all end?' Public and private medicine were beginning to conflict. At the same time entry into hospital was a mass of anomalies; the improved amenities, the reformed nursing and the growing middle classes all increased the demand. With the new 'scientific' medicine and anaesthesia people were now less frightened of hospitals, and by the beginning of the twentieth century both the Poor Law and the voluntary hospitals were complaining about the abuse of hospital beds. The problem of medicine being able to do more than it had resources for had begun.

THE ROYAL COMMISSION ON THE POOR LAW

In 1906 the Liberals obtained a landslide victory with a majority of 356 seats. They now had to show the rising support for the Labour Party that *they* were the party of social concern and a separate party was not necessary. Apart from industrial unrest below, there was a new concern from above. Michael Sadler, the Secretary to the Board of Education, had pointed out that England was 60 years behind its rivals; the armed services were alarmed as to whether the recruits of tomorrow would be fit for active service. Therefore, pressed by their Labour competitors the Liberals acted on two fronts: the young and the old. Under the guidance of Sir Arthur Newsholme, the Chief Medical Officer, they introduced measures to improve the health of school children (Chapter 8). As early as 1886 there had been suggestions that something should be done to take the old out of the stigma of the Poor Law; non-contributory pensions had been introduced in other countries, and a select committee under David Lloyd George (1863–1945) was set up to look at the possibility of a scheme financed by taxation. Opposition from the friendly societies defeated the committee's hopes, but the idea had taken root and as the Poor Law became more anomalous and surveys showed how many old people were in poverty the solution became more urgent. Despite attacks that this was a return to outdoor relief, the non-contributory Old Age Pension Act of 1908 was carried; this allowed people over 70 years old to claim a pension of 5 shillings a week (7/6d for a married couple), payable through the post office. Although it was a pittance, a blow had been struck against the principles of the 1834 Act, and the twentieth-century road to the Welfare State had begun.

The crux of the problem was the Poor Law itself. The outgoing Balfour government had set up a Royal Commission, but this Commission, whose monumental reports provide some of the most important source material of the era, did not report until 1909. The Commissioners included officials of the Local Government Board – who were in the position of judge and jury, leading churchmen and leaders of the COS including C. S. Loch and Octavia Hill, but they also included George Lansbury and two new-type social workers, Charles Booth and Beatrice Webb. Officials of the Local

Government Board giving evidence were clearly troubled at the present chaotic state, and admitted that they were trying to accommodate two systems with different aims – deterrence and welfare – but they pointed out, if the sick were freed from the less eligibility principle then the whole Poor Law philosophy would be undermined. On the other hand, if admission to the 'state hospitals', publicly financed, carried no stigma, what would happen to the donations to voluntary hospitals? And, above all, would this not destroy the impetus to the Christian duty to give? The possibility of a 'free service' was discussed but the cost would be enormous and it would certainly be opposed by the medical profession. The Majority Report, supported by the Local Government Board and the COS, favoured a solution whereby the poor would be allowed to see a doctor of their choice before seeing the Relieving Officer, then receive treatment at a District Provident Dispensary, be subjected to a means test, and urged to make better provision for their infirmities through a Sick Club. The evidence was confused by the fact that the medical experts pointed out that certain diseases themselves created pauperism, particularly tuberculosis, and a means test would deter patients from reporting who should be isolated and who needed treatment.

Mrs Webb, on the other hand, a sharp critic of the Poor Law, disagreed, and wrote her own Minority Report; Beatrice Webb (1858–1943), like her husband, Sidney, was a Fabian socialist who believed in the 'inevitability of gradualism' and reform through municipal socialism and improved labour conditions. Like her friend, Bernard Shaw, she was strongly opposed to the popular superstition about the value of medicine, and insisted that 'what the patient needed was not medicine but advice about the habits of life on which recovery depended' – a comment not without relevance some 80 years later. Mrs Webb was against the free choice of a doctor, as he could not be expected to give advice about 'the unwise habits that caused two thirds of the ill health of the poor'.[5] Although both reports now strike us as parental, the Minority Report was in fact to prove influential for many years to come. The Minority Report advocated the break-up of the Poor Law and the transfer of all health services to the counties and county boroughs, which could be enlarged or reorganised if necessary; the Health Departments of the Local Authorities would exercise single control over all preventive and curative services with all personnel working from Health Centres. The report, however, was damned by one totally unacceptable proposal – that the doctors should be employed by the Health Authority and paid a salary.

THE NATIONAL INSURANCE ACT

Meanwhile Lloyd George, now Chancellor of the Exchequer under Asquith, who had taken over the Liberal premiership in 1908, liked neither

Report and was on his way to Germany to study the insurance system there. Bismark (1815–98) had headed off the threat of socialism in Germany by a generous system of social benefits, and Lloyd George, backed by the young Winston Churchill, now at the Board of Trade, felt that a similar system in England might kill two birds with one stone: it would break the hold of the Poor Law and 'dish the Fabian socialists'.[6] Moreover, experience with non-contributory pensions had shown that general taxation could never do more than finance the most parsimonious scheme. Therefore the first thing to do was to find the necessary finance, and this was done by what was known as the 'People's Budget' of 1909, which increased duty on beer, spirits and tobacco, introduced a sliding rate of income tax and a heavier tax on unearned income, and was the first budget that deliberately aimed at redistributing wealth. This was a far call from *laissez-faire* and, not surprisingly, it produced a storm of protest in the House of Lords. Legislation could not proceed until after the Parliament Act, which limited the veto of the House of Lords.

The National Insurance Act of 1911 was a triumph for Lloyd George, although in the end it fell short of his original conception. He had to placate the insurance companies, which feared for their profit, and the medical profession who feared for their independence, but the fact that people were now living longer with an increased demand for benefits reduced the hostility of the friendly societies, which, having seen the demographic light, were not now so averse to state aid. The Act provided for manual workers to make a contribution of 4d a week to an approved society, the employers to pay 3d and the state 2d. Sold as a package of '9d for 4d', it entitled the worker, but not his dependants, to a free choice of doctor from those whose names were on a 'Panel' organised by local insurances commissions, and to get pharmaceutical services together with limited cash payments. The poor, instead of having thrift thrust upon them by the exhortation of a charity, were having it imposed on them by the state. The insurance aspect of the scheme gave it a certain respectability and, as Winston Churchill hastened to point out, the fact that the workers were paying their share gave the recipients of the scheme a certain self-respect.

Although national insurance was an important landmark in the evolution of the social services, ensuring as it did that 'insurance' would be the linchpin, at the time it aroused misgivings. On the one hand, the socialists regarded it as inadequate and wanted a non-contributory scheme; on the other hand, the hospital administrators were sure there would be a fall in the contributions to hospitals; and the doctors opposed the plan because they felt it would encroach on their professional freedom. In fact neither happened, but the Act had other repercussions. The male wage earner now had an incentive to go to a panel doctor rather than the out-patient department, and consequently trainee doctors and nurses saw less of the common complaints seen by the general practitioners, especially those caused by occupation. On the other hand, the general practitioner frequently referred his patient to hospital for treatment and as likely as not never heard of him again. When hospitals and general practitioners dealt with different categories of patients, continuity of care was ensured, but now they were dealing with the same patient for different reasons and referral started a communication problem that was to grow progressively worse. On the credit side, the general practitioner, whose very existence had been threatened by out-patient departments and bad debts, now had an assured income, and from this stability it was later possible to build up a peculiarly British concept of primary care.

Although the Act was regarded by its framers as only a beginning, it was many years before the worst deficiencies were rectified. The most important were the lack of cover for dependants and the failure to provide hospital care in a unified health system, and of course basically it was an illness and accident service. Some of those defects, though not the last, were later to be remedied by the Webb's new young friend, William Beveridge (1879–1963), who entered the Civil Service in 1908 and was now advising Churchill on the setting up of Labour Exchanges to deal with the problem of unemployment.

THE EMANCIPATION OF WOMEN BEFORE 1914

Society in late Victorian England was freer from legal restraint than it had ever been – and has ever been since – but this 'free' society was held together by a mass of restrictions of religion, family, status, class and, above all, the idea of women's role in society. However, even before the death of Queen Victoria, these restrictions were being loosened and challenged by writers like Ibsen (1828–1906), Shaw (1856–1950) and Wilde (1856–1900), who were advocating a new emancipation for women, and although they may not have understood the aims of women they at least recognised their right to play a full role in society. As early as 1857 a group of middle-class women founded the *English Women's Journal* which advocated the right of women to take up employment, to retain their property after marriage, more equitable divorce laws and the right to vote. At the time the movement was ridiculed by the press and found little support among women, but in 1865 John Stuart Mill (1806–73) gave the movement a new seriousness by his advocacy, and it was his wife who eventually persuaded Florence Nightingale to modify her views on the subject.

By the end of the century the Women's Franchise League had been formed by Emmeline Pankhurst (1858–1928) and her husband, and after her husband's death she and her daughters, together with stalwarts like Mrs Pethick-Lawrence and Mrs Fawcett, ran the movement, which in spite of internal rifts, grew in strength. By 1906, 400 Members of Parliament had pledged themselves to votes for women, and Campbell-Bannerman was sympathetic and received 350 representatives from delegations including some nurses, many of whom marched in uniform. Unfortunately, his successor, Asquith, was less sympathetic, and as the government – now worried by industrial strife and the threat of civil war over the proposed Home Rule Bill for Ireland – procrastinated, so the militancy of the suffragettes grew. In spite of the publicity this gained and the fact that it colours the image of the movement, the suffragettes expended more energy on their educational programme than they did chaining themselves to the railings, and the image was, of course, controlled by a male-dominated press. Seen in retrospect, it is possible to understand the government's problems, but it was a failure to act on a most fundamental liberal principle, and it is against this background that the calls for registration of nurses must be seen.

In the end it was to take total war, which was to depend largely on women's work, to break down the prejudice and produce the Representation of the People Act of 1918, when men and women of the age of 30 years were enfranchised.

THE EFFECT OF THE 1914–18 WAR ON THE HEALTH SERVICES

A factor in the delay of reform and the attitude to movements like those of the suffragettes was the general expectancy of war that pervaded Europe in the early years of the century, and throughout Europe and Russia there was social unrest as each nation faced up to the effects of the Industrial Revolution. All over the Continent there was a fall in the value of real wages, and in England in 1913, 16 per cent of the population were living in primary poverty.[7] The 1914–18 war was an entirely new kind of war, whose length and consequences no one had foreseen, starting with cavalry troops in red and ending with tanks and aircraft. The casualties were unprecedented, with 2 million on the Western front alone, and forward planning by the military medical services was hopelessly and totally inadequate. At home there was no central health authority, and all too late the Poor Law Commission had urged the unification of services. Now the War Office tried to persuade individual hospitals to give up beds for war casualties, persuasion that had to be backed by considerable subsidy. At the same time various charity organisations offered aid and stately homes, now difficult to run because of the call-up of servants; some recruited medical and nursing personnel, and auxiliary hospitals came into being without co-ordination or control. Inevitably there were disputes and conflicts, and it was not until the Joint War Organisation was set up under the tactful chairmanship of Sir Arthur Stanley that the disputatious bodies were brought together in something like a common effort (Chapter 12). Still there were not enough beds, and the next step was to commandeer accommodation in the Poor Law institutions. This proved difficult, but some were taken over and the displaced patients housed in even less comfortable conditions elsewhere, and for these the standard of care deteriorated. The movement of nurses and doctors into the armed services produced acute shortages and hardships in the civilian hospitals; but, in the general catalyst of war, doctors and nurses came into contact with the realities of life in the Poor Law world – a second-class world where staffing and equipment were far below the accepted standards in the voluntary hospitals. With bitter irony, this was a lesson that had to be learned again some 25 years later.

As the war dragged on with its increasing toll of wounded, the voluntary hospitals began to worry about their future, they were accepting a subsidy from the government and had been hit by inflation and were likely to be in dire straits if the subsidy were withdrawn. In short, the first step towards state control had been taken. Moreover many doctors serving with the forces had become used to a regular salary and looked with less favour on returning to the bad debts of general practice or the long wait for promotion in the hospital world. By 1917, there were 45,000 women doing nursing and a number of these were middle-class girls doing 'hard and rewarding work for the first time, and in many cases under conditions of unprecedented freedom'.[8] It was from these recruits, some of whom brought fresh qualities of leadership, that the profession was to find a new infusion into the ranks of administration in the inter-war years.

POST-WAR RECONSTRUCTION PLANS

New ideas about the land fit for heroes were formulated; a Ministry of Pensions was set up with more generous war disablement and pension cover and a system of allowances for dependent children, although it was not until 1925 that an insurance pension (that is, a contributory scheme) was provided for men at the age of 65 years and widows at 60 years. The Board of Education, pointing out that 'the war had brought a clearer recognition of the value of education', set up a committee under the chairmanship of H. A. L. Fisher, the distinguished historian, who in 1917 put forward proposals which provided the basis for the Education Act of 1918. This Act proposed a number of ancillary services such as nursery schools and centres for mental defectives; it abolished all fees to elementary schools and raised the standard in the higher classes. Unfortunately, the Fisher scheme for compulsory part-time education for all children between the ages of 14 and 18 years not receiving secondary education, was never adopted because of the post-war financial crisis. Unlike nursing, teaching had suffered a grievous manpower loss, and in order to make this good the salaries of teachers were greatly improved, which put elementary teaching into the category of a 'middle-class occupation' for the first time, and in terms of economic attraction it now outpaced nursing. Another result was the setting up of the University Grants Committee, which aimed at increasing university entrance, and although it was some years before women were able to take full advantage of the new opportunities, this in time would encroach on the recruits who once turned to nursing.

Not least of the reconstruction plans were those concerned with the more equitable distribution of the health services. A committee under Sir Donald Maclean, with Beatrice Webb on one of the subcommittees, now recommended the break-up of the Poor Law, and, in tune with the Minority Report, the transfer of all health matters to the counties and county boroughs. In 1918 Lloyd George was returned at the head of a Coalition government on a manifesto that included the implementation of the Maclean report; Dr Christopher Addison, a Liberal Member of Parliament was invited to take charge of the problem and a draft Bill was introduced at the end of the war. However, resistance from the medical profession and the Local Government Board was so strong that it was withdrawn, though something was salvaged, and in 1919 a Ministry of Health was set up with Dr Addison as the first minister, and the first and last doctor to be so until Dr Owen became Secretary of State at the DHSS. The next step was to ask Sir Bernard Dawson (1865–1945), later Lord Dawson of Penn, to be the chairman of a Council on Medical and Administrative Services and to produce an interim report. The Report, which appeared in 1920, bowed to medical opinion and set aside the more drastic measures proposed by the Maclean report; it recommended the combining of curative and preventive services and the setting up of primary and secondary health centres which were to serve as a base for general practitioners, nurses and health visitors. The primary centres were to be equipped with beds and the secondary centres were to contain diagnostic facilities and be visited by specialists. The problem of transfer to local authorities was avoided by the setting up of single Health Authorities, which were to be partly elected and with advisory councils at local level. This avoiding device was eventually put into practice some 54 years later, but without the democratic element.

The Dawson Report is remarkably in tune with modern thinking, and might be considered as foreshadowing the idea of the community hospital, but it was ahead of its time and in spite of early enthusiasm the report was not accepted. The medical officers of health felt, and with considerable justification, that the general practitioner's education did not equip him for preventive medicine – a chicken and egg situation that was to bedevil the scene for years to come. Moreover, some felt that the Maclean Report was more practical and urged waiting for the promised local government reform: they were to wait 50 years. Others settled back into the *status quo ante* and did not wish to be disturbed. But as unemployment rose to 16 per cent and strikes and social unrest became widespread, the worries of the doctors and administrators about professional independence were as nothing compared with the problems of finance. The Maclean and Dawson

Reports were quietly dropped – so too was Dr Addison; England had entered on the great post-war depression.

REFERENCES

1 Fraser, D. (1973) *The Evolution of the British Welfare State*, London: Macmillan, p. 86.
2 Cassells (ed.) (1910) *Text Book for Nurses*, London: Cassells.
3 Webb, S. and Webb, B. (1910) *English Poor Law Policy*, reprinted 1963, London: Cass.
4 Shaw, G. B. (1905) *Major Barbara*, in *Complete Works*, London: Odhams Press Ltd.
5 *The Poor Law Commission Minority Report* (1909), London: HMSO.
6 Fraser, D. (1973) *The Evolution of the British Welfare State*, (quoting John Burns the Labour leader), London: Macmillan, p. 151.
7 Bowley, A. L. and Burnett-Hurst, A. R. (1915) *Livelihood and Poverty*, quoted in A. Marwick *The Deluge: British Society and the First World War* (1965), London: Macmillan, p. 22.
8 Marwick, *The Deluge*, p. 93.

FURTHER READING

Marwick, A. (1965) *The Deluge: British Society and the First World War*, London: Macmillan.
Owen, D. (1965) *English Philanthropy, 1660–1960*, Oxford: Oxford University Press.
Rose, M. E. (1972) *The Relief of Poverty, 1834–1914*, London: David & Charles.

Chapter 12

Registration and the growth of nursing organisations

Miss Nightingale had accepted with reluctance two methods of entry for nurse training, one for special probationers and one for pupils, and, as she forecast, the former were invaluable in pioneering positions of nursing superintendents in other hospitals where they started similar training schemes. In 1858 the Medical Act had provided for the statutory registration of medical practitioners, and by the 1880s the new nurse leaders were beginning to ask whether nursing should not also be tested by public examination and the title 'nurse' restricted to duly registered candidates.

The leader of the registration movement was Ethel Gordon Manson (1857–1947), the daughter of a prosperous doctor, whose stepfather was a Member of Parliament. Intelligent and articulate, Miss Manson trained as a lady probationer at Nottingham, spending a further year at Manchester Royal Infirmary; later she was a sister at the London Hospital and in 1881, at the age of 24, she was appointed matron of St Bartholomew's Hospital where she became convinced of the need to raise the standard and lengthen the training, and of the necessity of protecting the young profession by state registration. In 1887 Miss Manson left to marry Dr Bedford Fenwick, who was himself active in medical politics and who shared his wife's aspirations concerning the registration of nurses.

About the same time Henry Burdett, later Sir Henry, who had founded the Hospitals' Association, was making similar suggestions in his publications, which included the *Nursing Mirror*, although he did not favour the high standards proposed by some of the nurse members, and this led to schism. Burdett (1847–1920) was by now a powerful figure in the hospital world. Having started life in a bank and then the Stock Exchange, he was now devoting himself wholly to hospital publications and surveys and, although the statistics in some of these are suspect, he has left a wealth of information. In 1887, the Bedford Fenwicks, who were to become Sir Henry's antagonists, invited to their house in Upper Wimpole Street nurses whose aims were the control of nursing by Act of Parliament, to join them in a 'breakaway' organisation from the Hospitals' Association, the British Nurses' Association. The response was good, and the committee included a number of matrons from London teaching hospitals, and Princess Christian Helena, daughter of Queen Victoria and married to the Prince of Schleswig-Holstein, consented to be the patron. Dr Bedford Fenwick persuaded the British Medical Association to pass a resolution in favour of nurse registration, and in 1889 a mass meeting was held at Mansion House to call for an official register of nurses.

OPPOSITION TO REGISTRATION

Opposition came from a number of quarters. Most important was Miss Nightingale herself, who was still an influence in the hospital world and who saw the idea of a central examination as likely to undermine her whole philosophy about nursing with its special emphasis on the right personal qualities and aptitudes. In a letter she wrote, 'Nursing has to do with living spirits and bodies. It cannot be tested by public examination, though it may be tested by current supervision.'[1] Apart from the fact that a public exam-ination could not test personal qualities, the profession was in the early stages of development and if a standard were set now it would be too low – though she conceded that such a safeguard might be necessary in the future. Anxious not to divide the profession and with good reason for disliking 'nursing camps', Miss Nightingale conducted her opposition from behind the scenes through friends in the hospital world and Parliament, and this influence was largely responsible for ensuring that the British Nurses Association did not obtain the right to produce a register on its own terms.

Resistance also came from hospital administrators. Sir Henry Burdett, still smarting from the defections from his Hospitals' Association, used his journals to belabour the registrationists. Other reasons for opposition were confused and complicated; provincial matrons and doctors feared control from London and saw the high standard to be set, and the high fees proposed, as denying them recruits. On the other hand, some of the less well-trained saw registration as a means of boosting their status, provided of course that *they* could register. Some doctors with fashionable practices supported registration because they saw the value of being able to ask for a trained nurse; others with less lucrative practices saw the new nurses as a threat and likely to take away some of their livelihood and prestige. Moreover, Mrs Bedford Fenwick was an ardent and outspoken supporter of women's rights, which many doctors were not. But these fears were nothing compared with the overriding problem of numbers. Of the 67,000 nurses and midwives recorded at the 1901 Census, probably less than 10,000 had received the 'reformed' training; if the remainder, who were obviously giving care, were denied the right to call themselves 'nurse' and forbidden to nurse, who would nurse the patients? It must be stressed that in spite of the talk about the 'growing middle class' this still formed only about 2 per cent of the population if an income of over £300 a year is taken as the criterion,[2] and even in 1934 about 75 per cent of the population were earning less than £250 a year;[3] on sheer logistics most nurses had to come from this group, and for this reason, if for no other, the purist registrationists were impractical.

In 1893 the British Nurses' Association, having failed to get Parliament to enforce registration, applied to the Privy Council for a Royal Charter and permission to produce its own register, but Mr Rathbone had been active behind the scenes in the Houses of Parliament and although the Charter was granted, the terms limited the Association to 'keeping a list of names of persons who may have applied to be entered therein as nurses'. This is not what the militant members wanted, and in the dissension that followed Dr Bedford Fenwick and his wife resigned, determined to pursue their aims by more forceful means.

EARLY NURSING ORGANISATIONS

As the factions grew more disputatious Mrs Bedford Fenwick looked for new ways of promoting her cause. In 1894 she founded the Matrons' Council of Great Britain and Ireland, which, although pledged to registration, made little headway. Then, while on a visit to the World Fair in Chicago, Mrs Bedford Fenwick conceived the idea of an International Council, and when the International Council of Women met in London in 1899 the opportunity presented itself, and the Matrons' Council took steps to promote an International Council of Nurses. Two years later the first Congress met in Buffalo, with Mrs Bedford Fenwick as the first President. In Buffalo she reiterated what she called her trumpet call to arms, that 'the nurse question was the Woman Question', and that 'our profession like every other profession needs registration'. Small wonder that people confused the two issues.

The registrationist now found a new ally in the Society for the State Registration of Nurses, which in 1904 amalgamated with the Matrons' Council, the league of St Bartholomew's Nurses and the Leicester Royal Infirmary League to form the National Council of Nurses of the United Kingdom; this Council now represented British nurses on the International Council and had as its aim the registration of nurses. The National Council was a loose federation of several organisations, most of which had social rather than political aims, and, as more 'leagues' were drawn in the structure, became increasingly cumbersome and, of course, totally unrepresentative of the great mass of nurses who did not work in teaching hospitals with 'leagues'. In 1893 Mrs Bedford Fenwick acquired the *Nursing Record,* which she used as a vehicle for her campaign for registration; in 1903 the name was changed to the *British Journal of Nursing*, with Mrs Bedford Fenwick remaining as editor, a post she occupied for nearly 50 years.

REGISTRATION BILLS

In 1902 the situation changed. The Midwives Act required all practising midwives to undergo training and register with the Central Midwives Board; registration of nurses was regarded as a logical extension, although perhaps not so logical as some thought, for the practice of midwifery is more easily defined and circumscribed than nursing. The aim of the Midwives Act was the protection of the public, which was not the aim of the advanced registrationists; they wanted to raise the status of nursing by limiting the intake. Now, re-rallying their forces the various organisations lobbied for registration, with the Royal British Nurses' Association again entering the lists.

In June 1904 the Select Committee on the Registration of Nurses was set up which, during the next year, examined witnesses and received written evidence, and finally reported to the House of Commons in July 1905. Allowing for the fact that the witnesses were pleading for or against registration and some of the evidence must be regarded as tendentious, it does give a reasonable picture of the state of 'reformed' nursing at the beginning of the century.

Miss Lückes, the matron of the London Hospital, who opposed registration because she thought it too early for the profession to be stereotyped, and in some cases 'a little training went a long way', gave a detailed account of training at the London Hospital. Candidates were carefully selected and spent six weeks in the Preliminary Training School, an idea that had been in vogue since 1890; then after this there were examinations and the successful candidates went on the wards where, apart from bedside instruction, they had four hours of theory a week and three courses of instruction a year; examinations were set and marked by outside examiners and consisted of written papers, practical tests and a *viva voce* interview.[4] The course lasted two years; 200 candidates were accepted a year and about 60 certificates granted, so it looks as if the 'wastage' rate was between 30 and 40 per cent. This is about the same figure that Burdett suggested for the Nightingale School, although he inferred that wastage was due to the fact that the probationers could not take it, whereas reading between the lines it looks as if at the London, in spite of 'careful selection', the candidates did not always come up to the standard required. Although there were a number of variations on the theme, with Miss Isla Stewart of St Bartholomew's reporting on a three-year training and others on trainings of four and a half years, it is clear that the reformed training gave a fair amount of formal education, and when considered in relation to medical knowledge at the time, the amount of theoretical understanding required was considerable. Giving evidence on behalf of the registrationists, Dr Bedford Fenwick estimated that about 60,000 persons would apply, but it is doubtful whether more than 6,000 had had the type of training described by Miss Lückes, and the question was whether these would be the only people who would be accepted for the register.

It is worth recalling a perspicacious comment by Miss Lückes; she was fearful of the uniformity of registration because she thought that different personalities of nurses were suitable for different types of work and it would be 'a waste to train all for everything' – a consideration that has dogged all attempts at devising a comprehensive basic training. It was prophetic, because nursing was soon to expand into many fields requiring different personalities and different levels of intellect, and much would have to be left to post-basic training.

The Committee, assuming the mantle of Solomon, reported in favour of registration but with the proviso 'that it is not desirable to prohibit unregistered persons from nursing for gain', and 'there should be a separate Register for nurses whose training is of a lower standard than that laid down by the Register of Nurses'.[5] Although the registrationists felt the battle was won, legislation was difficult to frame, and year after year Registration Bills were brought before the House and year after year they were blocked. In 1908 Lord Balfour introduced a badly drafted Bill in the Lords which was defeated; then another Bill received support in the Commons, but Mr Asquith could not find time to give it consideration. Now interested parties temporarily, and superficially, laid aside their differences and formed the Central Committee for the State Registration of Nurses, but there was so much dual representation that the strength of the lobby was doubtful and, as the war clouds gathered over Europe, the government, desperate about naval defence, had other and more pressing business than the registration of nurses, a subject of which they were no doubt heartily sick.

THE WORLD WAR, 1914–18

The war made a great impact on the nursing scene. Nurses were needed on an unprecedented scale, and the demand was largely met by the Voluntary Aid Detachment which had been founded by the British Red Cross in 1909. The 23 Army General Hospitals expanded, nurses left civilian hospitals, male nurses left the mental hospitals to join the forces, the 'TANS' were called up, and still there were not enough. Women in general, and nurses in particular acquitted themselves well, while a number lost their lives in the hell of Flanders; the nation was stirred by the shooting of Nurse Edith Cavell as a spy in 1915, and whatever the rights and wrongs of the assistance given by Miss Cavell in helping soldiers to escape, it enhanced the image of nursing.[6] In a spirit of patriotic fervour women, who had not previously thought of working applied to train, and once again matrons could be selective. But it was not long before friction broke out between the trained nurses and the VADs – both sides being unduly touchy about their status. Trained nurses were not united in much but they were at one in resisting any infringement of their hard-won professional position by VADs. The registration lobby was particularly acidulous, the *British Nursing Journal* commenting that 'young women with express training and assuming full nurses' uniform – with the addition of a red cross – were treated by medical men and society people as trained nurses'. As the acrimony increased, the Joint War Organisation Committee was left with the unenviable task of sorting out the squabbles.

In 1916 the War Office, anxious about the shortage of nurses, set up a committee under the chairmanship of Lord Knutsford to investigate the position; there was not a single nursing representative and the outcry was so great that Lord Knutsford resigned. Worried by the continuing disputes and the fact that such nursing organisations as there were embroiled in personality conflicts, Dame Sarah Swift, Matron-in-Chief of the British Red Cross and matron of Guy's from 1901 to 1909, discussed with the Hon. Arthur Stanley, the chairman of the Joint War Committee, the possibility of founding an organisation for nurses analogous to the Colleges of Physicians and Surgeons which could act as a national forum for nursing opinion. Arthur Stanley, who was also Treasurer of St Thomas's, discussed the proposition with Sir Cooper Perry, a member of the Army Medical Board and the Medical Superintendent of Guy's, and together they worked out a plan of campaign. A skilful letter was sent to all nurse training schools pointing out that although there was no unanimous feeling in favour of state registration, nevertheless it was obvious that something needed to be done to co-ordinate nursing interest. Arthur Stanley went on to propose that a College of Nursing be founded on the lines of the Royal Colleges of Physicians and Surgeons, pointing out that other professions organised themselves in this way. He succeeded where the former factions had failed; he was not associated with the undignified battle of the journals about registration, and was a layman of great tact and charm connected with the most highly regarded training school, but, above all, for the first time trained nurses were being offered a democratic organisation with the power in the hands of the members who would elect their Council themselves. The time was ripe, the war had changed the position of women, the vote was as good as won and it was increasingly obvious that regardless of the question of registration, trained nurses needed their own professional organisation.

THE COLLEGE OF NURSING

On 1 April 1916 the College of Nursing was registered with the Board of Trade as a limited company and a Council appointed to take care of its affairs until one could be elected by the members. The principal objects of the college were:

- To promote the better education and training of nurses and the advancement of nursing as a profession in all or any of its branches.
- To promote uniformity of the curriculum.
- To recognise approved nursing schools.
- To make and maintain a register of persons to whom certificates of proficiency or of training and proficiency had been granted.
- To promote Bills of Parliament for any object connected with the interests of the nursing profession, and, in particular, with their education, organisation, protection or for their recognition by the state.

The Articles of Association specifically prevented the college from imposing on its members or supporting with its funds 'any regulation which, if an object of the College, would make it a Trade Union', an article which the College, in common with other professional organisations, had eventually to change to meet the requirements of the changed and complicated Labour Laws. For the purpose of admission to its own register the college recognised for training those civil hospitals and infirmaries with at least 250 beds, a resident medical officer and at least one course of lectures a year. It was assumed that when registration came it would be based on general training, and it was therefore quite reasonable to limit membership to general nurses; and in the ethos of votes for women' and the sharp increase in the numbers of women over men and the fact that there were almost no general trained male nurses, it assumed that it would be an organisation for women.

By 1918 the membership of the College was over 13,000 and in an attempt to unite all nurses it made overtures to the Royal British Nurses' Association whose patron, Princess Christian, favoured amalgamation. But Mrs Bedford Fenwick objected and, although negotiations were started, the new committee of the association soon brought them to a halt, but by now the College had four times as many members and could manage alone. Now both the College and the association were pressing for registration, but not necessarily on the same terms. It had been generally agreed that, once a registering body was set up, two-thirds of its governing Council would be elected from the ranks of the first newly registered nurses; therefore the key to control lay with the Caretaker Committee because this committee would decide who should be registered and therefore who would have the right to vote, and in this each organisation had a strong vested interest. Both the College and the Royal British Nurses' Association presented Bills. The association wanted a limited entry with high standards and had as its ally the British Medical Association; the College, on the other hand, was prepared to be more flexible and had allies among the hospital administrators and wanted to include representatives from the Poor Law Unions. By 1919 the old Local Government Board had been replaced by the new Ministry of Health with Dr Addison as the Minister, who, looking at the Montagues and Capulets, decided, not unreasonably, to draft his own Bill. This was not to be the last time in nursing history that internecine dispute gave a hostage to fortune.

THE GENERAL NURSING COUNCIL

During the period of the Caretaker Committee the minister consulted not only organisations but also various sectional interests and the specialist hospitals which, like the general hospitals, were using probationers as at least half their workforce, and were only too anxious to be considered as 'training hospitals'. In spite of a strong lobby for a 'comprehensive basic training' – which meant different things to different groups – pragmatism prevailed and the 'supplementary registers were included rather as expediency than an educational policy. Some 'specialities' like paediatrics had a 'register; others, like orthopaedics or tuberculosis nursing, which at that time absorbed a large nursing force, did not.

The minister appointed the nurse members of the first Council; the College of Nursing had nine seats, the association four and the Poor Law Institutes two; within this Council Mrs Bedford Fenwick and the association members formed a minority party bent on a rigorous test for all applications, and after four months' work with more than 3,000 received, only 984 were registered. The Interim Act was due to end in 1922 and it began to look as if the first Council would be elected by a handful of registered nurses. As a protest 16 members of the Council resigned, and as the remainder were unable to form a quorum the minister had to intervene. Under his guidance a new checking procedure was devised and the protesting members withdrew their resignations. There were further unseemly rows, recalled by witnesses for many years to come, but by 1922 12,000 nurses were eligible for the first election and Mrs Bedford Fenwick lost her seat, and although she had questions asked in the House of Commons the decision remained.

In December 1919 the Nurses' Bill received royal assent and a General Nursing Council for England and Wales was established with the duty of setting up a Register of Nurses to consist of the following parts:

1 a general part containing the names of all nurses who satisfied the conditions of admission to that part of the register;
2 a supplementary part containing the names of male nurses;
3 a supplementary part containing the names of nurses trained in the care of persons suffering from mental diseases;
4 a supplementary part containing the names of nurses trained in the nursing of sick children;
5 any other prescribed part.

Under (5) was later added nurses of infectious diseases and nurses trained in the care of mental defectives.

The Nurses' Registration Act was passed for:

1 England and Wales;
2 Scotland; and
3 Northern Ireland (the Irish Settlement Act was passed in 1921).

Each country set up its own General Nursing Council with duties as follows:

1 to compile a syllabus of instruction;
2 to compile a syllabus of subjects for examination;
3 to compile a register of qualified nurses.

(These were to be people who had completed their hospital training within a stated period before the passing of the Act. After a prescribed time no nurse could be registered unless she had undergone approved training and passed the council's examinations.)

The first General Nursing Council consisted of:

16 nurses to be elected;
2 members appointed by the Privy Council;
2 members appointed by the Board of Education;
5 members appointed by the Ministry of Health.

This first syllabus was advisory only, but in March 1925 the first state examinations were held, after which no other applications were accepted; state registration was now by a three-year training in an approved hospital and by passing a written and practical examination conducted by the council. After 1925 the council ceased to recognise the Royal Medico-Psychological Association (Chapter 7) as an examining body for mental nurses, which in 1905 had reported to the Select Committee on its 'satisfactory system of nurse training', and for many years to come mental nurses boasted the possession of the RMPA certificate; however, after 1925 training for the part of the register for mental nurses was in the hands of the Mental Nurses Training Committee.

In 1921 the Council set up a Disciplinary and Penal Committee which had the power to deal with registered nurses who for some reason had shown themselves not to be 'fit and proper persons', and the council also had power to prosecute persons purporting to be registered nurses when they were not. The setting up of disciplinary machinery along the lines of the medical profession showed a recognition of nursing as a profession: two hallmarks were accepted, a standard of competence tested by examination, and a standard of personal behaviour 'more exacting than that required by the community in general'. The early council realised that not only could the nurse's personal conduct, including conduct outside work, bring odium on the profession, it could also be such that the trust of patients in the profession was lost; in such a situation technical competence was meaningless – a point Miss Nightingale had made some 50 years earlier.

In many ways the 'Thirty Years War' for registration was a Pyrrhic victory. The standard required, when the smoke of battle subsided, would have satisfied neither Miss Nightingale nor Mrs Bedford Fenwick, nor did it the College of Nursing: it was all an expedient compromise. By its own folly the profession had handed over the control of the standard of entry and the requirements for the basic training to the government, and of course to the ultimate control by people who had the responsibility for keeping the hospitals staffed as cheaply as possible.

Although the General Nursing Council did its best to mitigate this disadvantage, the statutory control was always there, and the first hallmark of a profession – that it controls its own standard of entry and training, was lost.

THE EARLY DEVELOPMENT OF THE COLLEGE OF NURSING

The college not having become the registering body as many had anticipated, was free to develop as an independent professional organisation. Previously the standard for admission had been more stringent than that required by the General Nursing Council, which is why the early founder members attached so much importance to their College membership. After the Registration Act the college decided to admit persons on the general part of the council's registers – a limitation in line with their main purpose which was to 'promote the better education of nurses' and, influenced by developments across the Atlantic, it was envisaged that the supplementary registers would be temporary and give way to a 'comprehensive' training with specialisation to follow, as in medicine.

From the start the College advanced on two fronts: the need for better and continuing education for nurses to fit them for new opportunities, and to improve pay and the conditions under which nurses worked. Armed with 20,000 members and a new headquarters, in 1919 the College started research into nurses' salaries and conditions, and published what was popularly known as the 'Nurses' Charter' which called for a 48-hour week – not to be achieved for over 20 years – improved training, better salaries, accommodation and, most important, a pension scheme for nurses. This work and the research involved soon started what was to become an ever-increasing aspect of the College's work.

The original letter to the training schools had offered members a say in their own affairs and this gave the College its greatest appeal. Under Article V, a council was eventually elected from the membership, and to extend participation 'centres' were set up throughout the country – later to be called 'branches'. Meanwhile, the special interests of nurses needed to be catered for, and to this end a sister tutor section was established in 1922 and a public health section the following year, thus beginning the quandary of so many organisations: local and geographical interests versus increasing specialisation. As in medicine, the pursuit of the esoteric and the particular may mean the loss of general principles and the totality of care; on the other hand, concentration on the general may mean a failure to push back frontiers and advance at important points in depth: the balance between the two is ever in need of fine tuning.

While the College was developing its branches and sections with the aid of paid officers in the areas and encouraging members to attend local meetings and send representatives to national gatherings, its Department of Education was pioneering post-basic education. At first it worked with the King's College of Household Science – now Queen Elizabeth College – and Bedford College of the University of London, with whom it had a special liaison, but soon it was offering its own courses, including a course for sister tutors, a 'housekeeping' course for matrons, and in 1928 the new health visitor's course. In 1926 Queen Mary, the patron of the College, opened the new building in Henrietta Place donated by Annie, Viscountess Cowdray, and in 1928, in recognition of its work in the field of nursing education, it was incorporated by Royal Charter and in 1939 George VI bestowed on it the title 'Royal'.

The early years included the founding of the Student Nurses' Association in 1925, originally independent of the college but associated with it. The title and the aspiration were euphemistic, for 'students' were probationers doing most of the work on the wards, and independence was not usually encouraged in hospitals. For this reason, and for others not unconnected with organisational rivalry, the college was regarded in some older and established quarters as a radical and subversive organisation and accused of sinister motives and of undermining authority. So begins the life cycle of many an organisation later to be considered orthodox.

The work of the College and its foundation structure must be seen against the social and demographic conditions of the times. The balance of females over the age of 14 rose from 595 per 1,000 in 1911 to 638 per 1,000 in 1921, and the proportion of widows from 38 to 43 per 1,000.[7] During the war the number of women employed had risen from 1.3 million to 7 million, but in the past men and women's work had been seen as separate and for the most part trade unions were for men only. If women did organise, it was usually in their own associations, which, because they were poor, were not effective. This situation did not change with the war, and although the Atkin Committee had recommended equal pay for equal production, there was little support for the proposal and the trade unions had insisted on safeguards about men returning to the jobs being done by women. In 1921 there were fewer women employed than before the war. As far as women were concerned, 'if the war represented a break with the past it was a break that was soon mended'.[8] On the other hand, women who had gone into 'women's work' tended to stay and between 1911 and 1921 the numbers in nursing rose by 76 per cent, unemployment for nurses was a possibility, and this tended to depress the market. Nurses certainly needed an organisation of their own.

But things were not the same, for now women had the vote and they tended to be more articulate and sought education and qualifications. The progress made by the College and other women's organisations in this respect was due less to female suffrage than to the fact that women had proved themselves in war, and because of the appalling loss of male lives many, who now would never marry, were bravely carving careers for themselves in a world very different from that of 1910.

REFERENCES

1 Woodham Smith, C. (1950) *Florence Nightingale*, London: Constable, p. 571.
2 Baxter, D. (1867) *The Distribution of Income* quoted in *The Common People* (1961), G. D. H. Cole and R. Postgate, University Paperbacks, London: Methuen, p. 354.
3 Aldcroft, D. H. (1970) *The Inter-War Economy*, London: Batsford, p. 382.
4 *Select Committee on the Registration of Nurses* (1905) London: HMSO, evidence of Miss Eva C. E. Lückes, pp. 15–24.
5 Ibid., p. 5.
6 Marwick, A. (1965) *The Deluge*, London: Macmillan, pp. 98 and 113.
7 Ibid., p. 290.
8 Davies, Ross (1975) *Women and Work*, London: Hutchinson, ch. 4.

FURTHER READING

Baly, M. E., (1980) *Nursing – Past into Present*, 2nd edn, London: Batsford (has useful illustrations of the period).
Braithwaite, W. J. (1957) *Lloyd George's Ambulance Wagon*, Bath: Chivers.
McGann, S. (1992) *The Battle of the Nurses*, London: Scutari Press.
Marwick, A. (1978) *Women at War, 1914–1918*, London: Fontana Books.

Chapter 13

Social change and nursing in the inter-war years

for you know only
A heap of broken images, where the sun beats,
And the dead tree gives no shelter, the cricket no relief,
And the dry stone no sound of water.

T. S. Eliot, The Waste Land (1922)

Some of the consequences usually attributed to the First World War were already in evidence in the Edwardian period, for by then the population growth was slowing down and much of Europe was entering the third stage of the demographic transition; the nineteenth-century economic expansion was losing its impetus and much heavy industry was in decline. The war, when it came, exacerbated these problems. The total number of dead in Europe is uncertain, but historians put it at between 12 and 13 million – this of course cannot be compared with the estimated 55 million dead in the total holocaust of the Second World War, but none the less it was sufficient to have repercussions on the population profile and untold psychological consequences. The loss of so many adult males, together with economic and social factors, such as the later age of marriage, which by 1930 was 27.3 for bachelors and 25.5 for spinsters, had the effect of lowering the birth rate which fell from 29 per 1,000 at the beginning of the century to 18.3 per 1,000 in 1921.[1] This fall certainly eased the pressure on maternity and child welfare services but it also meant that there would be fewer young people available 20 years later when the services needed to expand.

During the war, industries like munitions had flourished but these were not easily converted into peacetime use and in the meantime traditional markets had been lost, with Japan and similar countries becoming self-sufficient. The war stimulated new technology, especially electricity, which accelerated the decline of heavy industry and the old nineteenth century population drift was reversed, with London and the Home Counties increasing by 18 per cent and Lancashire by only 1 per cent, while the population of South Wales actually declined by 9 per cent. One result of this drift was that doctors looking for practices which they had to buy, and relying on fees from patients, were attracted to the South-East, and, in the absence of overall planning, the number of doctors influenced the growth of other medical services such as the setting up of nursing homes, cottage hospitals and clinics, thus contributing to the problem that would beset 'Resource Reallocation' nearly half a century later.

Apart from the alteration in the population profile and density there were deeper psychological and intellectual changes. At the beginning of the century writers like Shaw and Lawrence had questioned what appeared to be the outmoded values of society; now, after the excitement and shared values of the war, there was a sharper and more universal questioning of the system and in particular the class structure. The war had involved all groups as never before, and on the theory that groups which participate in a war expect to gain in proportion to their participation,[2] the war heralded a social revolution with a demand that services like health and education should be distributed more fairly and according to need rather than the mere ability to pay, and that other social services should be improved.

POST-WAR SOCIAL POLICY

The Coalition government of 1918 attempted to meet some of these needs. An effort was made to bring in a health service based on the Maclean Report and later the Dawson Report, but these had come to nought (Chapter 11). A similar fate befell Dr Addison's other great venture, the Housing Act of 1919, which floundered because of shortages of materials and grossly inflated building costs. On the other hand, the Fisher Act, though never fully implemented, did go some way to providing more equal educational opportunities. Then, in 1921, the Unemployment Act aimed at covering the hazard of unemployment by the insurance principle and taking unemployment out of the Poor Law; unfortunately coverage was limited, and for many the new 'dole' was indistinguishable from the old outdoor relief, and, as benefits were eroded by inflation the distinction became fainter. In 1925 the contributory principle was extended further, and the Widows', Orphans' and Old Age Contributory Act integrated into the National Insurance Act, a scheme giving workers the right to a pension of 10 shillings a week at the age of 65 years; this pension was payable until 70 when the pension transferred to the non-contributory scheme. The integration of the 1908 and 1925 schemes was complicated, but with a few extensions and amendments it remained in force until 1946.

Attempts were made to meet the demands for greater democracy by increasing the franchise in 1918, and by introducing some of the recommendations of the Whitley Committee in industry and furthering joint negotiation. However, the spirit of the times is perhaps best exemplified by the fact that trade union membership jumped from 4 million at the end of the war to 8 million in 1920. In 1925, the miners, who were suffering because of the decline in coal mining, asked the Trades Union Congress for support, and in 1926, when the miners were threatened with further cuts, the TUC called a General Strike. The trial of strength only lasted nine days because the government brought in the troops and special constables and in 1927 added to the legacy of bitterness by the Trade Disputes Act which made striking illegal. The miner's grievances were symptomatic of the Great Depression of 1929–33 which overtook much of the world. The world slump was largely caused by agricultural over-production and maldistribution, aggravated by a fever of speculation leading to the Wall Street crash in 1929 and a run on the banks of Europe. There was a fall in exports and in internal consumption due to a shortage of capital, which in turn led to a fall in production and massive unemployment. By 1933, 22 per cent of all insured workers in England were unemployed. However, for those who did manage to stay in work things were not so bad; because of the fall in world prices the cost of living fell by 14.5 per cent, whereas wages had only fallen by about 4.5 per cent.[3] It is against this background that the economic position of the nurse in the 1930s must be seen; the staff nurse, with her £50 to £60 a year after all her living needs had been met, was not as badly off as has sometimes been depicted. At that time women in industry were earning about 30 shillings a week, and Seebohm Rowntree in the *Human Needs of Labour* of 1937 put the 'poverty line' for a single woman living alone at 30s 9d.[4] In 1939 the cost of living was 11 per cent lower than it had been in 1924. In spite of this, Sir John Boyd Orr estimated that about half the population were too poor to afford an adequate diet and about one-third suffered from dietetic deficiences. By these standards nurses were not poor.

The psychological effect of the war, the inflation of 1922 to 1925 with its devastating effect on Germany, the terrible effects of the Depression did much to mould the outlook of people in a 'Waste Land' so poignantly described by Eliot as 'a heap of broken images'. There was a shaking of the old liberal values and a searching for new forms of political philosophy; some looked for more state control and the subordination of the individual to the needs of the state, which, taken to its logical conclusion, led to fascism and national socialism. Others looked to the left, to collectivist societies, for salvation. As Europe drifted into different ideologies the stage was set for renewed conflict and the shadow of expectation of war.

THE NURSES' CHARTER

It was not only the College of Nursing that was pressing for better conditions for nurses and calling for a new 'Charter'; in 1926 Mrs Bedford Fenwick re-entered the fray with her new British College of Nurses of which she was President and Dr Bedford Fenwick the Treasurer. By this organisation she hoped to undermine the College of Nursing, but as a forum for nursing opinion it made little impact and in the end only confused the issue. In the meantime, the upsurge of trade union membership in the 1920s was being reflected in nursing, and some trade unions now wished to include women or at least to have a 'women's section'.[5] Both the National Asylum workers' and the Poor Law workers' trade unions were increasing their membership, particularly in the mental hospitals where there were sporadic strikes in favour of a shorter working week. In 1926 the Labour Party issued a document on nursing; its main proposals followed those of the College of Nursing; namely, a 48-hour week, the separation of training school from the administration of the hospital and student status for probationers (*sic*); the great point of difference was that the Labour Party now advocated that nurses should be organised through the trade union movement. In 1930 Mr Fenner Brockway (later Lord Brockway), without consulting nursing organisations, introduced a Bill to limit nurses' hours to 44 a week and to impose a statutory minimum wage. The Bill received little support from any quarter and the profession itself was not enthusiastic. There had been arguments about a 'minimum wage' for over 150 years. One argument against it was that the 'minimum' tended to become a maximum, and of course from the trade union point of view it limited scope for negotiation; moreover, in his attitude to the 'wage' rate for probationers Mr Brockway seemed to be out of step with the Labour Party document. To most nurses the proposed reduction of hours seemed impractical and indeed many occupations worked similarly long hours, including young doctors. But most important as far as the College of Nursing was concerned was that it was anxious to negotiate salaries and conditions of service itself, deeming this to be a hallmark of a profession, and this was the main cause of rivalry with the unions. The college, however, was in a cleft stick, the majority of its early members being drawn from the general hospitals in the voluntary sector who, as the Depression deepened, were in dire financial straits: too much pressure about better salaries would force them to ask for government grants, and this would mean the end of independence, a spectre that hung like the ghost of Banquo over the teaching hospitals in the 1930s. Whatever their shortcomings, the main voluntary hospitals inspired their alumni with intense loyalty. The other dilemma that the college and other organisations faced was whether to demand the rate for the job for the probationer, and tacitly admit that this was the job she should be doing, or to refuse to ask for a 'wage' and to persist in asking for an 'allowance' in the hope that one day the shadow would become the substance.

What the professions or the unions thought was of little consequence, because as the slump worsened, probationers, far from getting a 'minimum wage', were asked to take a cut in pay. However, Mr Brockway's Bill had interested the proprietors of the *Lancet* who set up an enquiry under the

Earl of Crawford and Balcarres to study the pay and conditions of nurses and to investigate shortages, thus starting a long line of reports on nursing which were to be a feature of the nursing scene for the next 50 years.

The Lancet Commission, 1930–32 reported in 1932 and made a number of suggestions about improvements in nurses' conditions of service and living conditions; the Commissioners suggested that pay should be in accordance with the scales advocated by the College of Nursing – scales which in fact were not implemented until 1941, and, more controversially, that state subsidies be used for the education of nurses. The Report made some harsh comments about unnecessary discipline and petty restrictions suffered by probationers, and, while this was undoubtedly true in some cases, it must be remembered that the sample consisted of only 686 replies, and that questionnaire techniques were poorly developed. Since every hospital was a law unto itself there were enormous variations both in the standard of the nurses' home and the restrictions. Apart from the fact that many personal memories do not accord with the jaundiced view that 'nursing was falling into disfavour as an occupation', there is the solid fact that the numbers entering nursing were rising and the wastage rate of 28 per cent was lower than at the beginning of the century or any time since the Second World War. Between 1921 and 1931 the percentage of single women who were nurses aged 24 to 44 years declined slightly, though this was compensated for by an increase in the number of older nurses – probably due to the intake in the war; but between 1931 and 1951 – there being no census in 1941 – the proportion of single women in the 25–34 age group who were nurses increased from 4 per cent to 6.5 per cent. Moreover, nursing was now claiming more better-educated girls, and nursing was now competing with teaching for girls who had finished their general education between 17 and 19 years.[6]

CRISIS IN THE VOLUNTARY HOSPITALS

After the 1914–18 War, with increasing costs and a fall in donations the voluntary hospitals faced acute financial difficulties. A Committee on Voluntary Hospitals was set up under the chairmanship of Viscount Cave, which recommended an immediate grant of £1 million from the government; only half the amount was received, so every other means of raising money had to be tried. There were a wide variety of fundraising activities, with the Hospital Charity Ball becoming a feature of social life and the pages of the *Tatler*. Patients were now asked to pay towards their costs, and to ease the burden sickness would place on them, a number of funds were established of which the best known was the Hospital Saturday Fund; this fund had started as a workman's insurance scheme in 1870 but now changed its character and its membership. In return for regular contributions subscribers were assured of free, or at least reduced cost for, treatment in hospital. This gave the hospital a steady income rather in the way the old 'ticket system' had done, but it raised the vexed question of payment for doctors, for if the hospitals were charging for medical treatment why should some of this not be paid to the doctors? Some hospitals did pay their doctors and, as Abel-Smith points out, 'slowly the voluntary hospitals were ceasing to be voluntary and the doctors ceasing to be honorary'.

Just as free out-patient treatment had imperilled the income of general practitioners in the past, now 'free' in-patient treatment through the agency of insurance was depriving them of middle-class patients who tended to seek treatment at hospitals, and some doctors resented the insurance schemes. Another means of increasing the hospital income was by the increase in private patient accommodation, and many teaching hospitals built special 'wings', but with the virtual disappearance of servants and with smaller families the demand for private care was greater than the supply, and private nursing homes, good, bad and frankly dangerous, grew up without control. A few were purpose-built, but most were in private houses and frequently, in spite of the Registration of Nurses Act, most of the staff were untrained. The College of Nursing, concerned about the exploitation of the public and the undermining of the profession and its good name, presented a Bill to Parliament seeking the registration and inspection of nursing homes; the British Medical Association said that they were 'not aware of any abuses', but the Society of Medical Officers of Health were, and in 1927 the Registration of Nursing Homes Act was passed. This was a milestone in nursing history because it showed that a nursing organisation with a well-prepared case could change legislation in the face of considerable opposition and vested interest.

The voluntary system was expanding on another front. A matter of contention between the medical profession and the hospitals had long been that the general practitioners had no access to hospital beds. There had in fact grown up two classes of doctors – the hospital doctors, the purveyors of the new technology, and the others who, because of their exclusion from the world of drama and science, were somehow seen as lower in the medical hierarchy. Now general practitioners with the aid of local philanthropy and parochial fund-raising began to found their own hospitals. A few such hospitals had been in existence for some time, but the inter-war years saw a great expansion of this type of hospital so that when the National Health Service came into being there were over 1,500 hospitals with less than 100 beds and over half of these had less than 50 beds.[7] Like the voluntary hospitals, their growth was uncoordinated and unplanned; establishment depended not on the health needs of the community but on local pride or a fortuitous legacy. The facilities provided varied and the staff more so; in 1948 it was not unusual to find a hospital of 20 beds with an operating theatre, dealing with medical, surgical and maternity cases who might well include children and terminal cases and a few beds for 'private patients', where often the main nursing staff was made up of cadet nurses.

THE SANKEY COMMISSION

Not least of the problems of the voluntary hospitals was that they lacked any central organisation. The British Hospitals Association founded in 1884, was by no means universally supported, and at times it conflicted with the King's Fund, although both had aims in common. The King's Fund was originally the Prince of Wales Hospital Fund for London, which had been set up in 1896 to celebrate the Diamond Jubilee and which the Prince of Wales made his chosen field for charitable work. On his accession in 1901 the Fund was renamed, and the capital subscribed was used to encourage efficiency in hospital management, accounting and planning. The King's Fund was prestigious but was not always in accord with the Royal Colleges which tended to act as a forum for the teaching hospitals. In 1935 the Hospitals' Association, sensing the growing danger to the future of the voluntary system, resolved that an enquiry be set up under the chairmanship of Viscount John Sankey, now a member of the Cabinet. The Sankey Report is of significance because it influenced the Athlone Committee on nursing which had far-reaching repercussions, and also because in many ways it was seminal to the wartime organisation of civilian hospitals and hence to the National Health Service. The Commission recognised that the two hospital systems would have to exist for some time, the voluntary and the municipal, and that the voluntary system should be prepared to receive grants from the government; in particular 'the state should contribute to the treatment of the poor and to the education of doctors and nurses'.[8] In order to overcome the planning and co-ordination problem it recommended that no further specialist hospitals be built and that all hospitals should be grouped. Control should be by a Central Council with Regional Councils appointed by the hospitals in the designated Regions who would be responsible for the grouping and grading of the hospitals. In order to rationalise the beds and facilities, each group should hold some of its funds in common. Although it had not been worked out in detail the Sankey Commission had produced an exemplar for the structure of the National Health Service: a concept far from its thoughts.

The British Medical Association discussed the report and produced counter-suggestions at its meeting in 1938, one of which was the possibility of a whole time medical service; the resolution was lost but the idea had considerable support. In the light of events 10 years later this meeting is worth recalling, and it belies the theory that wars invariably produce a clamour for more radical measures.

CHANGES IN THE POOR LAW SYSTEM

The Ministry of Health Act of 1919 transferred the duties of the Local Government Board, the National Insurance Commission, the powers of the Board of Education in relation to health, and the responsibility for the Midwives Act to the Ministry of Health. From the start the ministry's duties were multifarious, though it could be argued that they were all interrelated, and all of them, including housing, impinged on health, an argument which accounts for the many vicissitudes through which this ministry, and later 'department', was to pass. Most of these duties were devolved to the counties and county boroughs on whom post-war measures like the Maternity and Child Welfare Act of 1918 placed new responsibilities, and there was an expansion of the duties of the medical officer of health in the field of personal health. During this period the more progressive authorities were improving their purpose-built hospitals, and were now employing consultants, training nurses and catering for a different type of patient. This made a mockery of the old 'workhouse test', and as the anomalies grew a commission was set up to investigate the function of local government and to make recommendations for its reorganisation.

The new Unemployment Act was being operated through the 'approved insurance' scheme, and the government was anxious to avoid confusing this with the deterring agency of the Poor Law, and to this end Neville Chamberlain, now Minister of Health, included the reform of the Poor Law in his Local Government Act of 1929. This important Act handed over the power of the old Boards of Guardians to the local authorities, which were urged to set up Public Assistance Committees, known as PACs, for the relief of destitution, and the local authorities were urged to allocate to their various committees all Poor Law functions not concerned with the able-bodied. These included the old Poor Law responsibility for welfare, health, the disabled, the orphans and pauper child care; thus it was hoped that some of the recommendations of the 1909 Minority Report would at last be put into effect. But before the new service could be implemented it was necessary for authorities to make a declaration of intent to acquire buildings. It was *not* mandatory for every institution to be appropriated, and while most urban authorities transferred all buildings containing sick persons to their Public Health Committees, rural authorities were often tardy and a number of 'mixed workhouses' were left behind to be administered by the PACs in a manner which appeared to be a continuation of the Poor Law. This is why it is true to say that the last vestiges of the Poor Law were not swept away until the National Health Service Act.

The central issue of the inter-war years was undoubtedly unemployment, and it was not until the end of the period when the theories of George Maynard Keynes (1883–1946) were accepted, which encouraged the government to intervene in regulating the economy by a programme of public investment, and there was an increase in spending power and thus a boost of trade which eventually got people back to work. Throughout the period, unemployment never fell below 10 per cent, and as in the nineteenth century it was the harbinger of sickness, and in spite of improvements in the public health services, in 1931 there were still 992 deaths per million population from tuberculosis – a purely preventable disease.

The new PACs were regarded as the old Poor Law writ large, and in 1930 when the 'dole' was cut the government resigned. The new National Government set up an enquiry which recommended that the insurance scheme be separated from the relief of destitution; the Unemployment Act of 1934 extended compulsory insurance coverage and restored the cuts in benefits, which were then to be administered by an independent statutory committee. The second part of the Act dealt with the large numbers who were not entitled to insurance and who were now to be the responsibility of the new Unemployment Assistance Board, the 'UCB', which would dispense relief on a national scale from Treasury funds, but when it was discovered that the old PACs were giving more generous relief the Poor Law suddenly became popular. Eventually, the PACs shed their responsibility for outdoor relief and remained as a 'last resort and refuge' for a considerable group of chronic sick still being maintained in the old workhouses, and finally handed to the care of the National Health Service.

However, the local authorities now had control of 180,000 hospital beds, almost all the preventive services and the welfare services, and as the public system continued to improve and classify its hospitals it became a challenge to the voluntary system which it now in many respects closely resembled. This resemblance, and the fact that people were beginning to ask whether there was a need for two systems and whether all hospitals could not be based on the local authorities as the Minority Report had suggested, was the driving force behind the Sankey Commission.

THE INTERDEPARTMENTAL COMMITTEE ON NURSING

In spite of the fact that high unemployment and lack of alternative careers for girls made it easier to recruit nurses, the wastage rate remained between 28 and 32 per cent, and although hospitals were employing 20,000 more nursing staff than in 1933, hospitals were reporting shortages, an indication of the increasing demands for care and the shorter hours[9] – and some might think suggested the wrong use of nurses. In 1937, the London County Council, with a total of 6,727 posts, had 355 vacancies, and in three years the *Nursing Times* increased its advertisements from 6,429 to 17,119.[10] Pressure from the profession, concern about shortages and wastage and the continuing debate about how nurses should be trained led the government to set up a committee on the nursing services under the chairmanship of Lord Athlone. Set up in 1937, the committee was disbanded at the beginning of the war, but because of the urgency of the situation an interim report was published in December 1938. The main difficulty facing the committee was the same as confronted the Lancet Commission – namely, the lack of statistical data on which to base recommendations. In order to rectify this position the committee set out to collect its own evidence, and though the task was never completed Professor Abel-Smith has traced the ledgers at the Ministry of Health and has pieced together the information that survives, which has given us an invaluable estimate of the state of nursing and the different categories employed at the outbreak of war.[11] It is estimated that in 1938 there were:

46,700   trained nurses and midwives ⎫
43,000   student nurses and 'pupils'   ⎬ a total of 113,700
24,000   'other nursing staff'   ⎭

It is by no means certain what these figures included and they should be used with caution. For example, were students doing a fourth year recorded as students or staff nurses? The only other known fact is that in March 1938 there were 89,254 names on the General Nursing Council's Register, and although in those days it was a 'live' register in as much as a fee was paid yearly, it gave no indication of whether these nurses were employed or in what capacity.

The Athlone Committee made certain recommendations to improve the staffing position and to encourage nurses to stay in the profession. These are important because they were ready to hand during the crisis of wartime. Some were implemented and became the foundation of future policy and have remained ever since. However, far-seeing as they were at the time, it is doubtful if the cautious proposals of 1938 were really sufficient to meet the changed post-war needs. Moreover, only the proposals with immediate relevance to the war situation were adopted; those dealing with nursing education were quietly forgotten. Among the main, and at that time highly controversial, recommendations was the setting up of a Nurses' Salaries Committee on the lines of the Burnham Committee for teachers. Other proposals included increasing hospital staff to relieve nurses of non-nursing duties, organising part of nurse training under general education and the recognition of the 'assistant nurse' who was to be on an official 'Roll' with the General Nursing Council. The reaction to the Report was muted; by 1939 England was under the shadow of war, and as Hitler occupied Prague in March and there was alarm from Danzig and Memel, there was little enthusiasm for changing the status of the 'assistant' nurse.

THE END OF AN EPOCH

The first 40 years of the century saw a great social change, especially in the desire for more democracy, equality and emancipation from the old restraints. Some of these trends were present before 1914, and indeed the conflicts they raised were part of the cause of the war, for although the 'occasion' may have been the shooting of the Archduke Ferdinand at Sarajevo, the real cause lay in the disintegration of the old structure of society. The war accelerated these changes, and the post-war reconstruction measures were an attempt to meet new demands; most of these measures failed to meet their objectives because of the lack of capital due to the slump and the crushing unemployment, which was itself a contributory factor to the Second World War, especially in the rise of national socialism. In one sense the Second World War was bound up with the consequences of the First, and many of the gains made in 1919 had to be won all over again in 1945.

Nevertheless, gains were made; because of the fall in the cost of living many people's standard of living improved; in fact, anyone who was in work was better off by 1939; the stock of the nation's houses improved, more people lived in suburbs, education had improved and children were better cared for. It was this, together with a better public health system, rather than advances in medical knowledge or more hospitals, that was instrumental in the continued lowering of the mortality and morbidity rates.

REFERENCES

1 *The Registrar General's Returns* (1960) London: HMSO.
2 Andreski, S. L. (1968) *Military Organisation and Society*, 2nd edn, London: Routledge & Kegan Paul.
3 Cole, G. D. H. and Postgate, R. (1961 edn), *The Common People*, London: University Paperbacks, Methuen, p. 64.
4 Rowntree, B. S. (1937) *The Human Needs of Labour*, London: Longman.
5 Davies, Ross (1975) *Women and Work*, London: Hutchinson, ch. 1.
6 Abel-Smith, B. (1960) *A History of the Nursing Profession*, London: William Heinemann, pp. 263–7, tables 12, 15.
7 *The Hospital Year Book*, 1951 count of hospitals, made by author, Institute of Hospital Administrators.
8 *Report of the Sankey Commission*, London: HMSO, p. 30.
9 *The Interdepartmental Committee on Nursing* (1938) London: HMSO.
10 Ibid.
11 Abel-Smith, *History*, Appendix I, i.

FURTHER READING

Mowatt, C. L. (1955) *Britain Between the Wars, 1918–1940*, London: Methuen.
Orwell, G. (1968) *Collected Essays, Journalism and Letters*, London: Secker & Warburg, see also *The Road to Wigan Pier* (1937).
Webster, C. (ed.) (1993) *Caring for Health: History and Diversity*, Milton Keynes: Open University.

Chapter 14

The legacy of the Second World War

> War and Revolution never produce what is wanted but only some mixture of the old evils with new ones; what is wanted is a peaceful and rational solution of the problems and situations – but that required great statesmanship and great popular sense and virtue.
>
> William Graham Sumner, *War and Other Essays* (1911)

When it comes to change war is the sorcerer's apprentice, and once released from the peacetime pot the genii are reluctant to return, but as Sumner points out, change produced as the result of crisis is often not the best long-term solution. In 1938, the Sankey Commission had suggested a compromise plan for the hospitals, but before the ink was dry people were urging more radical proposals. The *Lancet* was arguing that the medical services would have to be divorced from the insurance system and run like any other public service, and some medical spokesmen were advocating a salaried service. The Athlone Committee, which followed much of the Sankey Commission's thinking, had proposed there should be government grants for nursing education even though this might affect the independent status of the voluntary hospitals. By 1939 pressure was being put on the government to find a different method of financing nurse training, but disagreement in the profession and the advent of war saved the government the necessity of making a decision.

Perhaps, as Angus Calder suggests, the effect of war is not to sweep society on to a new course, 'but to hasten its progress along old grooves'.[1] This certainly seems true of nursing and the Second World War: instead of a new approach to nurse training and a rational assessment of nursing manpower to meet the changed health needs of the population, change as the result of war was piecemeal and pragmatic – each measure was conceded almost in desperation as the result of wartime pressure. True, there was the recognition of the 'assistant' nurse and the auxiliary force, but these were old grooves with an official face. The Nurses' Salaries Committee was a step forward, but because the scale started in wartime conditions and covered a conglomerate nursing force this led to problems later. Even the establishment of a Division of Nursing – usually regarded as a wartime success – could conceivably have been achieved without the aid of total war. Wartime atmosphere is not conducive to long-term planning, for in the dark days of 1941 it seemed possible that there might not be a long term. Nevertheless, it was the wartime legacy that formed the launching pad for the nursing service that had to meet the increased post-war demands of the National Health Service.

THE 1939–45 WAR: PHASE 1

The outbreak of war – meeting the needs

As long ago as 1927 the question of providing nurses in time of war had been considered and a Committee of Imperial Defence set up. In October 1937, during the crisis over the Austrian Anschluss, the committee was reconstructed under the chairmanship of Sir Arthur MacNalty, Chief Medical Officer of Health, and an Emergency Nursing Committee formed which invited the Royal College of Nursing, the Red Cross Society and the Order of St John to undertake the impossible task of compiling a register of assistant nurses and nursing auxiliaries. It was thought that the first weeks of war might involve massive aerial bombardment, and it was estimated that 67,000 nurses would be needed for First Aid Posts alone.[2] The armed services, then employing fewer than 1,000 trained nurses, said they needed at least 5,000. Clearly the target was unrealistic unless recruitment was increased sharply, or the service diluted with untrained staff, and/or drastic cuts made in the number of nurses employed in civilian hospitals. The endeavour to meet the target by *all three means* was to have important consequences in the future. Fortunately, bombardment, when it came, was less fearful than the prophecy, with the first severe test coming in September 1940 when London and the ports were badly bombed, but the highest daily average for casualties never rose above 7,380, a figure well below the estimates.[3]

The Emergency Hospital Service

In 1938 an Emergency Hospital Service was set up. The country was divided into Sectors, each with a 'Sector Matron' and administrative staff based on a teaching hospital – an idea that stemmed from the Sankey report, with the 'Sectors' as the forerunners of the original 'Regions' of the National Health Service. Urban hospitals were encouraged to discharge their patients, to evacuate others to rural areas and to cut their nursing staff by half, for it was assumed that, faced with a national emergency, many civilian patients would opt to go home. Large numbers of patients were discharged from sanatoria to make way for the casualties that never came – a policy that contributed to the increase in tuberculosis during the later war years.

The Emergency Nursing Committee was given the task of organising a Civil Nursing Reserve whose purpose was:

> To assist employing authorities to meet additional staffing *occasioned by the war*. Members were allocated to hospitals, First Aid Posts, evacuation trains, wartime nurseries and the district nursing service in reception areas and elsewhere.[4]

An appeal was made to all who had nursing experience, and by September 1939 7,000 trained nurses, 3,000 assistant nurses and about 20,000 auxiliaries had come forward. The Reserve, which throughout the war supplied upwards of 18,000 nursing staff, unwittingly played an important part in the development of nursing, for in setting up the Reserve the Ministry of Health had, unwillingly and unintentionally, become a direct employer of nurses. Furthermore, the Reserve consisted of large numbers of assistant nurses for whom there was no definition and no standard of training, and because of the lack of any manpower data at the Ministry there was no means of finding the potential strength of such a force. The Ministry of Health had therefore a vested interest in the resolution of the conflict in the nursing profession about a second grade of trained nurse. Moreover, to complicate matters, there was now a third grade: those who had received no training and who for convenience were called 'auxiliaries'.

In fact, pre-war hospitals had employed a wide range of auxiliary labour under an even wider range of titles; the tasks they did varied from the mainly nursing to the mainly domestic. Who did what depended not on suitability but on availability. However, within their own setting hospital authorities and wise ward sisters could, and did, exercise discretion over the allocation of tasks. Now there was little chance of discretion: a heterogeneous task force of 20,000 was registered with the Reserve ready to be sent to hospitals according to the category of registration. At the same time, because of the lack of activity in the early part of the war, members of the Reserve soon found themselves with little to do and were bored. Some hospitals had more staff than patients, while the ordinary staff in civilian hospitals had to close wards because of lack of staff.

The Reserve presented other problems. It had been hastily put together and it was not a cohesive force; many of the early recruits were unsuitable and added to the burdens of those who supervised them. Then there was the fact that the part-time members were generally tied to one place because of domestic commitments, and this added to the administrative difficulties. But on the other hand, the full-time members were partly paid by the Ministry and often received higher salaries than the permanent staff – a fact which hardly increased the popularity of the Reserve. As in the

First World War, when the Red Cross had the task of sorting out the embittered relationships between the Voluntary Aid Detachments and the regular trained nurses, so, in the Second World War, the lot fell to the Civil Nursing Reserve Advisory Council to find ways of healing the rift between the Reserve and the permanent service.

In the meantime the assumption that the needs of the civilian population could be subordinated to the emergency services for ever was being proved false. Many authorities reported a breakdown in the services and the Ministry received pitiable complaints about the hardships being suffered by the civilian population now largely deprived of a hospital service, which even before the war often seemed inadequate, and now, in some places, seemed non-existent. The need for nurses in the tuberculosis service was urgent; the Reserve might have helped but they were precluded because they were appointed to the 'emergency services'. The government now had to face the harsh reality, for the incidence of tuberculosis epitomised the problems facing the health and social services. In wartime civilian health needs did not just fade away, indeed, wartime conditions might exacerbate the need.

There were only two ways of dealing with the situation: one was to extend the area of government control; the other was by exhortation and added incentive to increase direct recruitment. But to add to the difficulties, during the winter of 1941–42 the country faced its first period of heavy bombing, and nurses were needed for the emergency services in greater numbers. Now the government, urged on by the professional nursing organisations, looked at the report of the Athlone Committee to see if any of the recommendations would help with recruitment. Meanwhile, a number of short-term measures were taken, measures that would have long-term effects. First, the function of the Reserve was extended and members were encouraged to volunteer for tuberculosis and mental nursing, which meant that the government was the part employer of *some* nurses in *all* types of hospitals. Second, in April 1941, the Ministry of Labour set up a Register for Women for National Service. If nurses were to be recruited by this means, then salaries had to be improved and a new scale offered to all recruits who came through the Ministry of Labour's nursing officers. There was now covert direction of labour and a mass of anomalies in the pay structure. However, the Ministry of Health was reluctant to solve the problem by implementing the recommendation of the Athlone Committee that there should be a National Salary Committee, preferring, as the government spokesman put it, 'to wait until the emergency was over'. The main reason for the reluctance was that the Beveridge Committee was sitting; a negotiated national scale for nurses presupposed the government as the future employer and a National Health Service, but it was not for the Ministry of Health to make this inevitable.

However, albeit unwillingly, the government was the largest employer of nurses and it could not afford the odium of recruiting exploited labour.

Therefore, in 1941 it recommended that *all* hospitals pay a scale equivalent to that paid to the Reserve. Not surprisingly, the hospitals asked to be reimbursed and the government agreed to meet part of the difference. It was now obvious that the hospitals could never return to the *status quo ante*, and in order to assist the government in its new role as an employer of nurses another recommendation of the Athlone Committee was implemented: a Division of Nursing was created at the Ministry of Health with Katherine Watt, later Dame Katherine, the first Chief Nursing Officer. The reforms recommended to meet the peacetime needs of 1938 were being accepted – piecemeal by *force majeure* – in wartime.

THE WAR – PHASE 2

In June 1941, as far as it is possible to ascertain from incomplete returns, there were about 89,000 nursing staff in the hospitals of England and Wales.[5] In the next two years, as the result of publicity and the Registration of Employment Order the numbers increased to about 93,000, but the increase was largely due to the recruitment of student nurses and increases in the numbers of assistant nurses and auxiliaries. The number of permanent trained staff remained static throughout the war at 23,000 – 24,000, a fact to be borne in mind when looking at the post-war difficulties. By 1942 the numbers in the Reserve had fallen due to better selection and the need for fewer nurses in First Aid Posts. The war did not produce a flood of recruits; they came, but more often than not they did not stay. Between 1941 and 1943 the number of vacancies remained more or less static, and of the 11,000 student nurses who qualified only *400 entered permanent hospital employment*. Nurses were still free to choose employment and they did not choose civilian hospitals. After joint discussions between the Ministries of Labour and Health an attack was planned on two fronts: attempts were to be made to control the movement of nurses and steps were to be taken to improve salaries and conditions of service.

The Report of the Nurses' Salaries Committee, 1943

This committee was set up in February 1943 under the chairmanship of Lord Rushcliffe, with a similar committee in Scotland under Professor Taylor. During its early deliberations the committee, which consisted of representatives from nursing organisations and employers, decided to widen their scope and cover not only the salaries of trained nurses and those in training, but also conditions of service and related matters, and at the same time include recommendations about salaries for assistant nurses and auxiliaries. Thus the Rushcliffe Committee became the starting point for negotiations, and for the first Nurses and Midwives Whitley Council in 1948 (see Chapter 16); the pattern set in wartime did not alter materially for a quarter of a century. Besides recommending scales for all grades[6] the Rushcliffe Committee proposed that the working fortnight be reduced to 96 hours, continuous night duty should not exceed three months for student nurses and six months for trained staff, and all nurses should be entitled to 28 days' holiday a year and one duty-free day a week, with sick pay graded according to length of service. For the higher grades salaries were paid according to the number of beds, a yardstick to be followed, *faute de mieux*, for the next 30 years.

The immediate result of these recommendations was that the economic position of the nurse was improved; when she was trained the nurse was now in a position comparable with teaching.[7] However, the vexed question of student status was left unanswered and the resolution of the problem made more intractable by the inclusion of the student nurse in the salary scales. This sudden economic improvement, some nurses doubling their salaries, made almost no difference to the recruitment figures, although it is possible that it had an influence on retention in the profession, but that is something impossible to measure.

The Nurses' Act 1943

There were two overriding reasons for this Act. First, the wide range of definitions made it impossible to calculate the potential of the assistant nurse. Second, the Rushcliffe Committee had laid down a scale of pay and it had to be decided who should qualify for this scale; the definition agreed by the profession was that nurses in *bona fide* practice should be allowed to apply to the General Nursing Council for 'enrolment'. By this Act, which to a large extent regularised existing practice, the enrolled assistant nurse now became subject to a professional code of behaviour and to the discipline of the General Nursing Council, and the Ministry of Health was empowered to restrict the title 'nurse' to those with recognised training and experience; a restriction it did not apply to its own presentation of nursing statistics (Chapter 18).

In spite of these measures there was still a failure to meet the needs of the civilian population, standards were falling and some patients were suffering hardship. Now the alarm bells sounded in another quarter – midwifery. After the fall in the birth rate at the beginning of the war it was now rising and in 1944 it was 17.7 per 1,000, the highest rate since the 1920s. There was no lack of recruits to train – the trouble lay in the few who wished to practise. Nurses regarded the certificate as the pass-port to promotion or to nursing abroad, and therefore the continual stream of pupils masked the true position. In order to encourage retention in midwifery, salary improvements were offered, but after the experience with the Rushcliffe award few believed that economic inducements would keep pupils tied to midwifery; the only solution lay in control and compulsion, a task that was given to The National Advisory Committee for the Recruitment and Distribution of Nurses and Midwives.

The idea of direction of nurses was distasteful and likely to be resisted; moreover, direction could be self-defeating since a dissatisfied service would be detrimental to voluntary recruitment, and in the end the Committee agreed on compromise measures:

1 *The control of nurses into the armed services.* There were now over 9,000 qualified nurses in the services of the Crown, and there were sharp exchanges between the Ministry of Health and the Directors of Medical Services about the level of requirements necessary to the armed services. In fairness to the services of the Crown, the personnel in the three services had increased tenfold and the war was being prosecuted on fronts all over the world. Eventually it was agreed, although not without acrimony, that certain categories should no longer be permitted to join the services.

2 *The registration of nurses and midwives, April 1943.* Under this order all nurses had to register, and if they were not employed they were urged to take a post in a shortage area. Strangely enough, hospitals for the chronic sick were not on the priority list, partly because it was thought that they could get by without public outcry, but more probably because it was tacitly agreed that exhortation was unlikely to persuade anyone to undertake this nursing without a sense of vocation. Indeed, this was the dilemma, the horns of which were the need for numbers, but the uselessness of numbers without proper motivation.

3 *The control of engagement order, September 1943.* This order, which applied to all women between 18 and 40 years of age was now applied to nurses and midwives. Employment had to be through the Ministry of Labour and nurses could only give up their posts in order to do further training; without this intention they were regarded as available for work in a shortage area and directed accordingly. In practice, few nurses were actually directed but the order had the effect, not surprisingly, of increasing the number of pupil midwives, since nurses with one eye on their professional prospects deemed a midwifery certificate of greater value than a spell in a sanatorium. As far as pairs of hands were concerned, the position in midwifery improved, but the ratio of trained to untrained was again adversely altered.

4 *Direction of labour, April 1944.* In spite of these measures the winter of 1943 was critical, and it was decided to direct nurses to priority areas. There was now not only control of engagement but also direction of labour; for the first time in history civilian nurses could be directed to posts not of their choosing. However, before the measure could be effective the course of the war had changed; in the summer of 1944 the second front was opened and the Emergency Service hospitals in the

south of England and the armed services were in dire need of nurses for casualties. In the end compulsory transfer was not effective, and in spite of propaganda it was clear that recruits were for the duration only. In 1945, with peace, the numbers in the uncontrolled groups of assistant nurses and auxiliaries fell sharply: it was said that there was an 'encouraging rise in the number of trained nurses', but of course this was due to the fact that student nurses recruited in the enthusiasm of earlier years, or to avoid some other form of war service, were now qualified and therefore controlled. Once the controls were taken off in 1946 the numbers declined (see Chapter 15). This produced a bitter inheritance for the National Health Service. War had not produced the solution that was wanted.

THE CONSEQUENCES OF WAR ON NURSING

War is a test of institutions. The inadequacies of the pre-war health and nursing services were aggravated by the strains of war, and, although there was no dramatic breakdown, the standard of care to the civilian population fell, especially to groups with little power to complain. The reasons for this decline in care were partly due to the increased demands made on the services, but more significantly, because in forecasting the needs too much emphasis had been placed on the emergency services, and the erratic ebb and flow of the war made manpower adjustment difficult. But above all, the Second World War, unlike the First, did not attract large numbers of recruits who would remain as part of the permanent nursing force. At the end of the First World War nursing was apparently so popular that people feared nurses would be unemployed. At the end of the Second World War 30,000 beds had to be closed because of lack of nursing staff.

The causes of the situation at the end of the Second World War were complex and largely bound up with the position of women and the social and economic changes of the previous decade. Because of unemployment and entrenched attitudes in labour relations, women had to win the rights they had won in the First World War all over again, but now they won them in much wider fields, not least of which was their participation in the armed services as a whole, and this opened up an enormous range of career possibilities for women, who, unlike their predecessors in 1914, had two decades of compulsory secondary education behind them. However, some of the wounds were self-inflicted. In the desire to get recruits at any cost selection was sacrificed and the age of entry was lowered, and this in turn caused frustration and irritation to the trained staff so that a kind of Gresham's law began to operate with the bad driving out the good. Moreover, recruitment was mainly to the ranks of students and auxiliaries so that the ratio of trained to untrained began to deteriorate, setting a pattern that was never reversed. Insufficient support and supervision and the movement and the exigencies of war had a deleterious effect on training, and many students felt their preparation inadequate. But the continual shortage of nurses meant that those who did stay and qualify were rapidly promoted to positions of responsibility for which they were ill-prepared, and all too often this gave them a sense of insecurity which could be passed on to the next generation. The wartime appeals by the Royal College of Nursing for further training for ward sisters fell on deaf ears, and the post of staff nurse was no longer one that was coveted.

Nevertheless, the war brought some benefits and the government acted on parts of the Athlone Report and there were improvements in salaries. Whether these would have come without the impetus of war is debatable; the chances are that the evolution of the health services and the demands for higher standards would have compelled action. 'What might have been is an abstraction', said Eliot, 'remaining a perpetual possibility.'[8] Some action really only dealt with the problems that the war itself had raised; for example, the cost of living rose by 41 per cent during the war so that the gains made by the Rushcliffe scale were hardly spectacular and it is doubtful if the staff nurse at the end of the war was as well off as the staff nurse in the 1930s. The war did nothing to solve the long-term problems of nursing, particularly the question of nurse training; in fact, it made them more intractable because even more reliance was placed on apprentice labour. The solving of these questions, said the government spokesman, 'must be left for calmer days'. Calmer days had gone forever.

However, it is salutary to compare the fate of the armed services with civilian hospitals. There was no difficulty in attracting nurses to the three services of the Crown: they could afford to be selective and often had long waiting lists. Yet the pay was as poor as in civilian hospitals and the conditions often much worse; discipline was strict and authority hierarchial, life laced with restrictions, and enforced posting – that condition the government longed to impose on the Civil Nursing Reserve – an accepted way of life. Setting aside the superficial answer that young women were attracted to a male world with all the possibilities of excitement in forward casualty areas – an illusory notion if ever there was one, for many spent their time nursing 'service families' in peaceful backwaters – there were other and more subtle reasons for this attraction. First, it is axiomatic that people strive to enter selective groups rather than unselective – and the longer the waiting list the greater the attraction. Secondly, the armed nursing services offered a cohesive corps with a tradition and a distinctive and becoming uniform, together with a status that was all too sadly lacking in the Civil Nursing Reserve. In the early years the nursing services of the Crown were comparatively small; before the war the Princess Mary Royal Air Force Nursing Service had only 80 sisters, and even when it expanded it had a cohesiveness and an *esprit de corps* that is given by a well-integrated institution. Perhaps recruits were seeking that sense of identity and 'belonging' that had once been given by their training hospital. Nor could status have been the only attraction, for male nurses fared less well than their women colleagues in this respect; this was largely due to the importance the services attached to the effect of women trained nurses in forward areas on the morale of the troops, and these nurses were therefore protected with officer status, a privilege many male nurses did not enjoy. Notwithstanding this, the services attracted a number of male nurses and this was one of the reasons for the fall in the numbers of nursing staff in mental hospitals. Again, the services could be selective, and many men returned from the forces to take positions of increased responsibility in civilian hospitals while the Reserve contributed comparatively few. In that montage of memories, sometimes rose-coloured, there is often a loyalty to 'service days' that somehow the Civil Reserve never inspired.

The effects of the Second World War compared with the First

The effects of war on nursing are complex and in need of more detailed study: why, for example, did two world wars have such different consequences for nursing? One obvious reason is that the two wars had quite different effects on the population profile. After the 1914–18 war the population balance was so changed that there was a considerable group of women who would never marry (see Chapter 12). At the same time the post-war depression made it necessary for more women to seek employment, and apart from necessity, the new status of women made more want independent careers. But there was little choice of careers and women were notoriously disadvantaged in both the educational and trade union world, so nursing, made respectable for half a century and its reputation enhanced by the war, was an obvious candidate.

The Second World War did not have the same demographic effect; the population balance was not altered except that the number of spinsters fell with the marriage rate increasing. Unlike the 1920s, after the Second World War, thanks to Keynesian policies and institutions like the World Bank, there was full, indeed over-full, employment. There were now an increasing number of occupations open to women, many of which offered better career prospects and status than did nursing. Moreover, the constant publicity about shortages, the lowering of the standard of entry, and the lack of an educational basis for training hardly enhanced the image of nursing.

However, there may have been another and more subtle reason accounting for the difference in the attitude to nursing. Was there some inherent factor in the nature of the casualties and in the state of medicine which attracted women to nursing in the First World War? Between 1914 and 1918 9 per cent of all men under the age of 45 were wounded or killed.[9] Of the 1.6 million wounded there were many for whom medical science could do little, but nursing could comfort always. In the absence of powerful drugs or advanced surgery, nursing was important and manifestly seen to be so. No matter the hardship, the nurses in Flanders knew that they were alleviating suffering; it was an intensely personal, if terrible, service.

In the Second World War, technology changed the nature of war and medical knowledge the nature of nursing. Aerial bombardment meant that the civilian population suffered often as much as the armed services, but in spite of the force of the explosives the number of casualties was in fact comparatively small. The greatest needs of the civilian population were not so much medical as social: the evacuation of children, marital breakdown, homelessness, hopelessness in the face of destruction, the plight of the elderly and the disabled all called for social rather than medical care. Even those nurses who helped with the terrible aftermath of war in Europe found that the skills they needed were those of a health visitor or social worker. Many nurses adapted because nurses are remarkably adaptable, but they were not the skills for which they were trained or that attracted people to nursing. Moreover, there were an increasing number of social workers specifically trained to supply the social needs of the community now often recruited from groups who would formerly have found an outlet in nursing. The ordinary medical needs of the community were still there but they had been relegated to make way for the emergency service which was under-used; there was shortage that begat shortage, with a sense of being lowly regarded in one, and boredom in the other.

In the armed services 369,267 were wounded and nearly as many killed; the ratio of wounded to killed was much lower than in the First World War; technology was such that death was more likely than wounds. The living conditions of the troops were better and medical casualties fewer. Inventions that had been on hand before the war were speedily put into use, and powerful drugs and advances in surgery changed the personal aspect of nursing; penicillin ousted poulticing and the ever-increasing spectrum of antibiotics revolutionised medical nursing. War led to all kinds of experimentation and the cutting of corners, some of which paid off, like early ambulation or saline baths for burns. Centres for plastic surgery were established, so that the nursing of burns was transformed, and in the orthopaedic wards the one-time rows of bedfast patients gave way to patients in 'hospital blue', hopping or wheeling themselves between physiotherapy and occupational therapy with the ward looking like a light industry workshop. Nursing was important, but there were times when it was not manifestly seen to be so.

Did nurses expect to nurse as in the First World War, and were they disillusioned? Within a decade the whole nature of nursing had changed. The personal service of providing relief and comfort was giving way to new technology and a multiplicity of other workers; the nurse it seemed was being ousted from her position of being the one person on whom the patient largely depended. There was alarm that nursing was losing its ineffable attraction; there were many debates within the profession on the future role of the nurse, for there was, it seemed, a need for a new sense of direction. That within a quarter of a century the health needs of the population would change and the wheel would come full circle so that nurses would again be needed for those for whom medical science and the new technology could do little was only dimly discerned at the time.

REFERENCES

1 Calder, A. (1969) *The People's War*, London: Cape, p. 17.
2 *Report of the Emergency Committee* (1938), London: HMSO.
3 *On the State of Public Health During Six Years of War* (1948), London: HMSO (tables of civilian casualties).
4 Ibid.
5 Titmuss, R. (1950) *Problems of Social Policy. the Emergency Medical Service*, London: HMSO and Longmans.
6 *Rushcliffe Committee Salaries Committee* (1943), London: HMSO:
   Students (1st year) £115 (emoluments valued at £75) net £40 pa;
   Students (3rd year) £125 (emoluments valued at £75) net £50 pa;
   Ward sisters £230–£300 (emoluments valued at £100) net £130–200.
7 Titmuss, R. *Problems of Social Policy*.
8 Eliot, T. S. (1959) *Four Quartets*, 'Burnt Norton', London: Faber & Faber.
9 Marwick, A. (1965) *The Deluge*, London: Macmillan, p. 290.

FURTHER READING

Ferguson, S. M. and Fitzgerald, H. (1954) *Studies in Social Services*, London: Longmans, (Second World War).
Titmuss, R. (1950) *The Problems of Social Policy* (History of Second World War – UK civil administration), London: HMSO and Longmans.
Women's Group on Public Welfare (1943) *Our Towns: Report of the Hygiene Committee*, Oxford: Oxford University Press.

Chapter 15

The National Health Service

> The report embodies a whole series of proposals, which would amount to setting on foot a systematic crusade against the very occurrence of destitution caused by Unemployment, the destitution caused by Old Age, the destitution caused by Ill Health and Disease and the destitution caused by Neglected Infancy and Neglected Childhood.
>
> Sidney and Beatrice Webb on 'The Minority Report of the Royal Commission on the Poor Law' (1910)

The 1942 idea of universal provision against the main causes of destitution was not new. As early as 1904 sociologists had been arguing that, although such a scheme would be costly, it could be justified by the greater expense it would save, for if emphasis was put on prevention rather than intervention after crisis, not only would human misery be averted, but also the money paid by the innumerable and often overlapping authorities dealing with pauperism would be reduced. This was the message of the Minority Report and the more radical reform groups of the inter-war years.

During the 1939–45 war the government was forced to play an ever greater role in providing for those for whom the national emergency had deprived of services, and in 1941 a Committee of Reconstruction was set up to plan for after the war. If the First World War forced social change as the result of citizen participation, the Second had an even greater effect. All had shared hardships, shortages and rationing and there was a determination that when the war was over there would be a more equitable distribution of goods and resources. The Welfare State when it came was, therefore, not only a reaction to Victorian poverty and inter-war unemployment, but also a response to participation in a national war effort.

THE BEVERIDGE REPORT ON SOCIAL INSURANCE AND ALLIED SERVICES 1942

Sir William Beveridge (1879–1963)* as a young man had played a part in the Liberal reforms of 1906 and was particularly associated with the setting up of labour exchanges; since then he had been a leading civil servant, the Director of the London School of Economics and the Master of University College, Oxford, and in all these capacities he had continued to put forward a wide range of ideas about social welfare. In 1940 he was invited by the War Cabinet to chair a committee to decide on the future policy for the social insurance and allied services, and the report associated with his name was virtually a one-man effort since the committee members were civil servants and not allowed to express opinions in public on controversial matters. Beveridge described his scheme as a 'revolution', but a 'British revolution that was a natural development from the past'.[1] The revolution lay in the acceptance by the state of fuller responsibility for social policy, for in future the state would determine policy rather than merely filling in the gaps left by private enterprise and charity. The new policy involved the final break-up of the Poor Law and the deterrent attitudes associated with it, and in order to do this provision had to be made for social services to be available to people *as of right*. Although Beveridge called his scheme a 'revolution' it was, in fact, a rationalisation of the existing insurance principle and was a typically liberal rather than socialist measure, for socialists would have preferred to have the social services financed by general taxation as in collectivist societies. Moreover, Beveridge was aware that the proposed 'flat rate' contributions would be a burden to the low-paid and that such a scheme could only hope to provide subsistence benefits. Thus, there would be ample opportunity for personal thrift, private schemes and for voluntary societies, which were to be encouraged; it was, in fact, a plan for a pluralistic society.

In planning the scheme four social services were crucial and legislation was to a large extent interdependent. These services were *The Education Act* 1944, sometimes known as the Butler Act after R. A. Butler, the then Minister of Education – the Act was based on the Haddow Report of 1926 which had never been implemented, and which was designed to provide equal educational opportunities for all children; *The National Health Service Act* 1946, which was based on reports from the political parties and various reports from the medical profession; *The Family Allowances Act* 1948, which provided universal allowances for children and which were designed to meet the needs of the family as a whole, and *The National Insurance Act and National Insurance (Industrial Injuries) Acts* 1948, which covered the proposals for a universal insurance scheme. For the purpose of this Act the population was divided into three classes of contributors – employed, self-employed and non-employed – with contributions varying with the class of contribution.

The principle behind the Act was that *flat rate* benefits would be paid to people provided a certain number of stamps had been paid or credited,

* Created 1st Baron Beveridge, 1946

or, in cases of long-term benefits like pensions, an average number of contributions made annually. For five years after retirement the pension depended on, and continues to depend on (although certain earnings are allowed) actual retirement from gainful employ.

The main benefits paid under the National Insurance Acts were:

- Unemployment benefit, payable for a maximum of one year;
- Sickness benefit, payable for as long as incapacity for work continues until retirement age;
- Retirement pensions, payable after a minimum age of 60 for women and 65 for men.

Other benefits under the Act included Widow's benefits, Guardian's allowances and Maternity grants, benefits for married women who paid the full rate of contributions and fulfilled the necessary conditions, and finally a death grant payable to the dependants of insured persons. The Industrial Injury Benefit was an updating of the old Workman's Compensation Act of 1925, was separately administered and was not dependent on the number of contributions. Injury benefits were, and are still, awarded at higher rates.

The Beveridge Committee envisaged that the proposed legislation would be comprehensive and sufficient to lay the five giants of Squalor, Ignorance, Want, Disease and Idleness – imaginative language that is redolent of the Webb's causes of destitution. Unfortunately, monumental and far-reaching though the Report was, it did not make sufficient allowance for post-war inflation, and consequently the early forecasts on costs were too low. As time went by more use had to be made of the Beveridge 'safety net', the *National Assistance Act* 1948, which was originally intended for those who were not covered by insurance, but had to be used more and more to supplement either benefits or wages that were below subsistence. In the ensuing years 'National Assistance' has changed to more euphemistic terms such as Family Income Supplement. The problem is the same as it was for the magistrates at Speen in 1795: should there be a minimum wage or an allowance? In 1978 more than 4 million people were receiving supplementary benefits.

As Beveridge himself was at pains to emphasise, the welfare services were a natural development from the past; the services that had worked were expanded while those, like the Poor Law, that were obsolete, were discarded. In spite of the shocked comments from reactionary quarters at the time, the scheme was an extension of the old National Insurance Acts, which were themselves a borrowing from Bismarck's paternalistic Germany, and many of the ideas in fact came from the Continent. However, the National Health Service, the fourth side of the Beveridge quadrant, was undoubtedly a British institution. The reason for this lay not so much in British waywardness but in the historical background of the

English health services (Figure 11.1) and the fact that 'state' medicine in England had been through a deterrent Poor Law. Contrary to popular belief, the National Health Service was not a 'revolution' but a pragmatic fusion of the health services as they had evolved by 1946. What was dramatic, and even reactionary, was that they were fixed by legislation at the point they had developed so far, as if they were caught by a flash photograph in a moment of time. The reason for this timidity and compromise was that there was more opposition to the National Health Service than to any of the other concepts contained in the Beveridge plan.

OPPOSITION TO THE HEALTH SERVICE

The general acceptance of a composite plan for post-war reconstruction gave a new urgency to plans for a 'National Health Service'. Various schemes from the past were examined, including the Maclean and the Dawson Reports and of course, the Sankey Commission. In 1941 the British Medical Association set up a Medical Planning Commission, which provoked considerable discussion. The main proposals were that the hospital services should be delegated to Regional Councils; that general practioners should work in groups of six to ten from Health Centres to be provided by the Regional Councils; that they should be paid partly by salary and partly by capitation fees; and that all insured persons and their dependants, which in practice meant about 90 per cent of the population, should be covered. The Report, although putting all hospitals under the Regional Council, left untouched the old problem of the dichotomy between the preventive and curative services, and between the hospitals and the general practitioners. The Royal Colleges of Physicians and Surgeons produced variations on the Report, and the debate was widened by people like Professor Ryle and Dr Harold Himsworth, urging that the whole system needed radical recasting on the basis of Exchequer funding and a full-time salaried service.[2] Meanwhile, both the Liberal and Labour parties published reports that were not dissimilar. As in 1918 there was a coalition government which, having accepted Beveridge's plan in principle, was committed to working out a scheme for a National Health Service. This it proceeded to do with the aid of the recently established Nuffield Provincial Hospitals Trust which had in fact been founded in 1939 to try and make possible the objectives of the Sankey Commission. The Plan was published as a White Paper in 1944 after a newspaper leak had caused a good deal of intemperate comment.

The government's plan, introduced by the Minister of Health, Mr Willink, was that a service for the whole population be operated through the *local authorities*. The government could not accept that there should be a central authority outside the accountability to Parliament or that there should be Regional Authorities not democratically elected (*sic*). But because most local authorities were too small, the White Paper proposed that for the purposes of a Health Authority the counties and the county boroughs should combine and the existing municipal services should enter into contractual arrangements with the voluntary hospitals, a scheme which had its roots in the Minority Report of 1909. There was to be a free choice of doctor and general practitioners would operate from Health Centres, but the fatal idea was floated that this might be on a salaried basis. Other proposals included an inspectorate service manned by doctors and nurses and other experts – a proposal sadly omitted from the service when it came.

The British Medical Association now suffered a change of heart: sinister motives were attributed to the government; Health Centres, so long advocated, were now suspect and a salaried service was equated with the end of clinical freedom. In this confused and stormy atmosphere with Dr Charles Hill, the Secretary of the British Medical Association, addressing mass meetings and keeping up what Calder described as 'an unedifying racket',[3] the Association conducted a poll of its members; 53 per cent were against the scheme but, strangely enough, 60 per cent favoured a scheme that gave full cover to the whole population, which is what most people understood the dispute was about, for full cover would reduce the scope for private medicine. The Minister was now in the position of having antagonised both the doctors and the voluntary hospitals who saw themselves as being 'taken over' by the local authorities; but to assuage their fears he would now incur the opposition of the equally powerful local government lobby. Here the matter rested, while the often unintelligible debate continued until 1945, when the General Election produced a Labour government and a new minister, Aneurin Bevan, and while, above all, public opinion demanded that something be done.

Bevan appeared to face three groups whose claims had to be reconciled. He wanted a 'prestige' service and could not afford to alienate the most powerful members of the medical profession, although his own natural inclination would have been towards a plan based on local authorities. He conducted a series of discussions with interested bodies, ably assisted by his Chief Medical Officer, Sir Wilson Jameson, then he proceeded to divide and rule. A scheme was drawn up that was generous to the voluntary hospitals, especially the teaching hospitals which kept their Boards of Governors and retained a good deal of independence and where consultants were allowed to have private patients and to work in hospitals on a sessional basis. The fears of general practitioners were partly alleviated by giving them a semi-independent organisation through Executive Councils and payment on a *per capita* basis. The problem of the hospitals was solved by the Minister taking over all hospitals, then handing them back to Regional Boards and Hospital Management Committees on which sat the appointed representatives of the voluntary hospitals, the municipal system and the doctors. As a compromise it was an ingenious device and was probably the only way to break the deadlock; the cracks, the schisms and the rivalries had been papered over to give what appeared to be a universal service, but which was in fact three separate services.

THE NATIONAL HEALTH SERVICE ACT 1946

The National Health Service came into operation on 5 July 1948. Originally it was intended that all treatment should be free of charge, but since 1948 there have been minor amendments to allow charges to be made for prescriptions and appliances. The Act set out to provide a comprehensive health service with the Minister empowered to take the necessary steps to meet all reasonable health requirements. To do this the existing health services were taken over by the Ministry of Health,* and the 3,600 hospitals welded into the Hospital and Specialist Services. The community health services previously administered by the counties and county boroughs became the Local Authority Services, and the services provided by the general practitioners and dentists the General Medical and Dental Services. Because of the complex nature of the services to be co-ordinated, and because in order to secure acceptance of the plan it had been necessary to devolve administration back to the many interests that had previously controlled the services, the administrative framework was immensely complicated (Figure 15.1).

The hospital services

The administration of the hospital services was delegated to 14 (later 15) Regional Hospital Boards in England and five in Scotland. The Boards consisted of members appointed by the Minister who controlled the general planning and exercised supervision over the hospitals in their respective regions; the day-to-day running of the hospitals was the concern of Group Hospital Management Committees. The teaching hospitals remained outside the purview of the Regional Boards and had their own Boards of Governors who were directly responsible to the Minister, except in Scotland where teaching hospitals were responsible to the Boards of Management. There were 36 Boards of Governors controlling hospitals, or groups, specially designed to provide facilities for teaching and research, each Board being associated with a medical school which obtained its funds through the University Grants Committee. London had 26 hospitals or groups designated as Board of Governor hospitals,[4] many of which of course undertook research or provided special facilities that overlapped with those of their close neighbours.

* Became the Department of Health and Social Security, 1969.

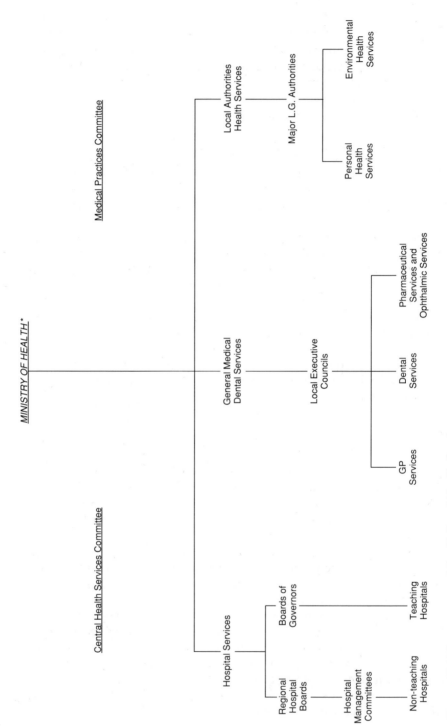

Figure 15.1 The structure of the National Health Service

The local health authorities

As defined in Part III of the Act local authorities continued to provide the same services as previously, including the Maternity and Child Welfare Services, whose main function was to give expert advice to mothers with young children and to expectant mothers; the local authorities also continued to supply a whole range of domiciliary and midwifery services, with the latter sometimes overlapping with, and at times conflicting with, the hospital and the general practitioner services. Other duties laid on the local authorities included the provision of vaccination and immunisation services, and they also had wide powers to engage 'in activities for the prevention of illness and the care and after care of persons who were sick or physically or mentally disabled'. Few authorities took up this challenge mainly because the burden would have fallen on the rates, whereas the hospital services were provided from Exchequer funds, an important factor in the use of hospital beds for social reasons.

The general medical and dental services

Under the Act, about 95 per cent of the population registered with the doctor of their choice and in theory were free to change if they wished, a freedom not always easy to exercise in practice. The general practitioner was paid a fee for each patient and, apart from this, there were complicated arrangements for remuneration from a central fund for such items as practice expenses, initial allowances and mileage allowances. Dentists were provided for differently; the dentist was paid a fee of service with certain fixed charges to patients at the time of treatment.

Organisation of the Hospital Management Committee

The greatest upheaval was in the hospitals, where those of varying traditions were grouped under one management. However, by pressure groups even this was mitigated; mental hospitals, and often specialist hospitals, were allowed to have single and separate committees – often consisting of the members of the old pre-health service committee. Moreover, in most cases the control remained largely with the people who have run the hospitals before, and the third schedule of the Act had found it necessary to lay down that at least half the Regional Board 'shall be persons other than medical practitioners'.

The day-to-day running of a group of hospitals was revolutionised in a way that had important consequences for the nursing services. The secretary of the Management Committee became the chief officer of the group, and it was his responsibility to organise and co-ordinate the various committees responsible for carrying out the overall policy; committees tended to proliferate, but in a typical group the main structure was as follows:

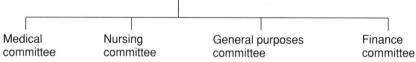

GROUP HOSPITAL MANAGEMENT COMMITTEE

(Secretary to the Committee – the Group Secretary)

| Medical committee | Nursing committee | General purposes committee | Finance committee |

The medical committee invariably consisted of medical practitioners, the nursing committee, on the other hand, was always predominantly composed of lay men and women. At the beginning of the service each hospital had its own house Committee, which, although it had no executive power, did act as an advisory body and formed a useful link between the hospital, the general public and the group.

The health service, therefore, was not only 'tripartite', representing three different sources of finance; there were also a number of bifurcations in the sub-structure. The mental hospitals were separate from the general, the chronic from the acute, the teaching from the non-teaching, and within the substructure itself there was a three-tier system of administration. It was devolution of authority downwards on almost Napoleonic Code lines, and bewildering to the average citizen whose needs the system had been set up to serve.

THE NATIONAL HEALTH SERVICE AND ITS EFFECTS ON NURSING

In 1948 the nursing service was suffering from the upheavals of war. Although the Nurses' Act had clarified the position of the assistant nurse there was no rush of recruits and the profession itself was lukewarm; the Civil Nursing Reserve had left an inheritance of part-time workers and the service had been diluted by auxiliaries about whom there was no agreement as whether they should receive training. The age of entry had been lowered, the educational test abandoned and a one-year 'crash' course for service personnel with nursing experience introduced. In search of ever more pairs of hands, and under the guise of 'bridging the gap' between school and nursing, a legion of 'cadet schemes' had come into being. The General Nursing Council stated, 'one reason for the wastage is known to be the very early age at which some candidates are accepted for nursing. A great number of girls below the age of 18, some 15½ years and even younger, have been recorded by the Council.' This same report goes on: 'another reason for wastage is the low educational standard of a proportion of the recruits accepted'.[5] The General Nursing Council as a statutory body inevitably took a cautious stance, and its report is probably an understatement.

Apart from these expedients, another wartime chicken had come home to roost. Recruitment in the war had mainly been to the ranks of students, who left when they were trained, and auxiliaries. Allowing for the fact that the hospital returns of 1949 were unreliable and the pre-war figures even more so, before the war there were probably two trained nurses to every three untrained; in 1949 it was nearer to one trained nurse to every two untrained,[6] but now, because of the advances in medical science and the shorter patient stay, a higher standard of supervision was required to ensure safe practice. By the end of 1946 the ratio of nurses to patients in sanatoria was *lower than it was in 1942* and the waiting lists were four times as long as they had been in 1941 – the darkest days of the war.[7] In November 1946 Aneurin Bevan described the situation as 'approaching the dimensions of a national disaster'.

Now there were other problems. First, because of the low birth rate in the 1930s there were fewer girls aged 18 years in the population; furthermore, improved infant care had altered the sex ratio – frail boy babies no longer perished but lived to be husbands, often in their early twenties or before. Not only were there fewer girls, but those there were were likely to marry early. Gone forever was that pool of devoted spinsters, who for nearly 100 years had been the main source of the stable labour force in nursing. Secondly, for those who remained unmarried the prospects were never brighter. Technological advance had created a new, if spurious, demand for labour, and under the influence of the Beveridge Report there was a large increase in the social services which needed recruits with the same attributes as nurses. The school-leaver was wooed at every turn. In comparison with the allurements of industry, the air lines, *haute couture* and the police force, nurses suffered from a number of disadvantages. First, they worked unsocial hours and, more important, then did not know when they would be off duty; unlike air hostesses and the women's services, the uniform was often drab, poor in quality and unbecoming. Second, although the Rushcliffe award had improved the economic position of the nurse, this was now being whittled away by inflation – especially as more and more lived out. Third, many of the opportunities offered to young people had educational programmes with the cachet of a university diploma or degree, or at least something which ranked as 'further education', which nursing did not. Finally, there was the elusive problem of the new nature of nursing. Medical advances had altered not only the diseases to be nursed but the age groups needing care. But as the hospitals seemed to be filling with the old and the long-term sick – once the despised groups of the Poor Law – so the new technology was changing the nursing of the acutely ill, and with the introduction of dialysis and apparatus like the heart lung machine the recovery of the patients seemed to depend less on the nurse.

On the horizon there were ever more machines and more powerful drugs and the age of computerised medicine; the role and function of the nurse, and indeed sometimes of the doctor, was becoming harder to define.

SUGGESTIONS FOR THE REFORM OF NURSING

In 1945 the air was thick with suggested panaceas for nursing. These came from the medical profession, the general press, trade unions, the nursing journals and the profession itself. Apart from those who believed that more money would solve all problems, or the *Spectator*, which proposed cure by 'the abolition of the personal and professional slavery that nursing has hitherto involved',[8] the serious reformers were divided between those who wished to shorten training, but make it intensive, and those who thought it should be longer but more comprehensive; the *Nursing Times*, for example, pointed out that hospitals who offered a four-year training had no difficulty in getting recruits, and that it was not the time that mattered but the way students were treated and regarded.

In 1947 the *Lancet* put forward proposals for a two-year training with a lower age of entry and a common portal of entry for all abilities who would 'eventually sort themselves out'. This scheme found little favour with the nursing profession who were, not without reason, wary of 16-year-olds of varying intelligence 'sorting themselves out'. Furthermore, the plan lacked any clear aim about the numbers to be trained, the objectives of the course or the numbers likely to require further training.

Before this, the Royal College of Nursing, foreseeing the National Health Service, which it welcomed, had set up a Nursing Reconstruction Committee under the chairmanship of Lord Horder. In 1942, Section I of the Report, taking up the threads of the Athlone Report, had dealt with the problem of the assistant nurse, and this had led to the Nurses' Act of 1943. In December 1943 Sections II and III were published, on Education and training and recruitment. On the first page the Committee posed the basic problem: 'It is obvious that the first essential in the establishment of true nursing education is the clear separation between the training of nurses and the obligation to provide nursing services for hospital patients.

Not everyone agreed. Nursing journals and their correspondence show that the profession was particularly sensitive to accusations, mainly from the doctors, of trying to produce an 'academic nurse' divorced from the practical situation. This was the last thing the Horder Committee was proposing, but it led to hedging the proposals with an ambience of imprecision:

> While the student nurse must be regarded as a component part of the hospital in order that she may cultivate a sense of responsibility, her status as a student should be fully recognised by the trained nursing staff, medical staff and the governing body and her work regulated accordingly.[9]

In order to meet these objectives there should be 'grants from national funds'; this is a borrowing from the Athlone Report, and in this respect the Horder Committee was working with its hands tied because the details for the financing of the health service were not then known.

However, the committee made a number of proposals, which included a drastic reduction in the number of training schools, the setting up of education committees in each Region, a higher rate of trained staff to supervise students, more ancillary staff to perform non-nursing tasks; and entry to the profession should be by the School Leaving Certificate, or a specially devised test by the General Nursing Council. The training would cover four years of planned study and practice, including experience in obstetric nursing and 'such branches as mental, fever and tuberculosis nursing with an elective six months in a speciality during the final year. Ward sisters in designated teaching areas should be encouraged to obtain the Diploma in Nursing, and men, as far as possible, should receive the same training as women. Once this wider training was available the 'other parts of the Register' should be closed and the General Nursing Council reorganised. One recommendation that was implemented was that the Council should appoint an education officer and set up a system of training for inspectors and examiners.

Eighteen months later the Committee produced *Minimum Standards for Nurse Training* and *Post-registration Nursing Education*. The supplements emphasised the interrelation of all branches of nursing and the need for nursing education to be seen as a continuing process having links with general education. The three months in an elective study would form the basis for the next step in post-registration study; a student who had done three months' public health nursing in her basic training would proceed to 'Specialist Training for the Public Health Nurse' and cover the course in nine months, probably at an educational college with other disciplines. Although the longer training was not acceptable to a generation in a hurry, the Horder Report enumerated a number of sound principles, not least of which was that nursing education should start with a basic foundation and the whole process of nursing education seen as a continuum and *all branches of nursing as interdependent*; principles that were to be restated 30 years later by the Committee on Nursing Education and later by Project 2000.

In December 1944, the General Nursing Council suddenly produced its own 'reform plan' which consisted of lengthening the training to four years and reorganising the present syllabus. The *Nursing Times* complained that the report 'had been hastily put together, there was too much emphasis on formal teaching and no regard was paid to the need for the student to have experience in the community'.[10]

The main criticism of both reports was that the training proposed was too long. Miss Pearce, a well-known educationist and author, wrote to the nursing press pointing out the folly of lengthening the training and arguing that the solution lay in getting back to the pre-war levels of domestic staffing: 'Before the war the best nursing schools had reduced the domestic work for students to nil, wartime shortages had changed the picture and nurses were doing more sweeping and washing up than they had done in 40 years.'[11] This was an over-simplification, but it was certainly true that there had been a fall in the numbers of domestic workers and in this respect many post-war students fared much worse than their pre-war counterparts, another example of things not necessarily getting better. But there was no way of 'luring back' the old style domestic workers – money would not buy them; it was all part of the changing scene paralleling the disappearance of servants from private houses after the First World War. Eventually the ward maid, around whom so much of the ward routine pivoted, would be replaced by machines and contract cleaners.

The advocates of the shorter training based their arguments on the premise that if nurses were to be taught good nursing there must be good nursing to study and this could only be achieved by an increase in the numbers of trained staff; a shorter training could be achieved without loss of quality if learners were given *student status and relieved of all domestic and ancillary duties*. The corollary of this argument was that the assistant nurse scheme be abandoned and all applicants accepted either as trainee nurses or auxiliaries. But this brought the argument full circle to the 'many different personalities and aptitudes' required in nursing; could they all be put through a common training programme, and in Miss Lückes' words, was it 'a waste to train all for everything'?

As in 1919, when the profession could not agree amongst itself, the government intervened and set up its own Working Party on the Recruitment and Training of Nurses under the chairmanship of Sir Robert Wood, which published its Majority Report in July 1947. The date is important; the committee started sitting in January 1946 and was taking its evidence that year.

It has been said that the Wood Report 'constituted the most outspoken and well-documented condemnation of the attitudes and behaviour of senior nurses yet published'.[12] Outspoken it may have been; well-documented it was not. The report is 100 pages long, half of which are devoted to the factual and statistical position of nursing in 1946. In order to ascertain the causes of 'wastage', the Working Party applied the comparatively new techniques of questionnaires and interviews; the relatives of 104 ex-students were seen and 55 ex-students interviewed and a further 400 letters examined. The Committee admitted that the sample was small and might be unrepresentative. What was far more unrepresentative was the fact that, because of the Control of Engagement Order, many students had come into nursing to avoid being drafted into factories or the armed services, and of course, in those circumstances there was practically no selection; when the controls came off in 1946 they not unnaturally abandoned training, a fact that both the Report and Professor Abel-Smith omit. Further, this was the great period of demobilisation, when the marriage rate soared and the birth rate was the highest for 25 years. No year could have been more atypical.

Of the students interviewed the research workers estimated that at least one third were unsuitable for nursing and 10 per cent were in intelligence category 'E', which they concluded 'established a prima facie case for better selection' – a conclusion with which senior nurses would not have disagreed. Although the students gave a wide variety of reasons for leaving, the Working Party stated: 'The conclusion that emerges clearly from the analysis is that the type of discipline that pervades the training schools is unquestionably the most important cause of wastage.[13]

This conclusion *may* have been correct but it did not emerge clearly from the evidence. The main cause could equally well have been the wartime lack of selection, the changed ratio of trained to untrained staff, or simply the higher marriage rate. Subsequent and more thorough analysis showed that among the many and complex reasons for learners leaving discipline was only one factor in a constellation of many others. The Report of the Working Party does not tell us much about hospital discipline – the sample is too small – but it does give some indication of the difficulties faced by nursing at the beginning of the National Health Service.

The hectoring tone of the Report hardly endeared it to the nursing profession. The plan for a two-year training, six months of which would be in a speciality, received a cautious welcome, but serious doubts were expressed about the possibility of giving a basic training in all branches of nursing in 18 months, and even greater doubts about letting a student so qualified practise in any field of nursing – unsupervised. Further criticism came from training schools for assistant nurses which the scheme would abolish, and neither the midwives nor specialities such as psychiatry would allow that the basic elements of *their* speciality could be imparted in a few weeks, and the General Nursing Council were not disposed to have their function curtailed.

The Minority Report

If the nursing profession could not agree, nor could the Working Party. One member, Dr Cohen, dissented and wrote his own report in which he pointed out that the Working Party had failed to look at the problem of the future demand for health services and the changing role of hospitals. Until these problems were examined it was impossible to say what was the *necessary and proper function of the nurse,* and on the answer to that question depended the type and method of training. Dr Cohen argued that until forecasts about health needs were put on a scientific basis, all recommendations about grades of nurses and the training these grades needed were useless. Thirty years later the Royal College of Nursing made much the same point to the Royal Commission on the Health Service.[14] Dr Cohen provided the profession and the government with the escape they needed; the debate could be shelved while research was conducted. But even without the Minority Report the Wood recommendations had little chance. Where were hospitals to find another 38,000 nursing staff to replace the students, of whom on their own findings one third were unsuitable? It was useless to suggest more part-time staff, hospitals were already using every pair of hands they could, and matrons were touring Africa, Asia and the West Indies in search of recruits. Over all there was the question of cost; by 1947 the health service estimates were rising, which was grist to the mill of the opposition to the service; the whole subject was political dynamite.

The training that had served the needs of municipal and voluntary undertakings before the war was no longer suitable, but as Dr Cohen pointed out, the future health needs were an uncharted sea; some believed that the demand for care would diminish, others foretold the need to expand the least favoured specialities like geriatrics, but the service and nursing were bedevilled by the wartime heritage of expediency where administrators often rationalised the possible into the desirable.

REFERENCES

1 *Social Insurance and Allied Services* (1942) (Beveridge Report) 'Introduction', London: HMSO.
2 Abel-Smith, B. (1964) *The Hospitals*, London: Heinemann Educational, pp. 446–7.
3 Calder, A. (1969) *The People's War*, London: Cape, p. 540.
4 *The Hospital Year Book* (1951) Board of Governor Hospitals, Institute of Hospital Administrators, London.
5 General Nursing Council (1949) *Annual Report for 1948*, London.
6 The Hospital Survey 1937–38 compared with the returns from the Ministry of Health, 1949, London: Ministry of Health.
7 Titmuss, R. (1950) *Problems of Social Policy*, ch. XXIV, London: Longman and HMSO.
8 *Spectator* (Oct. 1945), quoted by the *Nursing Times*, 15 Nov. 1945, London: Macmillan.
9 Royal College of Nursing (1943) *The Horder Report: the Nursing Reconstruction Committee* (Section II), 'Introduction'.
10. *Nursing Times* (1945). Leader (March).
11 *Nursing Times* (1945), Letter from Evelyn Pearce (26 May).
12 Abel-Smith, B. (1960) *A History of the Nursing Profession*, London: Heinemann Educational, p. 182.
13 (1947) *The Working Party on the Recruitment and Training of Nurses*, Ch. V, London: HMSO.

14 Royal College of Nursing (1977) *Evidence to the Royal Commission on the National Health Service*, p. 33.

FURTHER READING

Abel-Smith, B. (1978) *The National Health Service – the First Thirty Years*, London: HMS0.

Brucer, M. (1968) *The Coming of the Welfare State*, 4th edn, London: Batsford. .

Fraser, D. (1973) *The Evolution of the British Welfare State*, London: Macmillan.

Webster, C. (1988) *The Health Services since the War*, vol. 1, *Problems of Health Care, The NHS before 1957*, London: HMSO.

Willcocks, J. (1967) *The Creation of the National Health Service*, Library of Social Policy and Administration.

Chapter 16

Adapting nursing to new demands

The National Health Service took the services as they had developed by 1946 and fixed them with legislation in what was virtually a tripartite structure. When illness was largely episodic and attendance at a hospital or doctor's surgery an isolated incident in life such divisions mattered less, but it so happened that the National Health Service came into being as both the population profile and the health needs of the community were changing, and these changes affected not only the new need for continuity but also the cost of the service.

COSTING THE SERVICE

The Beveridge Committee under-estimated the likely cost of the health service because they were advised that once the backlog of untreated illness had been cleared the population would become healthier and make less demand on the service. Professor Titmuss, advising the government, calculated that the high users of the service were unmarried women living alone, and he prophesied that with the increased marriage rate and longevity of spouses, this problem would diminish. In preparing the first budget of £170 million the Beveridge Report said, 'a health service will diminish disease by prevention and cure'.[1] Professor Titmuss and the Report were wrong on several counts. Health services are self-expanding, good health care does not produce a fit population because reduction in mortality carries with it the likely increase in morbidity; the frail are kept alive to require ever more care. Furthermore, better education, greater affluence and new technical knowledge produce rising expectations for health care in all sections of the community. Again, the estimates have been confounded for, although the marriage rates have risen, so too have the divorce rates; the earlier the marriage the greater the likelihood of breakdown. Of the marriages made in 1961, 59 per 1,000 ended in divorce compared with the 21 per 1,000 for those made in 1921. Moreover, the gap between the survival rates of men and women has widened so that, contrary to the prophecy, the number of single households as a percentage of the total has risen from 10.7 in 1951 to 18.2 for the 1971 Census.[2]* These facts affect not only the cost of the service but also the nature of much nursing because people often come for institutional care, not so much because they want treatment, but because there is no-one to care for them.

The rising costs due to the new demand and post-war inflation could not have been foretold in 1948, but failure to make the correct forecast had some unfortunate repercussions and the estimates gave a hostage to the critics who over the years found many scapegoats for the increasing budgets. These have included the over-prescribing of drugs, the abuse of the service by the patients, too many administrators, the profligate use of wigs and fitted carpets on office floors. All, or some, of these may have been true at times and have had a marginal effect, but the main and abiding reason for the increase in costs is the genuine and legitimate demand for services as the *result of the lower mortality among the frail*; this, with an inflation rate that has been persistently higher than in competitor countries, outweighs all other factors. However, because there was little statistical material to indicate whether the service was giving value for money, the cost of the health service was the subject of uninformed dialectic and this hostile criticism rebounded in political decisions. But it was the other topic for debate, the structure of the health service, that was to have a profound effect on the nursing service, and most subsequent changes in nursing administration can be traced to its struggle to adapt to the health service.

THE STRUCTURE OF THE HOSPITAL SERVICE

Before the Nightingale reforms the chief administrator in a voluntary hospital was responsible for employing all staff except the doctors, who were honorary. Miss Nightingale's aim had been the control of nurses by nurses, and to achieve this it had been necessary to create a distinct nursing administration with the matron as head of the nursing service. By the end of the nineteenth century the management arrangements in voluntary hospitals were tripartite, with the house governor responsible for finance and the lay staff, the matron for nurse training and nursing service, and the medical committee for medical policy; this triple alliance was not always harmonious but generally a *modus vivendi* was achieved. The municipal hospitals, on the other hand, developed a different system. Having inherited their hospitals from the Poor Law they adapted the authoritarian system of executive power dispensed downwards, with a medical superintendent eventually displacing the Poor Law master, to whom both the lay and nursing staff were subordinate.

During the debate on the health service a crucial argument centred on the type of administration to be imposed on *all* hospitals. The medical

* See Chapter 19 for 1991 figures.

profession, which never looked kindly on the idea of one doctor exercising control over other doctors, favoured the voluntary system, in which of course they had all been trained. Nurses, who equally disliked the idea of doctors having control over nurses, shared this preference. The professional viewpoint prevailed, but the multilateral tradition of the voluntary system did not fit into the health service structure, which was linear and hierarchical.

In order to combat the criticism of bureaucratic control, authority had been devolved to the group, which soon became the most powerful committee in the service and were seldom overruled by a higher level. The group committee was responsible for upwards of 20 hospitals scattered over as many miles; this was a new concept, and the group administrators, who were mostly recruited from the municipal system, brought with them ideas of line authority, control and accounting that were often alien to the voluntary system, with the group secretary himself becoming the main spokesman for the group and in a position of considerable power. Matrons no longer had access to their governing bodies, and in large groups were often quite unknown to their employers. The group committee took its advice from its sub-committees, the most powerful of which was the medical committee, consisting of medical practitioners drawn from advisory committees who in any event usually had four or five of their colleagues on the governing body. The nursing committee was a different matter: it consisted of lay members, and nurses did not sit on the main committee, although pressure from professional organisations sometimes procured a place for a nurse 'not in the employ of the committee' – which was limiting. The matrons who found the system most irksome were those from the voluntary system who were used to direct access to their governors, and although, in spite of the Lancet Commission's recommendations, comparatively few voluntary hospitals had good staff consultation before 1948, most had been compact enough to ensure the adage that administrators 'should know many of their subordinates by name and the majority by sight'. Now, even if the group committee wished to hear the nursing viewpoint there were difficulties. First, there was the problem of time and transport in getting people together from a wide area. Second, the hospitals catered for different specialities which often had competing and conflicting needs. Third, the experience and qualifications of the matrons might vary widely, and in any event no matron had control over another.

A number of ideas were tried, including the election of one representative, a rota system, and even a group matron who had extramural duties – unpaid and unsanctioned by Whitley. No solution was satisfactory. Apart from hurt pride, there was a genuine waste of expertise among nurses who had trained for administration – often at their own expense. Because of the culminating dissatisfaction, the professional organisations made repeated protests to the Minister of Health, and in 1950 the Central Health Services Council, the advisory arm of the health service, set up a committee under the chairmanship of Alderman Bradbeer, to study the internal administration of hospitals. The task was formidable and the report was not ready until 1954; this in the end sailed cautiously between Scylla and Charybdis, and recommended that 'the matron was the equal partner and directly responsible to the governing body in matters affecting the training school and the nursing service, but in her less well-defined and non-professional duties she was directly responsible to the administrative officer'.[3] In order to overcome the problem of nursing representation the committee recommended the establishment of nursing advisory commit-tees to give collective advice.

Although the report was welcomed by the nursing profession it failed to tackle the cause of the problem which was the setting of the hospital tripartite and lateral system within the hierarchical structure of the health service. Nor did the distinction between the professional role and non-professional matters help much, for it was in those 'less well-defined duties', such as the responsibility for the patient's food, where failure to consult often affected the efficiency of the nursing service. Difficulties were aggravated by the fact that few employees understood the organisation in which they worked and personnel in the health service had been given almost no preparation for the new enterprise. It was the awareness of this failure that led to the almost over-insurance in consultation and prepara-tion before the reorganisation of 1974.

STANDARDISATION OF EQUIPMENT AND SUPPLIES

A first objective of the new service was the improvement of equipment and supplies by standardisation, mechanisation and interchangeability, for only in this way could the poorer hospitals be improved without excessive cost. An area where the need was paramount was sterilisation; reports were appearing showing the low safety level in many hospitals, and as the result of this publicity, the Nuffield Provincial Hospitals Trust set up a study on Planning and Organising Central Syringe Services, then, in 1958, the report *Supply Arrangements for Hospitals: Present Sterilising Practice in Six Hospitals*, caused further concern about sterilising practices. Increasingly the supply and maintenance of sterile equipment was taken from the wards and ceased to be a nursing duty. There were protests about the effect this would have on nurse training, but alarming disclosures about cross-infection eventually persuaded people that the old practices were not in the best interests of the patients. Central Sterile Supplies Departments were established with experiments in organisation and delivery and, although it was first thought it would be unnecessary to use nurses, those with a special aptitude quickly established themselves as Control of Infection Officers, demonstrating that nurses could adapt to the changing clinical and tech-nical demands of the new service.

Hospital catering was also affected by the new technology. Kitchens were centralised and experiments carried out with microwave cooking; new dietary standards were laid down and storage was assisted by better refrigeration and central planning. In the meantime heated trolleys, conveyor belts and central dish-washing machinery revolutionised the ward meal service and saved the time of nurses, or at least helped to make up for the loss of ward maids. Automation even spread to the out-patients' department where the vending machine and the paper cup tended to replace the Red Cross lady with the teapot.

What was true for catering applied also to the laundry service, where the individual hospital service was replaced by a central or contract service. In the pharmaceutical services new methods of packing and storage facilitated the move to centralisation and revolutionised the medicine round, particularly the once time-consuming, and often inaccurate, drawing up of hypodermic injections. Soon the hospital became an avid user of disposables and the new synthetics like polythene that were not so disposable.

In theory, centralisation and new technology saved the nurses' time, and this saving, it was argued, would help overcome the shortage of nurses. In practice it was not always so. There were 700 hospitals with fewer than 50 beds; the night sister making the porridge in the kitchen or boiling the instruments in a fish kettle was cheaper than microwave cooking and central sterile supplies. Moreover, at the end of the central system there was a patient wanting an individual service which frustrated mechanisation; some liked porridge with sugar, some with salt – some did not like porridge. Moreover, the needs of the patient were there for seven days a week, and the services of the new technology tended to be on weekdays only. Nor was bulk buying always an improvement; previously, thanks to voluntary effort, many hospitals were well equipped with glass and china that was superior in quality and design to bulk purchase. Nevertheless, the ineluctable conclusion of the 1950s was that the only way to save manpower – now becoming more expensive – and to give an efficient service, was to close all small hospitals and to build again, bigger and better. Outside the old sprawling slums were being replaced by high-rise flats which had not yet been called 'prisons in the sky'.

STANDARDISATION OF NURSES' UNIFORM

Nursing uniforms had evolved from the servant garb of the 1860s which was thought functionally, if not socially, suitable for work on the wards. Over the years it had been crossed with a strain of militarism, often to denote rank, and an occasional symbol from the ecclesiastical past, with nurses themselves doing their best to upgrade the original dull outfit. The cap, which started as a hygienic covering for late-Victorian hair styles, had become elaborate, decorative and useless; lace, bows, strings and streamers added to the charm and interest and probably brought more recruits to nursing than all the government appeals, but they did not fit the central laundry. Already costs had compelled well-known training schools to adopt a more utilitarian style, and there were now proposals for a 'National Uniform'. However, neither committees of distinguished men and women, nor *haute couture* houses, nor yet nurses themselves produced designs that were universally acceptable to nurses – or the central laundry. Some group managements did try to enforce standardisation within a limited area, but for the most part 'general issue' was of poor quality and uninspired, tending to support the idea that nursing was lowly regarded. Uniform had a psychological as well as a practical significance, with letters on the subject occupying much space in the nursing press, where unfavourable comparisons were made with the uniforms of the services of the Crown and indeed the individual uniforms of pre-war days.

THE UPGRADING OF HOSPITALS

Many groups inherited buildings still used for the able-bodied under Part III of the National Assistance Act. The chronic sick, who lacked interest for the medical profession, had always been unfavourably treated, but now their plight had worsened due to wartime shortages and evacuation. These prison-like buildings with their steep stone steps, high barred windows and dreary airing courts were quite unsuitable as hospitals, and to make matters worse, because of the stigma attached to the Poor Law, many were on the outskirts of the town, which made visiting difficult, and the patients, whose needs were often more social than medical, were made even more isolated. Perhaps the greatest benefit bestowed by the National Health Service during its formative years was the fact that it revealed this hitherto largely hidden, and conveniently forgotten, problem.

The situation called for a radical solution. With advances in medical science and increasing longevity, a new system for the chronic elderly sick was called for with properly dispersed small units firmly linked with the community health and social services in each neighbourhood. But a new system would cost money and the now rising estimates for the health service were under attack. Reluctantly, group committees prepared to spend ingenuity and money on these solid, grey, cheerless, nineteenth-century buildings. Laminated plastic partitions, cretonne curtains, coloured counterpanes and pastel-coloured paint transformed the overall drabness, while deodorants and potted plants masked the smell until new methods of treatment did much to remove the cause.

Improving the hospitals for the chronic sick meant a large increase in nursing staff, and it was the attempt to meet this need that put a new strain on nursing so that the shortage continued even when recruitment rose. The need had always been there but until the hospitals were grouped the disparities were not obvious and one answer to the question, 'How many nurses do we need?' was 'More than we thought'. It was in the chronic sick hospitals that the first assistant nurses made their notable contribution, for they were often the first trained nurses at the bedside that the patients had known, and for this reason those with responsibilities for such hospitals opposed any suggestion for closing the roll. The other factor affecting the demand for nurses was the increase in medical knowledge. The new geriatricians prescribed active and positive régimes, surgery was attempted at ages hitherto thought impossible and new drugs altered the prognosis for many bedridden patients. It was soon clear that 'treating the back-log' did not lead to vistas of health, but to more patients requiring treatment in higher age groups, and the greater the age the more exacting the nursing.

THE CONTROL OF SALARIES AND CONDITIONS OF SERVICE

A first essential of the new service was an agreed national salary scale and conditions of service for all employees. Before the war hospitals had been free to fix their own salaries and in fact bid against one another for scarce resources. During the war agreements like the Rushcliffe scale for nurses, and the Hetherington for domestics, brought some uniformity, but now all freedom was surrendered and national negotiating machinery extended to cover the whole service. The formula agreed was that instituted in the First World War under the chairmanship of John Whitley, the Speaker of the House, and used by the Civil Service since 1920.

The Whitley Councils of the Health Service were set up in 1949 and consisted of a General Council and nine functional councils (Figure 16.l). The General Council dealt with conditions of service as a whole and the functional Councils with salaries and conditions peculiar to particular groups. Each Council consisted of a management side appointed by the Minister after consultation with interested bodies, and a staff side of representatives from employee organisations chosen by the Minister. In 1948 Aneurin Bevan made it clear that 'While persons employed in the National Health Service would not be required, as a condition of service, to belong to a Trade Union or a Professional Organisation, it was hoped that employees would be encouraged to join their appropriate organisation'.[4] For many nurses this was something new, as in the past management had often frowned on employee organisations, or had decided to which organisations their employees would belong and they would acknowledge.

THE NURSES AND MIDWIVES WHITLEY COUNCIL

The staff side remained much the same as with the Rushcliffe Committee in England and the Guthrie for Scotland, with the professional organisations holding the majority of seats. Nurses, being mostly women, were not

GENERAL WHITLEY COUNCIL

Administrative and clerical	Auxiliary	Dental	Medical hosp. dental	Nurses and midwives	Optical	Pharmaceutical	Professional & technical A	Professional & technical B
MS17 SS33	MS19 SS16	MS9 SS12	MS19 SS21	MS22 SS29	MS22 SS27	MS19 SS26	MS20 SS25	MS20 SS21
Admin. Clerical staff in hospitals; Officers of RHB HMC BG Executive Councils	Domestic and analogous staff	Dental Officers employed by local authorities	Hospital medical staff; Medical staff of local authorities	Nurses and midwives in NHS and employed by local authorities; Some auxiliary grades	Ophthalmic or Dispensing opticians in NHS or employed by local authorities	Pharmacists in NHS & employed by local authorities	Social workers; Biochemists; Occ. therapists; Orthoptists; Physiotherapists Psychiatric social workers; Psychologists; Radiographers; etc.	Technicians Engineers

Composition of Management Side

RHB England Wales	4
RHB Scotland	1
Assoc. Hospital Management Committees	2
Boards of Governors of Teaching Hospitals	2
Boards of Management, Scotland	1
Association Municipal Corporations	2
County Councils Association	2
Inner London Education Authority	1
Scottish Local Authority Associations	2
Scottish Home & Health Dept.	1
Welsh Office	1
Department of Health and Social Security	3

*Negotiating Committee Organisation

Composition of Staff Side

*Association of Nurse Administrators	1
The Association of Hospital and Residential Care Officers	1
Association of Supervisors of Midwives	1
*Confederation of Health Service Employees	4
*Health Visitors' Association	2
National and Local Government Officers Association	2
*National Union of General and Municipal Workers	1
*National Union of Public Employees	4
*Royal College of Midwives	3
*Royal College of Nursing	8
Scottish Association of Senior Hospital Nursing Officers	1
Scottish Health Visitors' Association	1

N.B. Seats reduced later

Figure 16.1 Structure of the General Whitley Council

organisation-minded, but the minority who were joiners subscribed to a wide variety, and for this reason the staff side was large with 41 seats distributed between six professional organisations and six trade unions. This led to difficulties on the staff side, and there were rivalries about the allocation of seats which were not secured by membership alone but allowed for a number of other factors. There were also difficulties about the management side. The hospitals were under-represented compared with the local authorities, which were now not important as employers of nurses; but, more important, the ministry itself had five seats with the secretariat drawn from full-time officials who were in the position of being able to put pressure on the whole management side. Moreover, as the Minister appointed the members of the Regional Boards, pressure could be applied to those who stepped out of line.

With the first salary review of 1949, the Nurses and Midwives Whitley Council faced urgent problems. Staff had been transferred with a wide range of salaries and conditions which had to be fused into an equitable national scale. At the same time inflation, the new insurance contributions and income tax had eroded the wartime gains and there was considerable unrest particularly among student nurses. The problem was more complicated than a straightforward review. It was not only what nurses were paid, but *how* they were paid. Traditionally, hospital nurses 'lived in' and were paid a net salary with their emoluments valued at a nominal sum for superannuation purposes, so although the net salary looked absurdly low, in a period when rents outside were rising steeply, it was more valuable than appeared; nurses' pay defied comparison with other groups and 'emoluments' were over- or under-valued according to the standpoint-of the advocate. All this confused the public and sometimes the nurses themselves, but the reluctance to accept a gross salary suggests that in some cases there were delusions of poverty not justified by fact; much of course depended on the endowment of the nurses' home.

Both the management and staff sides wanted to change the system. Management wanted to encourage living out because there was not enough accommodation and there was an embargo on capital building; also earlier marriage and the new tendency of undertakings to employ married women[5] made it imperative that nursing be seen as an occupation compatible with domestic life. Professional organisations wanted to see nursing as parallel with occupations like teaching and this could only happen if salaries and expectations were seen to be comparable.

The first problem was the pay of students. The Wood Committee had recommended that student nurses should receive a training allowance and the report was awaiting parliamentary time. The Horder Committee had insisted that there must be a separation of the finance for nursing education, and the professional organisations were hopeful that nurse training would be put on a new footing and were fearful of anything that would jeopardise the discussions. The trade unions were concerned with practical issues; with student nurses as part of the labour force the low pay they received had the effect of holding down the wages of auxiliaries, and apart from the casuistry about the value of training there was the old problem of the low pay of women holding back the pay of men. Moreover, both sides had a vested interest in recruitment; if the student nurses became 'students' they would not be eligible for union membership; but if they remained 'employees' then the Student Nurses' Association was not a negotiating body and pressure could be put on them to join a union.

After a number of meetings it was concluded that nurses in training were students and they should be paid a training allowance, but it was a Pyrrhic victory with each side making words mean what they wanted them to mean and the students getting the worst of both worlds. The 'training allowance' was raised to £200 per year, which was £50 below the average wage of a manual worker: was this the value of the training? The whole 'allowance' was subject to insurance and superannuation deductions, and consequently the student nurse was not a true student and was debarred from the usual student privileges and contacts. The anomaly was brought forcibly home because since the Butler Act grants for further education had increased, and student nurses saw those who had left school with them obtaining grants for trainings that were apparently no more demanding than nursing.

In reviewing the rest of the scales the Council had a daunting task. Because they had always been poorly paid, nurses fought for small, complicated differentials; there were 250 scales in the consolidated Rushcliffe recommendations, with £750 as the highest salary for a matron with a hospital of over 1,000 beds, and the first-year student with £175 a year. In the hospital service alone there were 170 different grades packed within a range of £600 a year.[6] The objective of the staff side was to get the best increases and preserve the differentials that had been widened by Rushcliffe with the ward sister getting twice the pay of a student. Negotiations were protracted by a 'wages standstill' in 1950, and when the review was completed percentage increases were calculated on *net* salaries, which narrowed the differential and set a pattern that it was difficult to change.

Apart from reviewing all salaries when wages were frozen, there was the problem of fusing the two services and arranging superannuation transfers and options which were in fact very complicated. Before the National Health Service, many conditions were discretionary; now regulations had to be drafted to ensure that they were uniform and yet the existing staff safeguarded. Even the number of days allowed for compassionate leave, to see which relatives and for how long, were covered by precise regulation, and although uniformity brought a better deal for many, the situation was confusing, and as the regulations multiplied, fewer people understood them.

THE NURSES' ACT 1949

This Act put the legal stamp on nursing at the beginning of the health service. Although the Minority Report and the lack of enthusiasm for the Wood Report by the nursing profession had vitiated the recommendations of the Wood Report, they were finally debated in Parliament in April 1949. The debate agreed that the educational needs of student nurses were being subordinated to the service needs of the hospitals, but the government equivocated about giving the financial aid which the recommendations would require. The Bill, while paying lip-service to the need for a 'more radical and long-term solution', proposed instead a cautious updating of the present syllabus – words which echo down 30 years to the Rt. Hon. Patrick Jenkins and the 'need for more time for consultation' – presumably about that long-term goal agreed so long ago.[7]

The General Nursing Councils retained their previous powers and the English Council was enlarged to 34 members, half appointed by the Minister and the other 17 elected by nurses themselves; 14 from Regional Boards and 3 representing nursing specialities – and there was a new proviso that the Council members should be in active nursing. Other clauses provided for the reopening of the Register for persons who had previously failed to make application. The Register itself was still divided into parts but 'the part of the Register for Male Nurses' was closed and the Council was given the power to close other parts and did in fact finally close the Register for Fever Nurses in 1966.

Neither the government nor the profession had the united will nor the means to promote radical change, but a sop to Cerberus was offered in the form of the opportunity for 'experimental schemes of training'. The General Nursing Councils set up Area Nurse Training Committees which were empowered to initiate experiments in nurse training. In many ways the power was meaningless because, while the student was the main labour force, little real change was possible; the illusion of independence given to schools of nursing by financing them through Area Committees was not matched by reality. Nevertheless, there was experimentation and a number of schemes combining more than one training were implemented, early examples being the integrated schemes to include General Training and the Health Visitor Course between St Thomas's Hospital and the University of Southampton, and Crumpsall Hospital, Manchester, and the University of Manchester. There were a number of variations on the theme of combining two parts of the Register and by 1959 there were over 20 experimental courses.[8] The success of these schemes at least showed that there was much overlap in the different trainings and that some of the barriers between the different branches of nursing were unnecessary, and, given a higher standard of selection, many students could cope with a more comprehensive course.

In 10 years the nursing profession had probably been subjected to more change than in the previous 50. It was now clear that a kind of Malthusian law was going to operate with the public demand for nursing service increasing faster than ever nursing resource could hope to grow. Trying to resolve the conflict between demand and resource was going to be the main philosophical concern of the nursing profession during the next 40 years.

In the last analysis, much of the reaction to a reform of nursing education was bound up in the attitudes to the health service. In 1946 many people associated with the voluntary system were resentful about the loss of autonomy for individual hospitals, and in the massed chorus of protest the suggestion that nurse training might be removed was seen as another manifestation of bureaucratic interference. Moreover, nurses themselves, while generally sympathetic to the aims of the health service, were often fiercely attached to their training hospital. The more militant students who had demonstrated in Whitehall about their pay showed by their letters to the nursing press that they were by no means sure that they wanted to exchange their martyr's crown for the freedom offered by Sir Robert Wood.

REFERENCES

1 *Beveridge Report* (1942), Social and Allied Services Cmnd. 6404, London: HMSO, p. 437.
2 Office of Population Censuses and Surveys (1975) St Catherine's House, London: HMSO.
3 *The Internal Administration of Hospitals* (1954). Report by a Committee of the Central Health Services Council, London: HMSO.
4 Rt Hon. Aneurin Bevan (1948) *Hansard*, 29 Jan.
5 *Report on Pensionability of Unestablished Civil Service Parliamentary Papers*, Appendix XII, Cmnd. 6942, (1945–6) London: HMSO.
6 *Nurses Salaries Committee Consolidated Recommendations*, (1947) London: HMSO.
7 Vaughan, G. (1979) Letter from Health Minister to the General Nursing Council, 2 Aug., *Nursing Times*, 16 Aug. p. 1,380.
8 General Nursing Council (1959–60), *Annual Report*, Appendix B; Experimental Schemes approved under Section 12 (I) of the Nurses Act 1957, p. 30.

FURTHER READING

Annual Reports of the DHSS (then the Ministry of Health) 1948–60. Forsyth, G. (1973) *Doctors and State Medicine*, London: Pitman.

Chapter 17

New demands on nursing

Although the architects of the National Health Service had envisaged a comprehensive and unified service, it was in fact a conglomerate of sectarian interests and a compromise between competing demands. The service was rather like three old houses that have been joined together but have kept their dividing walls, whose inhabitants only communicate with one another through the distant landlord. The strain on the structure was made worse by the new demands for care and the fact that the services were unequally distributed, for the mortality and morbidity patterns were the same as in Chadwick's day,[1] and the health service made no provision for their redistribution. The other problem was that it was an 'illness' service with the most prestigious part of the building occupied by the hospital services whose mechanistic philosophy dominated all policy and expenditure.

However, although compromise had been the only way out in 1945, the service was soon under attack, and as early as 1951 speakers at conferences were suggesting that Regional Boards were unnecessary and the priorities for health care were wrong.

THE CENTRAL HEALTH SERVICES COUNCIL

This Council, set up under Part I of the National Health Service Act had a number of standing committees advising on all aspects of the service. The reports of these committees indicate the subjects for discussion and what seemed in the 1950s the appropriate solutions, and it will be observed that many of the problems besetting the 1990s were already being discussed 40 years ago.

In 1952 the Central Council urged the need 'to secure closer and more lively co-operation between the branches of the service'[2] and because this was so pressing the Council issued a separate report on the need to set up a network of joint liaison committees. It was quickly made clear to the Council that more committees would not be welcome, and in 1953 the Council advised the government to set up a Committee of Enquiry into the Cost of the National Health Service to make recommendations and modifications 'such that a rising charge can be avoided while providing an adequate service'. The committee, under the chairmanship of Mr C. W. Guillebaud, had little room in which to manoeuvre because with every year that passed the health service was lifting the iceberg of hidden sickness further out of the water. The committee, aware of the structural defect of the service, examined the possibility of setting up *ad hoc* Health Committees, or of reverting to the keystone of the old Minority Report and placing the health services under the local authorities. Conscious of the disturbance of the former, and the fact that there was no hope of the medical profession accepting the latter, the committee concluded that a service now costing over £400 million a year must be accountable to the responsible minister, and bowing to the inevitable, pronounced that the structure laid down was on 'broadly sound lines'.[3] One member of the committee, Sir John Maud, dissented and was of the opinion that if local government were reformed it might be possible to transfer local responsibility for health matters to the new authorities – a point made by Beatrice Webb in 1909.

The economic advisers to the committee, Professors R. Titmuss and B. Abel-Smith, pointed out that in spite of the rising cost of the service expressed in terms of the gross national product, it had in reality fallen. No change was suggested about the way the service was financed nor about the provision of private or amenity beds, but the economic report threw a surprising light on the users of the service, for, contrary to popular belief that the service was now dealing with untreated sickness in those previously denied care, it was shown that men between 26 and 64 years old in social groups I, II and III were making full use of the service, while Groups IV and V, in spite of their higher mortality rates, used the service less – in other words, it was the middle classes who used the service. Moreover, in spite of the changing demographic profile, a higher proportion of cost was devoted to the under-15 age group than to those over 65 years old; figures that should have made it clear that the service was not sufficiently accessible to those with the greatest need.[4]

The Guillebaud report singled out the midwifery service for special enquiry because it was the most affected by the divisions in the service; the lying-in woman came under the care of all three services and not infrequently suffered from the lack of communication between the services. The enquiry into the Organisation of the Maternity Services under the chairmanship of the Earl of Cranbrook is important because it dictated the future of midwifery training.

By 1957, 64 per cent of all births were taking place in hospital but the percentage varied widely between regions, with those in the greatest need getting the poorest service. The committee recommended increasing hospital confinements to 70 per cent in all regions, and to do this it was necessary to provide more maternity beds and midwives in hospitals. Before the war 60 per cent of births took place in the home, so there were proportionally more domiciliary midwives for whom the new policy would mean less work – although since the Midwives Act of 1936 which established a salaried service, few remained as private practitioners. To overcome the problem the committee recommended that 'some could be persuaded to return to hospital until interchangeability could be made a condition of service'.[5] The writing was on the wall for the domiciliary midwife. The committee examined the possibility of a single maternity service, but came to the conclusion that it would be impractical to have one unified service as an island in the tripartite sea.

While the Cranbrook Committee was deliberating, another committee was looking at the care of children in hospital. New ideas about the effect of deprivation on children and the work of pioneers like Dr John Bowlby caused paediatricians and others to consider the harm done to children when separated from their parents by admission to hospital, and the enquiry, *The Welfare of Children in Hospital*, under the chairmanship of Sir Harry Platt, became a landmark in the care of children. The Report, published in 1959, recommended that hospital care should only be used as a last resource – thus, of course, making the nursing of children in hospital more intensive, and all children should be nursed in special units under the supervision of a sick children's nurse and a paediatrician. In order to meet the mental and emotional needs of children parents should be encouraged to visit at all times and to help with the nursing, and children should be allowed to bring and keep their favourite toys. For many nurses these recommendations ran counter to their training where the first consideration had been the avoidance of infection. Now old notions of hygiene and isolation had to be superseded by a new understanding of child psychology, and, above all, nurses had to learn to understand their own emotional attitudes to children and their own natural desire to gain a child's affection. All this had important implications for nurse training – psychology had to oust hygiene.

This report threw up another problem. The Wood Report said that a nurse could be trained in two years and practise *in any speciality*; now it was being suggested that children should only be nursed by those who had undergone a rigorous and special training. Moreover, any idea that such a training was not necessary was further dispelled by the realisation that the frail children, once so easily killed, now survived to need more specialised care. The better midwifery postulated by the Cranbrook Committee would mean that premature and handicapped babies would survive to require intensive treatment. Everything was moving towards a new intensity and specialisation of nursing care.

Another problem considered by the Central Health Services Council was the reception of in-patients in hospital. The report, originally produced by the Scottish Council in 1953, was subsequently adopted in England and recommended to all hospitals. The traditional reception of patients in hospital had evolved out of the requirements and attitudes of charity and the Poor Law, and in spite of modifications it was often outmoded. The Report recommended giving the patient as much information as possible before admission, and on arrival a leaflet containing a description of the hospital, its routine and welfare services, the names of the chief officers and an explanation as to who should be contacted about what. Other proposals included better signposting, more flexible visiting times, later waking of patients, improved facilities for ambulant patients and better arrangements for patients and their relatives to contact the sister and the doctor in charge of the case. Finally, the recommendation which subsequent research showed to be neglected, 'that there should be good liaison between the hospital and the patient's own doctor who should be informed as soon as possible of his discharge'.[6] If these recommendations were carried out it meant that greater social skills were being demanded of nurses and added responsibility for giving information.

THE DISABLED PERSON

The problem of crippling was not going to fade away as people had prophesied. Now the child with Pott's kyphosis was being replaced by the adult with the intervertebral disc lesion and the older person with arthritis. Consideration was now given to the idea of a separate service for the disabled, and in 1953 the government set up a committee under the chairmanship of Lord Piercy, 'to review and make recommendations on all aspects of rehabilitation and resettlement of disabled persons'. The Disabled Persons (Employment) Act of 1944 and school health regulations had set out to give continual care to the disabled, and centres of rehabilitation like Roffey Park had been set up but the service remained uncoordinated. The Piercy recommendations are important, because yet again emphasis was placed on intensive care and the need for special staff with particular skills, and again there was a call to plan a continuum of care which was made more difficult because of the divisions in the health service. Many parts of the Report, such as the training of resettlement officers, the better use of the Disabled Person's Register and the need for local authorities to play an active part in helping with structural alterations and appliances, found their way into later legislation, such as the Chronically Sick and Disabled Persons Act of 1970, which required the new social services departments of the local authorities to meet the needs of handicapped persons and to provide, or give assistance in obtaining, certain services. Section 4 of this Act made it mandatory for local authorities to ensure that public buildings allowed access to the disabled. New attitudes to rehabilitation, especially in the elderly, had implications for nurses in hospital, but they also brought new responsibilities to the district nursing service and to the health visitor, who needed to be aware of the increasing range of help and appliances available to disabled people.

ADAPTING NURSING TO NEW NEEDS

Meanwhile, as the result of reports, articles in the nursing press, conferences and meetings, the nursing profession was looking for ways of improving nursing care and making better use of the nursing manpower, which statisticians were warning could not be much expanded. People began to question some of the hallowed ward routines and tasks allocated according to rank, and although the apprenticeship system does not readily produce iconoclasts, once the questioning started it gathered momentum and many time-honoured practices were discarded; beds were no longer made and temperatures recorded twice a day as routine, and with the shorter patient stay the blanket bath book went into the waste paper basket. With visiting at all times the ward became more informal and mundane with the television news replacing evening prayers. Physiotherapists, technicians, occupational therapists, the library, the shop, students doing a thesis, work-study experts all made the ward noisier, and often dirtier. Now nurses began to question the wisdom of trying to nurse patients with varying degrees of dependency in one area, and was not trying to do so a waste of skill.

Progressive patient care

The nature of the hospital was changing, as Dr Cohen had predicted. On the one hand, new knowledge and technology like heart lung machines, respirators and dialysis made it possible to save lives that would have been lost and to operate where before surgery would have been impossible. On the other hand, the rising cost meant that it was imperative that the patient's stay was short; rapid bed turnover was already the administrator's talisman in measuring health care. But different types of patients needed different amounts of care, and in America attempts were being made to measure nursing activity and dependency.[7] The logical conclusion was that expensive equipment be placed together and patients with a high dependency nursed as a group in one area by a high ratio of trained staff. When the patients no longer needed intensive care they could progress to medium care and then to self-care. However, by the time the hospitals had prepared their plans, a new philosophy was developing about the effects of hospitalisation and this, together with the escalating costs, ensured that self-care units were never developed.

The idea of 'progressive care' was not new; hospitals had often separated their very ill patients and in the armed service, because of the low ratio of trained staff, and the fact that servicemen often remained in hospital longer than civilians, there had always been a system of progressive care with the ill patients nursed by the trained staff. However, this system of nursing raised problems for nurse training, for it was agreed that in the interests of the patients and the students themselves, nurses in training should not be sent to intensive-care units as part of the workforce. Increasingly, there were areas where the student could not just 'learn on the job' as the price of error was too great. The new 'technical' nurse clearly needed more knowledge about what she was doing and *why* she was doing it than could be picked up in the routine work of the wards, and the classroom was still divorced from the ward situation. But as the potentialities of intensive care were realised further specialities like 'coronary care' and 'renal care' were developed, for which nursing staff needed special training and skills. For many years this need was met by various specialist units offering courses, but these were uncontrolled and some were of doubtful value, and eventually after much pressure from the Royal College of Nursing the Joint Board of Clinical Studies was set up in 1970.

Patient and team assignment

While hospitals were developing 'progressive patient care', the profession was discussing patient assignment and its modification, team assignment. Hospitals with favourable staffing ratios had always attempted to allocate patients to particular nurses, but generally it was a practice more honoured in the breach than the observance; in a crisis job allocation was quicker. Moreover, the idea that the *nature of the task defines the status of the worker* was deeply ingrained in the hospital world with its roots in the nineteenth-century work philosophy. Studies in Scandinavia and America showed that job allocation in fact gave the student little work satisfaction, and in its policy statement in 1956 the Royal College of Nursing developed the theory of *team nursing* and called for more investigation and research into the subject.[8] But although it was much discussed, many things militated against the development of team assignment. First, intensive-care units seemed to make the problem less urgent, for when the patient's needs were greatest he was nursed by a team. Second, there was still hostility to the assistant nurse, and the insecurity of the student nurse, inter-professional rivalries and antagonisms all operated against the team concept. Third, repeated financial cuts and staff shortages meant a reversion to task allocation for the sake of speed. Finally, in many cases the will was not there, and those who aspired to higher status had no wish to return to the sluice.

The patient's day

The pattern of ward work was a legacy from pre-war institutions with routines dictated by the early rising habits of most hospital patients, the working times of hospital cleaners, and the times when the doctors, who were honorary, could fit in their ward rounds and operating sessions. When the doctors and nurses were the only footsteps of ones that disturbed the ward, suitably rubber-heeled, this early waking did not matter because the patients usually had two hours' undisturbed rest in the afternoon. Now, as Miss Muriel Powell* put it succinctly, 'there is no rest in the patient's day', and it was becoming an irony that patients needed to be fit to stand a spell in hospital. In 1958 the Central Health Services Council set up a working party with Miss Powell as chairman to study the pattern of the in-patient's day. The committee in its report expressed concern at the lengthening of the patient's day and pointed out that the routine no longer reflected the mores of the world outside and, as far as possible, life in hospital should be arranged along the lines of the patient's home life – a statement that foreshadows the philosophy of the nursing process. Early morning bed-making should not begin before 7 a.m. and the patient should have at least an hour and a half of undisturbed rest in the day.[9] Nearly 20 years later a survey of patients' attitudes to the hospital services shows that the main complaint is that they are woken too early, 44 per cent of the survey before 6 a.m.[10] Reports come and go, but there seems to be some ineluctable reason why hospital patients will always be wakened with the first streak of dawn.

Noise in hospitals

Another cause for rising concern was the increase in noise in hospitals. Hospitals with notices outside saying 'Hospital, Quiet Please' became a cartoon joke, and with more staff, visitors and noisy equipment Miss Nightingale's dictum that 'unnecessary noise is the most cruel absence of care that can be inflicted on either the sick or the well', seemed forgotten. On the advice of the Nursing Advisory Committee, the Ministry eventually issued a circular on control of noise in hospitals[11] which was largely based on a survey conducted by the King Edward Hospital Fund in 1957 and followed up two years later. The follow-up showed that some progress was being made with regard to equipment, but there were still complaints about noise from other patients and a number of complaints about the noise made by nurses.

The night duty span

Linked with the pattern of the patient's day was the question of the work load carried by the night staff, especially at the end of their duty span. Attitudes to night duty had grown up when patients who were post-operative stayed in bed for three weeks and medical patients were

* Dame Muriel Powell, 1970; died 1978.

probably bed-fast for six weeks. Since nature and authority dislike a vacuum, the time of the night nurse was fully occupied making dressings, cleaning equipment, testing urine, doing the flowers or any other task that might be suggested. Now that the wards were no longer full of semi-convalescent patients and the new therapy tended to be continuous throughout the night, there was a call for a reappraisal of the numbers and seniority of night staff. In 1959 the Royal College of Nursing published a report on *The Problem of Providing Continuous Nursing Service Especially in Relation to Night Duty*, which was issued to employing authorities. The report urged that ward routines should be rearranged so that the night duty span of 12 hours was genuinely reduced and that no nurse should spend unduly long periods on night duty with the inevitable professional and social isolation it entailed, and although there was a case for leaving a third-year student in charge of a ward, all students on night duty must be properly supervised and supported. Again, in the interests of safety and of the students themselves, limitations were being suggested to the use of student labour. However, it was not until 1972, when the 40-hour week was introduced and extra payment for night duty made more realistic that the night staff made any real gains. Then, ironically, they were the first to be cut during periods of retrenchment because they were comparatively expensive.

WORK STUDY AND THE NURSING PROFESSION

Dr Cohen had said, 'we must ask what is the function of the hospital before enquiring what is the function of the nurse', and he pointed out that if custodial care gave way to more positive treatment the duties of the nurse, and her training requirement, would be that much transformed.

This was happening in almost all forms of nursing, and it seemed reasonable to ask the question again. In trying to show, a priori, that value could be placed on nursing 'productivity', the Wood Committee had done a tentative 'job analysis', but this only showed what the nurse was actually doing; what it did not show, and could not show, was what the nurses *should* be doing to meet the needs of the community.

In 1948 the Ministry of Health asked the Nuffield Provincial Hospitals Trust to set up an advisory panel to carry out a complete job analysis of the work of the nurse and other members of the hospital team in order to obtain the necessary data so that an answer can be given to the fundamental question, 'What is the proper task of the nurse?' For practical reasons, the terms of reference were changed so that the unit became not the hospital but the ward. *The Work of Nurses in Hospital Wards*, which was published in 1953, has since been criticised for its research methods and the conclusions it drew from the data gathered; the survey was, however, breaking new ground and subsequent research benefited from the fact that the soil had been turned over. The value of the report lay not so much in its findings, which the observant could have predicted, nor in its conclusion – 'no mere statement of fact can bridge the gap between the present and the proper task of the nurse' – which was hardly a revelation; but in the fact that Mr Goddard and his team sold the scientific method with missionary zeal: things would never be the same again. Conferences were arranged up and down the country, and although some audiences were hostile and denied the fact that students received as little as seven minutes' ward teaching a week and that much bedside care was given without supervision, few quarrelled with the findings that nursing was impeded because of lack of equipment and the shortages of such simple things as matches.

The Nuffield analysis introduced nurses to the mysteries of flow and string charts, and some, fired with enthusiasm, trained as work-study officers themselves, and Regional Hospital Boards started to employ work study teams which in turn produced their own surveys. The other value of the analysis was that it dispelled some of the fallacies cherished by the public, and nurses themselves, not least of which was that the student nurse spent her time on domestic duties. Although the profession had a long way to go before it was research-minded, a start had been made.

CHANGING STAFF RELATIONSHIPS

There is no doubt that the nursing profession had a poor image as far as personal relationships were concerned. Every report, especially those concerned with wastage, seemed to carry an appendix of letters from those claiming to have left because of 'petty discipline'. Letters from the dissaffected do not constitute historical evidence unless they are properly balanced; moreover, the wastage rate, although higher than for women in further education (which nursing was not), was lower than for most women's occupations.[12] However, there were reasons why authoritarian attitudes existed and why they were now resented. First, like the army, crisis tends to be normal, and the operating theatre and the battlefield are notorious for not lending themselves to sweet reason. Second, the ratio of trained staff to untrained was low, and simple authoritive rules had to do duty for leisurely supervision, but perhaps more important, the process of democracy was delayed because technical knowledge advanced with such rapidity that each generation was stranded on the beach of its own insecurity, and insecurity breeds aggression. This situation did not apply to nurses alone; the whole health team, including administrators and doctors, were stranded on the same beach as they were swamped with new ideas that often ran counter to their training and education. One of the effects of insecurity was to specialise. As Richard Titmuss put it, 'the generalist occupies a world of uncertainty and it is safer (and easier) to specialise than generalise'.[13]

As specialisms increased, this created problems of communication, and as each new group carved out its career and status pattern so the organisational pattern and the chain of command became more complicated. There were now supervisors and their deputies for catering, domestic services, engineering, supplies and the pharmacy services, each with their own hierarchical ordering, and while at ward level clerks and ward hostesses may have saved nursing time there were now more people to be co-ordinated, to have their off duty arranged, to go off sick and to have personal problems that needed a listening ear.

Within 10 years of the inception of the health service public demand and new thinking on all aspects of care, from intensive-care units to geriatric departments, were moving faster than staff could be adequately prepared for, even had there been an investment in staff education; without this investment staff had to prepare themselves as best they could. The fact that many did adapt and meet the new challenge was a tribute to innate resilience in nursing which may owe something to the early, versatile, and sometimes maligned, training where nurses performed a multiplicity of tasks, many of which were non-nursing.

REFERENCES

1 Chadwick, S. E. (1842) *Report on the Sanitary Condition of the Labouring Population of Great Britain* Edinburgh: Edinburgh University Press.
2 *Central Health Services Report for the Year Ending 1951* (1952) London: HMSO, p. 3.
3 *The Report of the Committee of Enquiry into the Cost of the National Health Service* (the Guillebaud Report) (1956) London: HMSO.
4 Abel-Smith, B. and Titmuss, R. (1957) *The Cost of the National Health Service in England and Wales*, Cambridge: Cambridge University Press.
5 *The Report of the Maternity Services Committee* (the Cranbrook Report) (1959) London: HMSO.
6 *Reception and Welfare of In-patients in Hospitals in Edinburgh* (1951) London: HMSO.
7 Abdellah, F. G. (1955) 'Let the patients tell us where we fail', *Modern Hospital*, 85: Abdellah, F. G. and Levine, E. (1957) 'Developing a measure of patient and personnel satisfaction', *Nursing Research*, 5, New York.
8 Royal College of Nursing (1956) *Observations and Objectives,* London, p. 5.
9 The Pattern of the In-patient's Day (1961) Report by a sub-committee of the Standing Nursing Advisory Committee.
10 *Royal Commission on the National Health Service*, (1969) Research paper submitted by the Social Survey division of the Office of Population Censuses and Surveys (Janet Gregory), reported in *Nursing Times*, 25 Jan. 1979.
11 King Edward Fund for London (1960) *Noise Control in Hospitals*, report of a follow-up enquiry; also HM Circular (61) 68.
12 *The Committee on Nursing* (Briggs Report) (1972) London: HMSO.
13 Titmuss, R. M. (1968) *Commitment to Welfare*, London: George Allen & Unwin, p. 208.

Chapter 18

Who will nurse the patients of tomorrow?

> Some confusion has been caused by differences in the interpretation of the title 'nurse'. The term has been used rather loosely in the tables previously supplied by the Department, and in fact covers all grades from nursing auxiliary and nursing assistant upwards.
>
> Extract from a letter from the Ministry of Health
> (Statistics), June 1963

If there was confusion at the Ministry of Health about who should be recorded as a nurse it was little wonder that official spokesmen, including the Minister himself, often gave misleading answers about nursing manpower.[1] Apart from the muddle over the title 'nurse', in an attempt to improve the statistics there had been different arrangements and presentation of the figures every year or two and it was impossible for an investigator to compare like with like. In 1948 Dr Cohen said, 'the statistical resources of the Ministry of Health are lamentable',[2] and even by 1962 they were still often meaningless. One of the difficulties lay in the fact that part-time staff were not shown as whole-time equivalents (wte) until the mid-1960s, and no one knew how many staff were doing four hours a week and how many 40 hours. Later, in an effort to make a comparison with earlier years, an equation of two part-time staff equalling one full-time worker was used, but this was only an estimate and could be misleading when comparing grades, and areas, where part-time working was high compared with those where it was low. Other problems arose over the inclusion, or exclusion, of midwives, or of pupils subsumed in the total, and the double count where 'home nurses' were also midwives, or even the triple count where they were also health visitors, or the fact that the number of sessions that counted as a full-time consultant changed in 1972. Nevertheless, such figures as are available do indicate certain trends, even though every tabulation should carry an official warning and this warning continues into the 1990s.

THE CHANGING NURSING TEAM

In 1962, which is a suitable mid-point at which to examine these trends and the effect of the health service on nursing, the number of 'nurses', full and part-time, had risen from 148,336 in 1950 to 213,132 – an increase of 40 per cent – which, even allowing for a heavier work load, might look as if all was well. On closer analysis, however, it was obvious that the composition of the team was changing: a trend had been set in train, which, if continued, raised doubts about the answer to the question posed by the editor of the *Nursing Times*, 'Who will nurse the patients of tomorrow?' In 12 years the proportion of auxiliaries had risen from 16.6 to 24.3 per cent of the total, and the proportion of registered nurses had fallen from 46.5 to 42.1 per cent, and although in 1962 the proportion of learners was slightly down, until then they had been the same as in the 1930s – about 35 per cent of the total (Table 18.1). Perhaps more significant for those who supervised the team was the fact that part-time staff had risen from 18 to 26 per cent. In 1950, before nursing became so intensive, roughly 70,000 trained nurses supervised some 80,000 untrained staff; in 1962 it was 93,000 trained staff supervising 123,000 untrained.[3]

From the point of view of manpower there was a strain on two counts; first, grateful though the service was to part-time staff, they created administrative difficulties especially when the times the staff were available did not fit in with the needs of the patients. Second, the team was more complex, with a wider range of ability and understanding, and this took more time and skill to organise. But apart from the changing pattern of the ward team, there were other factors which did not appear in the parliamentary answers. The working week had decreased to 44 hours, holidays had been lengthened; in fact, the value of the manpower figures could be reduced by 10 per cent compared with 1950, and above all, but difficult to quantify, was the changing value of student labour – *a third of the total nursing force*. In 1962, after years of striving, the General Nursing Council had reintroduced an educational test for candidates for the General Register (but not the Mental Register), and a new and more demanding syllabus was introduced. Although the student was still cheap labour, training demands were increasing year by year, and even though no one was sure how much time was taken up with 'education', the time was coming when the student could no longer be regarded as the main labour force of the wards; this, however, was how the student nurse was shown on the manpower returns.

There were other anxieties about the manpower situation. During the early years of the service, in order to deal with the post-war shortages, there had been a deliberate drive to recruit candidates from overseas, and

Table 18.1 Nursing staff in hospitals (England and Wales)

Grade	1937 Number	% of total	Grade	1950 Number	% of total	Grade	1962 Number	% of total
Registered	39,668	39.0	Registered } Enrolled }	46,985 16,595	46.5	Registered } Enrolled }	64,135 13,772*	42.1
Students	35,781	37.0	Students } Pupils }	48,713 2,248	36.9	Students } Pupils }	55,066 7,277	33.6
Other nursing staff (inc. assistant nurses)	25,577	23.1	Auxiliaries	23,339	16.6	Auxiliaries	45,059	24.3

* Lower figure for enrolled is accounted for by the increase in the number of part time ENs

Source: Returns to the Inter-Departmental Committee, 1937, quoted by B. Abel-Smith in A History of the Nursing Profession

Source: Ministry of Health Returns. For the sake of comparison an estimate is made of the manpower value of part-time staff by calculating 2 pt as 1 wte

Note: The figure for ENs remained almost the same from 1949 to 1964

in the period 1959 to 1965 the number of overseas students as a percentage of all students rose from 12 to 21 per cent. Entering the usual caveat about the reliability of the Ministry's figures, researchers estimated that 35 per cent or more of the nursing staff were non-British.[4] From the data available it was impossible to tell how many of these would be a permanent addition to the workforce and how many would return, when trained, to countries whose need was even greater than that of Britain. There was further concern about the tendency of immigrant staff to concentrate in certain areas and types of hospitals; in some places it might be as high as 80 per cent, a situation as unfair and unhelpful to the immigrant staff as it was to the patients and the hospital administration.

But if the immigrants were helping to keep the service afloat, the exits were a counterbalancing force. It was estimated that during the early 1960s between 2,000 and 3,000 newly trained British nurses left for America and the Commonwealth; many would return, but the exits just about cancelled out the gains from overseas students who qualified and stayed.[5]

Not unrelated to the changing ratio of the nursing team, the lack of supervision and the high percentage of overseas staff in some areas, was the continued high wastage from training. In 1961 it was 39 per cent, but again the average concealed the fact that in some hospitals it was well over 50 per cent. Ever since the Nightingale School withdrawals from training had been between 25 and 33 per cent, and there are probably intrinsic factors in nursing that mean a certain level must be accepted without too much concern, in fact it is better that those who find they have not the aptitude do leave, but a figure of nearly 40 per cent indicated that something was wrong. By 1962 the nursing attrition rate had become the subject of many research studies, usually by people working in the social sciences but even without these it was clear, as the General Nursing Council had always urged, that the lack of an educational standard of entry in many hospitals was a paramount cause, and students who could not cope with the requirements of the syllabus, such as the calculation of medicines and lotions, worried those who supervised them and added to that general anxiety referred to by Professor Revans when he wrote of hospitals as places 'cradled in anxiety'.[6] The other outstanding reason for wastage was the conflict the student endured as the result of the duality of her role as learner and nurse.[7] Another, though lesser, cause of wastage was the fact that now more than 1,000 students left every year to get married (Figure 18.1).

As the public and the professional press became more critical, the more thoughtful urged the need for a method of training nurses that did not impose such a conflict on the learner, was flexible enough to allow for early marriage and at the same time accommodated students with different educational backgrounds and career aspirations. In 1961 the Royal College of Nursing set up a committee under the chairmanship of Sir Harry Platt

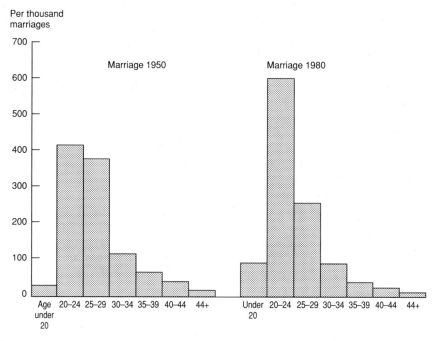

Figure 18.1 Proportional age distribution of first marriages (the second graph represents projected figures)

'to consider the whole field of nurse education in the light of developments since the Nursing Reconstruction Committee completed its work'. During the three years the committee was sitting it had to contend with many changes. 'The Hospital Plan' was published in 1962, and threw doubt on the future of the mental and the smaller hospitals;[8] the Robbins Committee on Higher Education[9] reported in 1963, and urged expansion in further education particularly to meet the needs of women whose educational potential had always been underexploited; the corollary of this for nursing, if it was to compete for able school-leavers, was that it should offer a course that was intellectually stimulating and could be regarded as further education. Then, during a sterling crisis in 1962 a wage freeze denied nurses any improvement in salaries over 2.5 per cent; nurses who had not done so well in the 1959–60 'boom' and free-for-all were falling behind other workers, and some with families to support were at subsistence level, a fact which had an adverse effect on morale and recruitment. In these circumstances nurses made their first organised protest and mass lobby – a venture for which success depended on the novelty and the dignity with which it was conducted. Nurses were now campaigning on two interrelated fronts, to improve education and training so that nurses could meet the more sophisticated demands of the service, and to obtain salaries that would attract recruits with the education, aptitudes and personal skills best fitted to meet those demands. On both counts the campaign was only partially successful, and it is no accident that ten years later the 'Raise the Roof' campaign would be associated with the setting up of the Briggs Committee.

THE SOCIAL CONSEQUENCES OF DEMOGRAPHIC CHANGE

The health needs of the community were changing because the whole pattern of family life, housing, work and recreation had altered. The victims of infectious diseases had mainly been the young, and at the end of the nineteenth century one-third of the population died before the age of 20, so that the population profile looked like a Christmas tree (see Figure 1.2). The most spectacular decline had been in the infant mortality rate (the IMR), from 156 to 21 per 1,000 live births in 1962.* This, together with the fall in the death rate for all children, had a profound effect on the population structure and set in train a number of consequences for which the health and social services were ill prepared. Figures 18.1, 18.2 and 18.3 probably illustrate one of the most significant demographic changes in modern history, only to be compared with the population growth in the time of Malthus.

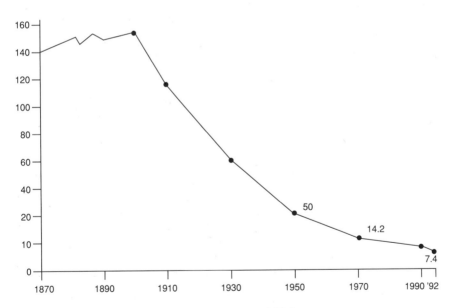

Figure 18.2 Infant mortality rates in England and Wales

* Now 7.4 (provisional) per 1,000, 1992.

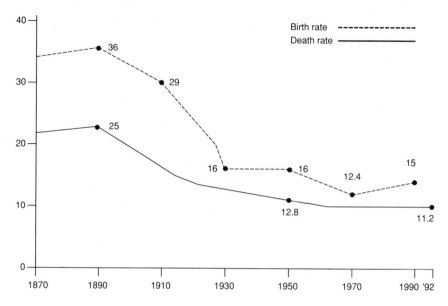

Figure 18.3 Birth and death rates per 1,000 population in England and Wales

By 1962 there were more than 6 million people past the age of retirement compared with the 1.5 million at the beginning of the century, and of the 6 million one-third were over the age of 75 years. This increase not only had implications for the pension funds and social services, it also created a demand for nursing service of greater, not less, skill and care.

In the early part of the century, except for the paupers, most, but by no means all, of the comparatively few old and frail were contained in their own families. Charles Booth (1840–1916), when advocating Old Age Pensions, argued that giving old people an independent income – lost if they claimed poor relief – would 'exercise a healthy influence on family relations'.[10] The young would accept the old, not as a burden, but as a contributor to the household. At a time when the labourers in York were receiving 21 shillings a week as a wage, this inducement no doubt worked.[11] In the higher income groups the plenitude of servants, or even one faithful housekeeper, often enabled the enfeebled old person to remain at home.

By the second half of the twentieth century this situation had changed. After the First World War there was a sharp decline in the number of servants, a class that was soon to become extinct; one of the side effects of a more egalitarian society is that many old people move into institutional care for lack of simple domestic and housekeeping help. But more important was the fall in the birth rate (Figure 18.3): the start of this decline seems to have coincided with the Education and Factory Acts at the end of the nineteenth century, which made children more of a liability than an economic asset, which of course coincided with the pioneers in birth control like Dr Marie Stopes (1880–1958), who began to make women see that unwanted pregnancy could be avoided. However, it seems likely that the over-arching reason was the realisation that better sanitation and nutrition, together with improved child care, had led to fewer infant deaths and now fewer births were needed to cover the loss. Linked with these improvements was the generally higher standard of living, which in turn gave people greater hopes for their children, and these aspirations could only be achieved in a smaller family. None the less, these standards were relative, and it is important to remember that one-third of Edwardian England lived in poverty, and for these people, there was one way of mitigating hardship – to have fewer mouths to feed.[12]

The fall in the population caused almost as much controversy as the rise a century before had done. Writers of letters to *The Times* suggested that the nation was becoming decadent and there was a decline in fertility, the signatories usually being men who attributed this to the fact that women were being educated and were developing 'a pernicious tendency to move into spheres of work for which they were emotionally and physically unsuited'. But as the serious investigators said, this was a 'volitional regulation' and that family limitation was at work in all social grades except the poorest

The fall in the infant death rate and the birth rate had consequences that the writers of letters to *The Times* did not foresee. There had always been more boys born than girls, but the boys died more easily, and in the adolescent years there was always a surplus of girls. The boys, being in a buyer's market, could afford to wait for marriage, and in the days of long apprenticeships and marriage actually forbidden before a certain age for many posts, often had to do so for economic reasons. Now, in the second half of the century the frail boys had survived, and once they were outnumbering the girls they could no longer afford to wait for marriage, and this started to take place earlier, a trend assisted by post-war full employment and the apparent, if illusory, affluence. The family size was low with an average of 2.4 children, which meant that the families were often complete by the time the parents were 25 to 30 years old; this of course brought the generations closer together and in turn influenced the population structure; it also meant that grandmothers were very often working women and great-grandparents more common. Early marriage and the small family had two other effects: the stock and size of houses, and the position of women in the workforce and society.

One result of the higher standard of living and the smaller family was that households increased faster and contained fewer people. The commonest type of house to be built since the First World War has been the three-bedroomed suburban house, which, while it accommodated the nuclear family comfortably, seldom allowed for the prolonged stay of parents. But this small house and the increase of labour-saving devices (necessary with the disappearance of domestic help) freed women from the bondage of the kitchen sink, and with perhaps 30 years of useful working life before them they looked for an occupation outside the home. Unfortunately, because of past attitudes of schools and parents to the education of girls, and often the low expectations of the girls themselves, many housewives were not equipped for occupations requiring educational qualifications, a fact that had to be recognised by professions which normally looked for school-leavers, and special arrangements made for housewives with the right potential. On the other hand, some women merely wanted an occupation outside the home and were happy to take, or accept *faute de mieux*, traditionally low-paid women's work. But the rise in the number of working housewives created a whole cycle of new needs such as 24-hour laundrettes, convenience foods, crèches, and nurseries and arrangements for the care of other members of the family once thought to be a family responsibility. But even if married women had not worked outside the home the clock could not have been turned back with regard to the care of parents and other elderly relatives.

First, there was the sheer problem of longevity. With women living to 90 and beyond, the consequences of taking in grandmother might well be a guest in the spare bedroom of the semi-detached house for 25 years; it was not uncommon to find daughters, well past retirement themselves, coping with parents whose nursing requirements were extremely heavy. Moreover, not only had the life style of the daughters changed, so had the expectations of parents. Parents were younger in outlook, more physically fit and independent than earlier generations, and after the comparative prosperity of the post-war years with adequate, if not princely, pensions, they moved to 'retirement' areas and their bungalows by the sea. Unfortunately, the discrepancy between the male and female death rates meant that these areas soon had a preponderance of widows living alone, who, as they grew less mobile, were cut off from their families, and now probably had neither the will nor the means to move again.

The other factor militating against family support was, as in the Industrial Revolution, a technological revolution that altered the working habits of many people. Old industries died (see Chapter 13), and new ones, often requiring different skills, had grown up in different parts of the country; the universal car meant that more workers were peripatetic and the new families tended to move away from the parental base. With the proviso that the 'extended family' is a convenient label and only relatively true in historical fact, there is no doubt that the modern small families tend to be more isolated than the families of some of the old industrial communities; there were fewer people to bear one another's burdens in a time of crisis, a fact that was to have significance for health workers in the community. Now there was no going home to Mother round the corner –

and coming back, or a tearful journey up the street to Auntie. Maiden aunts had their uses, but maiden aunts were on the way out.

NEW HEALTH PROBLEMS

By the second half of the twentieth century the social and demographic changes outlined above were producing new health needs. The elimination of the infectious diseases had increased life expectancy and revealed the non-infectious diseases, and there was now a movement into a period of general survival into ages where degenerative diseases appeared. These diseases were complicated, and by the time they were manifest the individual had had a long exposure to the environment and a variety of different agencies, some of them like smoke pollution and chemicals, insidiously harmful. Apart from this, there were also the habits of a lifetime such as drinking and smoking or the taking of medicines once hailed as panaceas. In the past bacterial diseases had mainly attacked the young and the weak and this must have had some effect on natural selection so that breeding was from the survival of the fittest. Now the frail were surviving to reproduce. Genetic disease is comparatively unimportant if it produces a fatal defect before the reproductive period since death occurs before the disease can be passed on.[13] But from the point of view of heredity there was now a new factor; namely, that people were living to ages where the genetic component might play an important part and indeed might well determine the way of death. For this reason many of the new health problems were not susceptible to preventive measures and there was no chance of repeating the strategy so successful in the first half of the century; there would be no second bonus.

The captains of death of the nineteenth century were soon replaced by new killers. By 1960 cancer and heart disease already accounted for a third of all deaths, with arterial disease playing an important role in the higher age groups – proportions that would soon increase. In the younger male age groups an important cause of death was the motor vehicle accident and other external hazards, but although accidents seem to figure largely in this group, deaths from violence have in fact not increased in this century; this is because there are no other major killers of the young, and although accidents are prevalent and take much skilled time, improved resuscitation, intensive care and surgery mean that the victim now has a high chance of survival. However, if the 'diagnosis' of the admissions to the average charity hospital in the first half of the nineteenth century are examined, a remarkably high proportion will probably relate to accidents; death from accident or violence was just as likely before the motor car.

While it was not denied that modern scientific medicine and the age of antibiotics had in many cases improved the quality of life, and the death rates for age-specific groups below the age of 45 years had improved, by 1960 it was clear that the millennium had not come. Male life expectancy, which had been improving, became static and in fact started to decline for all ages after 45 years; middle-aged men had little more life expectancy at the age of 45 years than male babies had at the beginning of the century (Figure 18.4).[14] One reason for this trend is that, just as the killers of the past were eliminated by determinants outside medicine like better sanitation and food, so also the modern killers, the neoplasms and ischaemic heart diseases, have their causes outside the realms of mechanistic medicine.

However, the health service is largely a service of intervention and cure; it deals with what has happened. But if there is to be a reduction in the death rate for middle-aged men it will not depend on an increase in the number of transplants, the use of new drugs or more doctors and nurses, but a modification of the adult male's life style and habits. There are workers in social medicine who argue that the adult nation will not be healthier until it ceases to be obsessed with the gross national product and 'keeping up with the Joneses',[15] and point to Norway where, they think, the standard of living is too high for comfort. Undoubtedly, pressure at work, which sadly often only has meaning as a way of earning money, the habits of affluence, and indulgence in an unwise diet and too little exercise – themselves often the concomitants of modern work – were largely responsible for the disappointing mortality trends in the 1960s. Twenty-five years later the lessons have not been learned and still 'at a certain point more and better food appears to mean an increased demand for medical services.'[16]

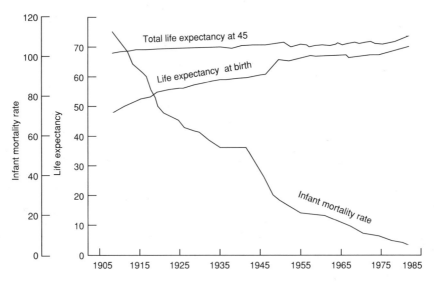

Figure 18.4 Trends in male life expectancy and infant mortality in England and Wales (Crown copyright)

THE NURSING WORK LOAD

In order to convince the government that the nursing service was short of manpower, and the corollary that the pay was not enough to attract recruits, nursing organisations tried to draw up a balance sheet of the demands set against the resources, but unfortunately there was so much that could not be quantified and there was no research into quality. Of the demands that could be measured, perhaps the most striking was the 25 per cent increase in the number of in-patients in 10 years, although the number of hospital beds had only increased by 4 per cent, an indication of the new pace on the wards. Out-patient attendances had risen by 16 per cent, midwives were dealing with 3.7 per cent more births, and the ageing population was placing new strains on the community staff.

Behind the figures there was a new intensity of care that mere percentages could not reveal; as pointed out in Chapter 17, all nursing including geriatric care was becoming more dynamic, while specialised and esoteric surgery required more highly trained nursing assistance. In the wards the patients were more knowledgeable and expected more information and explanation, which the nursing staff, being the most approachable, were expected to supply. Treatment and drugs were more powerful and potentially dangerous, and the supervision of the largely untrained staff became more important; it mattered little if the student nurse gave too much potassium citrate – a double dose of steroid was another matter. But the ward sister was also an administrator and the bureaucratic demands of the service took up more time, sometimes to the detriment of supervision and teaching. The threefold task was becoming too much and training hospitals began to use 'clinical teachers' to give bedside instruction to the students.

However, perhaps the greatest strain on the trained staff came not from the patients, but from the remarkable increase in the number of consultants, whose numbers were determined by the output from the medical schools. By 1962 the number of consultants had increased twice as fast as the number of registered nurses, and every consultant had a manpower consequence and most had a nursing consequence. The increase in specialisms led to a demand for specialist nurses who had to be trained and was an opportunity welcomed by many nurses who wanted to stay in the clinical field. But one consultant's complement of nurses for a special project soon became another's necessity, and more than one enquiry into the competence of the nursing administration turned on the matron's ability to produce the number of nurses each new consultant required.

Although the demand for skilled nursing was greater, nevertheless some jobs had been shed. In some hospitals, though not all, nurses no longer prepared the breakfasts, made the dressings, packed the drums, arranged the flowers or sorted the laundry; they were no longer responsible for special diets or supervising the cleaning, except on Saturdays and Sundays.

Ward clerks and messengers had removed some of the chores, and in theory the nurses had more time to give to patients, but they were not always trained to use time for this purpose. Apart from the fact that many hospitals were so small that the theory did not work in practice, there was another side to the coin. It was soon discovered in intensive-care units and on geriatric wards that the walk to the pathological laboratory, specimen in hand, had a therapeutic value – it was the necessary breathing space, a recharging of batteries which were all too soon run down when faced with long stretches of intimate care for those who had no control over their mental and physical reflexes, and whose incessant cries frayed the nerves. Eliot wrote, 'humankind cannot bear very much reality', and nurses were no exception. When the work-study experts denied them the non-nursing duty of a walk in the fresh air away from the cries and the smells, they needed more frequent tea breaks, and eventually shorter hours. Perhaps those who suggested that the night nurse should arrange the flowers when the vital spirits were low were wise in their generation.

STANDARDS OF CARE

In the ferment of the 1960s the most emotive cry was that 'the standards of care were being lowered'. But what was the standard by which care was measured? The best of pre-war nursing or the worst? There had been little research into standards of care, and it was not known whether patients in the same condition 30 years earlier were more or less likely to have a bedsore. Each generation has its own standards. It was possible that a generation inured to the chilly ablutions when on service with the ATS or even Civil Defence were less worried about privacy than their mothers. On the other hand, there is evidence to suggest that pain and discomfort were less well tolerated. Nevertheless, there was a sense of unease among many nurses that, because of pressures and the changing ratio of the nursing team, the number of people on the wards and the noise and the dirt, the patients were less well nursed. After 15 years of the health service it was difficult to say whether the actual giving of care was improving, and all that could be said with certainty was that in certain areas such as the long-term sick, the care was manifestly better, although better care was bringing terrible problems in terms of numbers. The other certainty, less comforting, was that acute patients seemed to get well whether they were well nursed or not. In the past when people were desperately ill with pneumonia or typhoid, medicine could do little and nursing was paramount. Now the patient was cured by antibiotics whether he was nursed or not; if his meals were badly served and he had no opportunity to wash his hands after using a bedpan he would soon be home and cured – and probably grateful. The fact that nursing had 'lost an Empire but not found a role' was more worrying to the nurses in the 1960s than the question of status or even pay. The answer to 'What is the proper task of the nurse?' seemed as elusive as ever.

In the last two decades the profile of nursing staff has changed; there are several reasons for this. First, the advent of Project 2000 has meant a reduction in the number of learners. The total number of learners for all courses (see Tables 18.2 and 18.3) is now 51,756 as compared with 55,000 in the 1970s, but the discontinuation rate has fallen from 30 per cent to 11 per cent for traditional courses and to 8 per cent or less for Project 2000. We do not need to recruit so many learners to produce the same number of registered nurses. Presumably, as more candidates start on Project 2000 this trend will continue. This is a bonus. At the same time this means that learners are now only 8.6 per cent of the total nursing service as compared with 33 per cent in the 1960s. At last we have broken the pattern of a third of all nursing being done by learners.

Second, the health service reforms with their internal market have been looking at the skill mix. Qualified nurses are now expensive, and there have been numbers of reports suggesting that nursing can be done with fewer trained nurses and more auxiliaries and health-care assistants. Trust hospitals, struggling for contracts, have closed wards and there have been a wave of redundancies (see Table 18.4). At the same time the recession has hit nursing. It is difficult to be precise about its impact, but it looks as if nurses have attempted to re-enter the labour market or to increase the hours they do in order to maintain household earnings. At the same time, fewer nurses have been inclined to leave their jobs; as a result, there have been fewer vacancies, and qualified nurses have difficulty in finding posts and nurses are becoming increasingly concerned about job security and career prospects.

An analysis of the figures for Great Britain shows that the number of whole-time equivalent qualified nurses working in the NHS fell by 5,235 between September 1991 and March 1992, and the total nursing staff fell by 2.4 per cent.

Although according to the figures (Table 18.3) the numbers of unqualified staff fell by 1.23 per cent, the Department of Health do not have the number of care assistants and we do not know if there is a fall in the total number of support staff or whether the skill mix is being altered.

What will happen to nursing when the economy improves? One suggestion is that there will be a growth in the service sector, particularly in jobs for women. However, a note of warning must be sounded: with hospitals struggling for contracts there will be a temptation to dilute the skill mix and use a higher proportion of health-care assistants or find different ways of organising and delivering care. It is up to the nursing profession to prove, by research, that quality care pays. Perhaps the exposure of a few tragic accidents where there have been too few staff of the right calibre will add grist to the mill.

Table 18.2 Pre-registration nursing in training populations in relation to recruitment and wastage, traditional and Project 2000 courses by speciality, as at 31 March 1992

Levels 1 and 2	In training as at 31.3.92	Entries 1991/92		Discontinuations	Discontinuations as a % of in training total	Discontinuations as a % of 1991/92 entries
		Initial + re-entry	Post-registration			
General/adult	39,667	12,554	3,983	1,842	5	11
Mental health	6,808	2,195	1,133	479	7	14
Mental handicap	2,329	799	232	155	7	15
Children's	1,663	556	628	65	4	5
Common Foundation Programme*	1,141	760	4	46	4	6
Comprehensive (RGN/RSCN)	152	0	0	16	11	-
Totals	51,756	16,864	5,980	2,603	5	11

* In certain colleges, the choice of branch is made near completion of the Common Foundation Programme (CFP).
Note: Discontinuations which occurred during the period shown do not necessarily relate to entries which occurred during the same period.
Source: Figures by courtesy of the English National Board

Table 18.3 Pre-registration nursing in training populations in relation to recruitment and wastage, as at 31 March 1992

Levels 1 and 2	In training as at 31.3.92	Entries 1991/92		Discontinuations	Discontinuations	
		Initial + re-entry	Post-registration		as a % of in training total	as a % of 1991/92 entries
Level 1						
General	30,071	6,390	3,969	1,312	4	13
Mental health	4,865	898	1,113	332	7	17
Mental handicap	1,583	282	229	97	6	19
Sick children	866	53	628	21	2	3
Comprehensive (RGN/RSCN)	152	0	0	16	11	–
P2000 Adult	9,523	6,164	13	497	5	8
P2000 Mental health	1,939	1,297	20	141	7	11
P2000 Mental handicap	742	517	3	56	8	11
P2000 Children's	797	503	0	44	6	9
P2000 Common Foundation*	1,141	760	4	46	4	6
Level 2						
General	73	–	1	33	45	–
Mental health	4	–	–	6	150	–
Mental handicap	4	–	–	2	50	–

* In certain colleges, the choice of branch is made near completion of the Common Foundation Programme (CFP). These student numbers are therefore included under CFP.

Note: Discontinuations which occurred during the period shown do not necessarily relate to entries which occurred during the same period.

Table 18.4 NHS nursing staff: numbers by grade as of 1 September 1991 and 1 March 1992

Great Britain	1/9/91	1/3/92	Change	% change
Senior nurses	2,420	2,258.1	−164	−6.77
Educational staff	6,790	6,562.7	−227	−3.35
Qualified clinical nursing staff	301,350	297,015.2	−4,335	−1.44
Other qualified staff	590	81	−509	−86.27
Total qualified staff	**311,150**	**305,915**	**−5,235**	**−1.68**
Learners	47,940	40,734.8	−7,205	−15.03
Unqualified nursing staff	113,810	112,408.6	−1,401	−1.23
Other unqualified	790	555	−235	−29.75
Other nursing/midwifery	9,870	12,340.1	2,470	25.03
Total staff	**483,550**	**471,953.5**	**−11,597**	**−2.40**

Source: *Nursing Standard*; figures released by Department of Health, Aug. 1993.

For over 40 years the NHS has been dominated by the acute general hospital, which has absorbed over half the budget. Perhaps with the Tomlinson enquiry there is a chance of a shift towards preventive medicine and community-based facilities. Now Project 2000 nurses are being trained partly in the community and in the social sciences, and they are coming to realise that in terms of nursing care needed, as Coriolanus said 'There is a world elsewhere'.

REFERENCES

1 *Hansard* No. 553, (21–29 March 1962), p. 1097, Rt Hon. Enoch Powell, London: HMSO.
2 *The Recruitment and Training of Nurses* (*Minority Report*), (1948) ch. III, para. 66, p. 17, London: HMSO.
3 Ministry of Health (1963) *National Consultative Council on the Recruitment of Midwives and Nurses*, NCC 79.
4 Gish, O. (1969) 'Nursing and midwifery migration in Britain', *Nursing Times*, (1 May), p. 69.
5 Ibid.
6 Revans, R. W. (1964) *Standards for Morale: Cause and Effect in Hospitals*, Oxford: Oxford University Press.
7 MacGuire, J. (1969) *Threshold of Nursing*, London: G. Bell & Sons.
8 *The Hospital Plan for England and Wales* (1962), Cmnd, 1604, Ministry of Health, London: HMSO.
9 *The Robbins Committee on Higher Education* (1963), Cmnd. 2154, London: HMSO.
10 Booth, C. (1902) *Life and Labour of the People of London*, final vol., London: Macmillan, pp. 143 ff.
11 Rowntree, B. S. (1914 edn) *Poverty, a Study in Town Life*, London: Nelson, pp. 167–72.
12 Bowley, A. L. and Burnett Hurst, A. R. (1915) *Livelihood and Poverty*, London, p. 46.

13 Smith, A. (1968) *The Science of Social Medicine*, London: Staples Press, p. 110.
14 McKeown, T. (1976) *The Role of Medicine*, ch. 1, London: The Nuffield Provincial Hospitals Trust.
15 Draper, P. *et al.* (1978) *The National Health Service in the Next Thirty Years*, London: Unit for the Study of Health Policy, p. 43.
16 Galbraith, J. K. (1969) *The Affluent Society*, London: Penguin Books.

FURTHER READING

Owen, D. (1976) *In Sickness and in Health*, London: Quartet Books.
Smith, A. (1968) *The Science of Social Medicine*, London: Staples Press.

Chapter 19

New problems for old in the community

In that world elsewhere there was the world of the mentally sick, also the health problems associated with work and, above all, the vast and often unmet needs of the community. The community services, like the hospitals, had grown up unplanned from charitable endeavour and the Poor Law services, and by a chance of history the nursing services in the community had been placed under the aegis of the Medical Officer of Health who had been appointed to deal with sanitation and communal health problems (see Chapter 8). As the twentieth century advanced, with the teaching hospitals absorbed in the interesting and the acute, the importance of community health and preventive medicine seemed to be forgotten.

Apart from sanitation, the great contribution made by the early public health doctors and nurses was in child care, and although it is difficult to say which was cause and which effect, there is no doubt that the smaller families, the better health of mothers and children, and the lower infant mortality rate owed much to the first health visitors, who broke through the cycle of apathy and child neglect that all too often accompanied under-nourishment and too frequent pregnancies. But by 1950 the circumstances that had called the health visitor into being were for the most part no longer there, and some wondered if the health visitor had not worked her-self out of a job. Although there were still problems with special groups like immigrants and the new 'socially deprived', generally speaking school-children, though they were often unwisely fed, were seldom starving or ragged and in the clinics babies were more likely to be overweight than marasmic. As in the case of demand for hospital services where illness had not just withered away, so in the community new and more complicated medico-social problems took the place of the old poverty – ill health depri-vation of cycle of former years, and many of these new problems arose from the social and demographic changes discussed in Chapter 18.

In 1891 the average family size was 6.2 children, of whom two would probably die in infancy, a fact poignantly borne out in many a Victorian churchyard. Birth and death were the common experience of family life, and the elder children, so vividly depicted in the novels of Dickens, frequently brought up the younger, and in their turn, when they married, knew all too well about childbirth and its problems. Now after two generations of small families, only children were marrying only children of whom probably neither had seen birth or death, and on their housing estates or blocks of flats were divorced from family links and had no one to turn to for advice. Responsibilities that had once been shared by a large family now had to be borne by young parents alone and in some cases it was more than their shoulders could bear.[1]

DEMOGRAPHIC CHANGES

The strain seemed to be one of the reasons for the increase in the divorce rate. Of women born in 1900, only 49 per cent married before the age of 25 years and of marriages made in 1921 only 5 in 1,000 ended in divorce; now over 150 per 1,000 will be divorced. Since 1971 the marriage rate has fallen by one-third and divorces have doubled. The whole attitude to marriage has changed. According to the 1991/92 figures, one couple out of five living together is not married. One family in seven is headed by a lone parent, and one family in 12 includes at least one stepchild and only one-quarter of all households include both parents and a quarter of them are not married.[2]

All this has a relevance for the community services and social workers. Single parents are usually young; two out of three are under 30 and half under 25 years, and they generally have few qualifications with less ability to find a job, and nearly half have a gross income of less than £100 a week. This has doubled the need for low-cost housing, which is not available, and the need for child care has mushroomed. Two out of three families with children under 5 use some kind of regular care with nursery schools or unpaid family and friends and England is poorly supplied with work place crèches.[3] Some single families manage magnificently, but the strain is considerable, and the families are vulnerable and make high demands on the health visiting services.

At the other end of the scale is the rise in longevity. In 1948, when the National Health Service began, 3 per cent of the population was over 75 years; now it is 5.4 per cent, and by the year 2000 1.9 per cent will be over the age of 85 years (see Table 19.1). While the young old, the newly retired, are fitter than they have ever been, those over 85 and living alone and handicapped are growing in numbers.[4] The current emphasis on community health care is to keep people in their own homes as long as possible. This will mean an added burden on district nursing and call for skills in communications and co-ordination of the services.

Table 19.1 Elderly persons as a percentage of UK total population
(males and females)

	>65	>75	75–84	>85
1948	10.7	3.4	3.0	0.4
1950	10.7	3.6	3.1	0.5
1960	11.7	4.2	3.6	0.6
1970	13.0	4.6	3.8	0.8
1980	14.9	5.7	4.6	1.0
1990	15.6	6.9	5.4	1.5
2001*	15.5	7.4	5.5	1.9
2011*	16.1	7.4	5.3	2.1
2021*	17.9	7.9	5.8	2.1
2031*	20.4	9.1	6.8	2.3

* Projections based on 1989 mid-year estimates.
Source: OPCS.

THE DEVELOPMENT OF THE ROLE OF THE HEALTH VISITOR

In 1891 Frederick Verney said, 'a health visitor is not a nurse and does not pretend to be one', and the early health visitors were not nurses. In 1907 both the Bedford and Battersea Colleges were offering courses for candidates without nursing qualifications, but the concern about child health after the publication of the report of the Interdepartmental Committee on Physical Deterioration in 1904 (see Chapter 8) and the legislation that followed tended to concentrate the health visitors' work on mothers and children, health visiting seemed an aspect of nursing and nurses soon outnumbered other applicants. The Maternity and Child Welfare Act of 1918 made it the responsibility of local authorities to establish Maternity and Child Welfare Committees. In 1919 the new Ministry of Health defined entry requirements to health visiting as a

- one-year post basic course for a person already qualified as a nurse (after 1925 that meant a registered nurse);
- a different one-year training for a person already a university graduate;
- a two-year training for non-graduates who were not nurses.

Some observers have seen the variety of roads of entry to health visiting as a lost opportunity which might have enabled health visiting to develop different branches of social work and thus avoid much of the subsequent controversy. However, with an infant mortality rate of 75 per 1,000 it was inevitable that health visiting would emphasise mothers and babies.

In spite of the economic difficulties, there was an improvement in child health by the 1930s, although, as McKeown and others have pointed out, this was a trend already begun with better nutrition and sanitation.[5] Improved health owes more to the water closet and the turnip than to the whole armoury of drugs. However, once the diseases of malnutrition and the infectious diseases had been laid low the health visitor faced the obstinate problems of peri-natal death, genetic disabilities and behavioural health that would not yield to the old community health strategies.

In 1948 the National Health Service made the local authorities responsible for employing health visitors. It clarified their duties and confirmed the concept of the health visitor as being an all purpose family visitor. In 1945, the Royal College of Nursing started a one year course for the training of health visitor tutors and this facilitated the expansion of training courses in establishments of further education. However, apart from her statutory functions for infant care, school health and duties under the Child Life Protection Act the health visitor's role remained indistinct; she was seen as the 'well baby nurse' and babies were manifestly well.

In 1953, concerned with the failure to use the service fully, the government set up a working party under the chairmanship of Sir Wilson Jameson to advise on the proper training of the health visitor in the National Health Service and the School Health Service. The report, published in 1956, emphasised that the health visitor was in touch with a wide range of families and would be 'a general purpose family visitor'.[6] At the same time a similar working party under Miss Younghusband was set up to make recommendations for the training of the social worker. The result of these two reports was that in 1962 the Health Visitor and Social Work Training Act set up a council for training health visitors and a similar council for training social workers. The new council replaced the old Royal Society of Health as the examining body for the Health Visitors Certificate and issued a syllabus; the entry requirements were the General Certificate of Education with at least five subjects at O level.

The new Council had implications for nursing. First, the entry requirements with a specific educational standard meant that not all nursing students could proceed to health visiting. Second, with a complementary council for social work, health visiting was firmly placed in the 'medico' side of the work, and health visiting was clearly a branch of nursing. Third, the council was an independent educational body and had implications for professional status that would not lightly be given up.

In 1972 the Committee on Nursing under the chairmanship of Professor (later Lord) Asa Briggs recommended a reform of nursing education in a system of progressive education and that the multiplicity of training bodies be replaced by one central body.[7] The midwives and health visitors disagreed; both had a tradition of separate training bodies, and without their agreement there was no hope of progress. Eventually, in 1979 the Nurses, Midwives and Health Visitors Act became law, which made provision for delegated power in the case of health visiting and midwifery, and, after much lobbying, a last-minute amendment to allow for a joint committee for district nursing. Although the health visitors and midwives kept their independence and the district nurses gained the independence they had long sought, it was at the expense of unity and the implementation of the Briggs report. Since then the baton for reforming nursing education has been taken up again (see Chapter 23), and Project 2000 is a reality. Here the programme is linked to higher education, is progressive and comprehensive including models on social and preventive medicine and health promotion, and this has implications for the curriculum for health visitors and district nurses.

In 1986 the Department of Health and Social Security set up a working party under Julia Cumberledge (later Baroness) which reported as *Neighbourhood Nursing*.[8] The recommendations included the harmonising of some of the basic education for community health workers, the enhancing of the team with specialist nurses and that practice nurses be integrated into the neighbourhood nursing scheme, that greater use be made of suitably qualified nurses as counsellors and that patients could choose between seeing the doctor and the nurse.

Today the health visitor's role has changed. The funding arrangements for general practitioners has altered, and the doctor's perception of the health visitor varies. Someone in the practice is now responsible for child surveillance, and the Health Promotion Banding of general practitioners affects the work of the health visitor. Now health outcomes have to be measured by such considerations as accident prevention, breast feeding, stroke programmes and immunisation programmes; good outcomes means a higher band and more money.

In 1989, the Children's Act increased the need for care case conferences and for a closer relationship with social workers. There is now an open dialogue and parent participation and this affects record-keeping. At the same time, health visitors are now more concerned with group work, and teaching parenting skills and accident prevention in the home. But the greatest demands now made on the health visitor come from areas of high deprivation and the problem of homelessness. A hundred years ago the first health visitors at the time of the Booth Survey (see Chapter 8) were concerned with the submerged tenth of the population living in dire poverty; today, in areas of high unemployment with a high percentage of homelessness, numbers of people in ethnic minority groups and people like new age travellers, the wheel has come full circle.

DISTRICT NURSING

Although there have always been nurses visiting patients in their own homes, including parish nurses employed by the Poor Law before 1834, the modern concept comes from the experiment set up by Mr Rathbone and Miss Nightingale in Liverpool in 1861 and the founding of the Queen Victoria Jubilee Institute in 1887. The Queen's Institute was a voluntary organisation run by local District Nursing Associations which collected subscriptions and donations. As time went by the Queen's Institute was increasingly used by local authorities to provide a home nursing service; different authorities had different practices, and some used other organisations like the Ranyard Mission founded in 1868, but it is a good example of statutory authorities taking over a service pioneered by a voluntary organisation.

During the inter-war period people increasingly used hospitals (see Chapter 13), and the district nurse tended to be associated with the poor sick and chronic illness and this is how doctors and colleagues saw her.[9] The National Health Service made it obligatory for local authorities to provide a district nursing service, which they did in a variety of ways. However, district nurses were soon caught in the maelstrom of change, with the problems of working wives, early discharge from hospital, increased longevity and the use of sophisticated equipment in the home and powerful drugs that called for new skills and further training. In 1955 the Ministry of Health set up a working party to look at the work and training of district nurses, which ended with the setting up of a panel of assessors and the National Certificate of District Training. Many nurses continued to get their certificate through the Queen's Institute, which was of a higher standard; then, as the pressure for short courses increased, the Queen's Institute withdrew from training and each authority organised its own scheme. There was considerable criticism of this scheme because it tended to be vocational rather than educational and district nurses felt at a disadvantage compared with health visitors.

In 1975, as the result of the debate on the Committee on Nursing and the new duties imposed on the district nurse, a working party was set up under Mr A. Carr which published a new curriculum. It recommended a six-month course in a college of further education, and in 1979 district nurses finally got their own District Nursing Joint Committee under the aegis of the Central Council for Nursing, Midwifery and Health Visiting (UKCC). In 1983, when the National Boards replaced the training bodies previously responsible for further education the committee became operative. The new curriculum was based on educational concepts, the nursing process, nursing models, the extended role of the nurse and the correlation of theory and practice. Unfortunately, in a time of financial stringency, because of the cost of the mandatory course and new ideas about the skill mix, the number of places offered for district nurse training has fallen by one-third – this at a time when the role of the district nurse is expanding because of the high demands of the elderly, the hospital at home, new problems of chemotherapy and the nursing of AIDS.

Now the NHS Community Care Act 1990 aims to allow vulnerable people to live as independently as possible in their own homes or in a homely setting.[10] As from April 1993 social service departments are responsible for assessing the needs of all in society who need social care. They will assess any individuals who may be in need of residential or nursing-home care and will be responsible for putting together a care plan. Nurses in all settings have an important contribution to make if community care is to be successful, and they may be asked for specialist assessment which will contribute to the care management process.

Care in the Community is the responsibility of local authorities, and, although it will not be cheap, the emphasis on keeping patients at home is not unconnected with the escalating cost of residential homes, which have mushroomed in the last few years. In 1979 social security payments direct to claimants in residential care were a mere £10 million; today the bill approaches £2.5 billion.[11]

How the district nurse operates varies from authority to authority and from budget to budget; the service provided depends on what the purchaser wants. In some authorities there is a move away from a district nursing service to a more specifically orientated service with nurses as specialists such as the stoma therapist, the paediatric nurse, the post-stroke specialist, the community psychiatric and the AIDS specialist.

THE SCHOOL HEALTH SERVICE

It is just over 100 years ago since the Metropolitan and National Nursing Association appointed a nurse to look after the health of schoolchildren in Chancery Lane, but it was the report of the Interdepartmental Committee of 1904 (see Chapter 8) that caused the real concern. In 1905 the London County Council set up their own school medical service with their own nurses, and in the following year the Education (Provision of Meals) Act was passed. The other measure, the Education (Administrative Provisions) Act provided for school medical inspections, thus beginning the school health service. However, in order to placate the vociferous general practitioners only limited treatment was provided, and most children were referred, but, in practice, most parents could not afford a doctor, and the diseases and dysfunction discovered by the school nurse and the doctor went untreated.

As part of the post war Reconstruction Plan in 1918, the Fisher Act extended the duties of education authorities to provide medical inspection and treatment for all children in elementary schools and medical examinations for all children in secondary schools. In 1919 the new Ministry of Health took over the school health services, with the Chief Medical Officer, Sir George Newman, as the Chief Medical Officer to the Board of Education. By 1939 the standard of health to recruits in the army had improved, but all was not well, the incidence of preventable disease was still high and in 1943 *Our Towns* and similar publications revealed that many children were ill-fed and verminous and that poor health was often compounded with behavioural problems made worse by evacuation. In 1944 the Education Act (the Butler Act) made it the duty of all authorities to provide treatment, medical inspection, school meals and milk to all children.

Since 1944 there have been many debates about the school health service. First, it was argued that now all parents had free access to a doctor and it was no longer necessary. Second, the take-up of the services tended to be by the middle classes who knew how to use the services, and this raised the debate between the universalists who argue that restricting the services to those in need creates a sense of stigma, and those who maintain that welfare services should be restricted to the most needy. Third, the argument that the services were costing too much led to cutting down on such things as milk, school meals and medical examinations, while those working in the field challenged these assumptions. Now, new problems were replacing the old. Children were staying at school longer, they were maturing earlier and having emotional and sexual problems. The old hazards had been replaced by new ones like drug-taking, smoking, teenage pregnancies and sexually transmitted diseases and later, glue-sniffing. Added to these problems are those raised by the growing ethnic mix with different cultures and customs and the ever present problem of keeping a look-out for the abused child.

In 1976 the Committee on Child Health Services (the Court Report) drew attention to the fact that Britain had been overtaken by other countries in infant mortality rates and child health.[12] It pointed out that group attachment (see below) had diverted health visitors from primary prevention to secondary or even tertiary prevention, which is concerned with limiting and containing something that has already happened. The report showed that visits to the under-5-year-olds had fallen and that children in need were slipping through the net, and it recommended that there should be an integrated child health service with one practitioner in each group medical practice with a special paediatric training. The conclusions for the health visitor were radical; there was to be a child health visitor (CHV) with paediatric training who would have the oversight of other child visitors and the school nurse, and who would have an added and defined geographical responsibility. The committee also recommended that each school should have a specially nominated school doctor and nurse trained in educational medicine, who would have time to know the schools, and there should be increasing encouragement for older children to consult the school nurse and doctor for themselves.

Although the report was accepted, it was not implemented because of cuts in the health services, and it has now been over shadowed by other changes and the education reform. Where schools have opted out and hold their own budget it depends on the ethos of the school as to what services they decide to purchase. Where the school health services are developed, the school nurse has a higher profile and she takes over health interviews and health education in the schools. There is more emphasis on sex education and the problem of AIDS and the growing awareness of child abuse, both physical and sexual, with all the attendant problems of confidentiality. Since the Education Act 1987 school nurses have been involved in 'statementing' children with special needs.

THE ORGANISATION OF THE COMMUNITY SERVICES

Originally the community health services came under the Medical Officer of Health (see Figure 11.1, p. 133). However, with the coming of the National Health Service in 1948, the preventive and community services were divorced from the curative services, which were under the control of the Regional Hospitals Board and the Boards of Governors (Figure 15.1, p. 186). In 1974 the Local Government Act reorganised local authorities and the Health Service Reorganisation Act organised the health services into Area Health Authorities and District Authorities. This structure proved too cumbersome and, in 1982, there was further reorganisation into District Authorities, which were now responsible for all the hospital and community health services in the district. Now, at last curative and preventive services were under one authority and communication should have been easier, except for the fact that general practitioners remained independent.

However, while one breach had healed another had widened. The social services with whom the community services had links through the Medical Officer of Health were now torn asunder. The Seebohm Report of 1968 had put the social services under a Director of Social Services in the local authority. While the health services were under the local authority all was well, but once the community services were under the district the boundaries were no longer coterminous and the old link was lost. This was to create difficulties in families with medico-social problems and was to have repercussions both professional and legal, particularly in cases of suspected child abuse. Another problem was that the general practitioner was independently employed and the relationship of the social services with the primary care teams was, at times, anomalous.

At the same time both health visitors and district nurses were independent practitioners but local authorities are bureaucratic, and develop hierarchies into which doctors and nurses have to be fitted. It is important that professionals order and control their own practitioners, and some professionals assumed managerial positions. The same problem arose in the health services as in the hospitals; numbers of professional people were doing jobs that were neither managerial nor professional. In 1968 a working party was set up under Mr E. Mayston to advise on senior nursing posts in the community. The committee took into consideration the growing practice of group attachment and the coming unification of the health service, and came to the conclusion that the principles enunciated by the Salmon Committee were applicable to the community, and they recommended that the grades should be reconstructed to reflect the levels of management. Although most authorities implemented the recommendations, they were quickly overtaken by other developments, but the district nursing officer proved to be a common point of reference for all group practice nurses. However, with the coming of Trust Hospitals and Districts, different authorities have adopted different management arrangements. The history of the organisational arrangements in the community in the last two decades illustrates the number of changes inflicted on the staff and the resulting amount of stress.

PRIMARY HEALTH CARE

The concept of primary health care teams sprang from *ad hoc* experiments in the 1950s in group attachment. Instead of working in isolation from the health authority, selected health visitors and district nurses were attached to group practices and worked with general practitioners. The experiments proved mutually beneficial and educative to both doctors and nurses, both becoming more family orientated. In 1964 a sub-committee under the chairmanship of Dr Annis Gillie found that the elderly living alone took up much of the general practitioners' time, and they often needed a variety of services of whose existence they were unaware, and that many of their problems stemmed from the fact that they did not know what help was available. From then on Medical Officers of Health and Chief Nursing Officers began to lay plans to extend the scheme and, within ten years, some 60 per cent of all health visitors and most district nurses were attached. In 1985 the World Health Organisation emphasised the importance of primary health services in the Declaration of Alma-Ata which aimed at achieving health for all by the year 2000.[13]

A British Medical Association working party on primary health care teams listed the advantages of team care as:

1 Care given by the group is greater than the sum of individual care.
2 Rare skills are used most appropriately.
3 Peer influence and informal learning within the group raise the standards of care and the corporate status of the team.
4 Team members have increased job satisfaction.
5 Team working encourages co-ordinated health education.
6 Team working lowers the prevalence of disease in the community.
7 The individual gets a more efficient and understanding treatment when ill.[14]

Members of the team

Teams have evolved in a variety of ways to suit different neighbourhoods and practices. Some are more successful than others. In 1986 the Cumberledge Report[15] noted that 'nurses are at their most effective when they and the general practitioners work together in an active primary health care team'.

The size and composition of the team has been widely debated. The British Medical Association has distinguished between the nucleus team composed of doctors, nurses, health visitors, social workers and medical secretaries, and the wider team which includes the allied professions such as physiotherapists, pharmacists and other services provided by hospitals, local authorities and voluntary services. Within the multidisciplinary team is the primary nursing team, which consists of the health visitor, the district nurse and the practice nurse. The practice nurse may be employed by the health authority and attached to general practice, or she may be employed directly by the practice.

The rise in the profile of the practice nurse has been a significant change accompanying the focus on GP practices. Many have been ill prepared for their new role in health promotion and are now attending courses, supported by practice facilitators who have been instrumental in raising standards and acting as the practice nurses' advocate. Practice nurses have increased their role in family planning since many health authorities have closed clinics.

The wider primary health-care team includes midwives and specialist nurses like school nurses, community psychiatric nurses, paediatric nurses, and occupational nurses and Macmillan nurses who work outside the health service. Apart from community-based nurses, contact must be maintained with specialist nurses, such as stoma therapists, cerebral vascular accident specialist nurses and the AIDs nurse. The district nurse cannot be a specialist in everything, and there is a tendency for her either to specialise or work more closely with specialist nurses, and this is a challenge. The Group of Primary Health Care Nursing of the Royal College of Nursing has identified two groups whose needs can best be met by specialist intervention: those where a different training is required, such as the community psychiatric nurse; and those where the problem is relatively rare, such as stoma care and AIDs.[16] The Cumberledge Report suggested that, wherever possible, specialist nurses should be part of the neighbourhood nursing service, and where this was not possible the relationship between the services should be made specific in a written contract.

The extent of interdisciplinary co-operation in primary health care varies greatly from one part of the country to another. Development is poor where the numbers of nursing staff are inadequate, where general practitioners do not accept the concept or where they work single-handed, as is often the case in London. Removing these defects is going to be a major challenge when the Tomlinson Report advocating the reduction in the number of acute hospitals in London and other urban areas is implemented.[17] To reorganise the services into primary health care teams is going to take much resource and years of patient work.

CONCLUSION

Beveridge set out to slay the giants of disease, squalor, ignorance, idleness and want, but like the dragon's teeth sown by Cadmus they have sprung up to fight again. Homelessness, ignorance, unemployment and poverty are still giants to be slain. The first edition of this book, in 1973, mentioned the film *Cathy Come Home*, which drew attention to the plight of the homeless. The second edition, in 1980, commenting on the fact that there were 1 million unemployed, said, 'Cathy has still not come home'. Now, 14 years later, the situation is worse, there are nearly 3 million unemployed, there are 3 million people without their own homes and more than 50,000 living in temporary accommodation; and there are a million unfit houses. Between 1981 and 1991 statutory homelessness by court order nearly trebled. During 1991 local authorities spent £122 million on bed and breakfast accommodation alone.[18] Forty-three per cent of the homeless were so because parents or relatives were no longer able or willing to keep them, and the problem has been exacerbated by the precipitate discharge from mental hospitals where ex-patients fail to take their drugs. Those sleeping rough or in night shelters are prey to the health hazards of yesteryear – vermin, malnutrition, tuberculosis, skin diseases and chronic chest infections. Unfortunately, being without an address often means being without a doctor, but where they do receive help they make heavy demands on the services. Not only are they in physically poor shape, they are prone to drug-pushing and -taking, dirty needles and, of course, AIDs.

It is strange that the government's Green Paper on Health Promotion,[19] which aims to reduce deaths from heart disease and strokes in people under 65 years, to reduce smoking, increase exercise and cut fat consumption, should have nothing to say about poverty. In 1980 Professor Sir Douglas Black reported concern about continuing inequalities in the health care of the nation .[20] The chances of a pregnancy ending in a dead baby for the wife of a manual worker was twice as high as that for a doctor, lawyer or for a university professor, and these discrepancies, and others like them, have continued unchanged for the past 50 years. This has been confirmed since by the report *The Health Divide*.[21]

Florence Nightingale wrote: 'the connection between health and dwellings of the population is one of the most important that exists?[22] The fact that there are a million unfit homes must be a factor in the health of the community and the district nurse and health visitor work against Sisyphean odds in such housing. Housing is no longer considered a social issue but a market commodity. Local authorities were told that they no longer needed to build, it was all being left to the private sector. The lack of low-priced rented housing is the stumbling block to mobility and to the health needs of a sizeable section of the community. If Shelter had not been born in 1966, it would need to be invented in the 1990s.[23]

In the past 50 years the problem of the health needs of the community have changed out of all recognition. Some of these problems are caused by demographic change, some by changing attitudes to marriage and the family, some by the advent of safe contraception, other by attitudes that are the by-product of a more materialistic and secular society. The new problems will be more intractable than defeating bacterial disease with immunisation programmes or nourishing schoolchildren with healthy meals and milk. One ray of hope lies in a realistic implementation of the Tomlinson Report, which will entail, eventually, reducing money spent on expensive hospital beds and diverting to a universal programme for first-class primary health care.

REFERENCES

1   Brockington, C. Fraser (1958) *World Health* London: Penguin Books, p. 91.
2   *Social Trends*, 23 (1993) London: HMSO.
3   Ibid.
4   Office of Population Censuses and Surveys (1991) *General Household Survey*, London: HMSO.
5   McKeown, T. and Lowe, C. R. (1966) *An Introduction to Social Medicine*, Oxford: Blackwell Scientific Publications.
6   *Inquiry into Health Visiting (Jameson Report)* (1956) London: HMSO. p. 302.
7   *The Report of the Committee on Nursing (Briggs Report)* (1972) Cmnd 5115.
8   Department of Health and Social Security (1986) *Neighbourhood Nursing: a Focus for Care (Cumberledge Report)*, London: HMSO.
9   Hockey, L. (1966) *Feeling the Pulse*, London: Queen's Institute of District Nursing.
10 Department of Health and Social Security (1993) *Caring for People*, London: HMSO.
11 *Social Trends*, 23 (1993) London: HMSO.
12 *The Future of Child Health Services* (Court Report) (1976) London: HMSO.
13 World Health Organisation (1985) Declaration of Alma Ata, Geneva: WHO.
14 British Medical Association, Board of Education and Science (1979) *Report of the Panel on Primary Health Care Teams*, London: BMA.
15 Department of Health and Social Security, *Cumberledge Report*.
16 Royal College of Nursing (1980) *Primary Health Care Team Appraisal*, London: RCN.
17 Department of Health and Education (1992) *Report of the Inquiry into London's Health Services, Medical Education and Research (Tomlinson Report)*, London: HMSO.
18 Social Trends, 23 London: HMSO.

19 *The Health of the Nation: a Consultative Document for Health in England* (1993) London: HMSO.
20 Black, D., Morris, J. N., Smith, C. and Townsend, P. (1980) *Inequalities in Health: a report of a Research Working Group*, London: HMSO.
21 Health Education Council (1987) *Inequalities in Health in the 1980s: Health Education Authorities*, London: HMSO.
22 Nightingale, F. 'On the Census Return 1861' in *As Miss Nightingale Said . . .*, M. E. Baly (ed.) London: Scutari Press, p. 39.
23 Field Frank, *The Times*, 1 April 1993.

SUGGESTIONS FOR FURTHER READING

McKeown, T. and Lowe, C. R. (1966) *An Introduction to Social Medicine*, Oxford: Blackwell Scientific Publications.
Owen, G. M. (ed.) (1977) *Health Visiting*, London: Baillière & Tindall.
Nash, W., Thruston, M. and Baly, M. E. (1985) *Health at School*, London: Heinemann Nursing.
Charles Webster (ed.) (1993) *Caring for Health: History and Diversity*, Milton Keynes: Open University Press, Health and Disease Series.
Social Trends, 1993. London: HMSO.

Chapter 20

Mental health nursing – origins and developments

Peter Nolan

Mental health nurses have been ill served by historians. Virtually ignored by writers both in the field of nursing and that of psychiatry, they appear to have been judged to be not part of the health-care system for all of the nineteenth and most of the twentieth centuries. A number of reasons might be put forward to explain why mental health nurses have been thus consigned to the historical side-lines. Salvage[1] suggests that they have been overlooked because they worked in isolated institutions, apart from the mainstream practitioners of medicine and nursing. Florence Nightingale herself regarded asylum nurses as on a par with the least important domestic servants, and gave neither their training nor their work any recognition when the School of Nursing at St Thomas's Hospital was established in 1860. Her great ally, Mrs Bedford Fenwick, was equally adamant that asylum nurses were not 'real nurses', but rather a part of the penal system, more concerned with confining people than caring for them.

The psychiatrists who have written histories of their profession have also failed to acknowledge the role of nurses through the decades. So complete has been this omission that Dr Alexander Walk, addressing the Royal Medico-Psychological Association in 1961, commented that unless a history of mental nurses was written, a comprehensive understanding of the development of psychiatry could not be achieved.[2] Walk's challenge prompted a modest response from mental health nurses, who began at last to try to reconstruct their past and bring it to the attention of their own profession and of other related disciplines. They did not furnish their readers with a sweeping overview of mental nursing history, but instead painted a series of more intimate pictures. Adams'[3] account looked at the early struggles to create unity within the ranks of asylums nurses and their efforts to achieve the status of a profession. Carpenter[4] chronicled the problems along the path to respectability: the poor pay and conditions of service endured by asylum nurses, the high-handed medical superintendents to whom they were subject, and the inhuman routines tailored to the demands, not of patients, but of institutions above all anxious not to allow inmates to escape and to keep running costs to a minimum. Since

Carpenter, an increasing number of authors have added to the body of knowledge concerning the history of mental health nursing, unearthing along the way some valuable primary source material which has yielded insights into how mental health nursing has developed into what it is today.[5, 6, 7, 8] The work of the mental nursing historians is still 'work in progress', but the commitment to it is now considerable.

A greater understanding of the history of mental health nursing would alert those who hail the rise of community care in Britain as something progressive and innovative to the fact that it is, in essence, a return to the situation which existed prior to 1845. Then, care of the insane was largely carried on in the domestic context by women. It was the values of family life that William Tuke tried to incorporate into the Retreat, his justly famous, purpose-built establishment for the insane at York, opened in 1796. A wealthy tea merchant, Tuke was revolted by the conditions under which a young relative of his in the York Asylum was being cared for, and vowed to provide in his establishment the best that a civilised society could give to the disenchanted and sick at heart. Care at the Retreat was based on the family life of Mr and Mrs Jepson, the Head Attendant and Matron, who provided for the residents wholesome family meals, musical entertainments and readings, tea parties and trips to the seaside.[5] The Jepsons saw themselves as spiritual guides to those who were enduring the 'dark night of the soul', just as the guides depicted by Brueghel had accompanied the mad in the Middle Ages on their way to healing shrines. The Retreat became so renowned for the quality of its care that the great humanitarian reformer, Lord Shaftesbury, was inspired to take up his cudgels on behalf of the mentally ill and campaign for specialised institutions that would provide care for all the nation's mentally ill along the same lines as at the Retreat. His efforts resulted in the Lunatics Act of 1845 and the establishment of the asylum system, a national network of institutions caring for the insane. Within these institutions, mental nursing took shape.

During all the detailed and lengthy debates in the House of Commons prior to the passing of the Lunatics Act, no politician was heard to enquire who it was that would run the institutions and care for the patients on a day-to-day basis. Nor was the fundamental philosophy behind the inauguration of the asylum system ever clearly defined as being Shaftesbury's stated aim to imitate the provision for the sick made at the Retreat. From the start, the medical superintendents appointed to head up the asylums were divided as to what purposes they considered their institutions should serve. A few thought the asylums should be centres of learning where large numbers of insane patients could be conveniently studied; others saw them as refuges for the sick from an uncaring world; yet others saw them as centres for the distribution of welfare to lunatics and paupers. Within a decade of their opening, 90 per cent of asylum residents were, in fact, former inmates of workhouses, and a large number of workhouse attendants had found work within the asylums. The attendants were not looking for a career in the asylums, but rather a job that offered agreeable working conditions during the winter months. In the spring, there was a considerable exodus of male staff, moving on to take up agricultural work which provided better pay and excellent perks in the form of vegetables, fruit and dairy produce.

The workplace which the asylum attendants entered offered little in the way of induction or guidance as to what constituted good practice; attendants were largely left to their own devices to decide what nursing care they should provide. They had no training to help them understand the conditions suffered by the patients, many of whom had progressive diseases which manifested themselves in behaviour more akin to that of animals than that of humans. The institution stated only that attendants must ensure that inmates were supervised at all times and kept as busy as possible, on the principle that 'Satan finds work ...' and that patients would benefit from hard labour in preparation for their return to the new industrial community.

TRAINING – CONTROL OR EDUCATION?

Once the asylum system was established, it soon became obvious that there would be a need to rethink or to start thinking about its social and therapeutic aims, and the role and training of the health professionals working within it. In order to bring about a coherence of purpose among the various institutions, the dissemination of standardised information and the introduction of in-service education were seen, by some progressive doctors, as essential. Even before the 1845 Act, Dr Alexander Morrison had considered it important to educate doctors in a better understanding of mental disorder and had started a course of lectures for colleagues at the Bethlem Hospital in 1823; John Connolly followed his lead at the Hanwell Asylum in 1842, and Thomas Laycock in Edinburgh in the 1860s. However, it was not until 1885 that a national training scheme for doctors leading to the Certificate in Psychological Medicine was inaugurated. In the same year, a first effort was made to draw together the 40 years of experience in practice of the asylum attendants in a book entitled *The Handbook for the Instruction of Attendants on the Insane*. The first edition contained 64 pages, was bound in red hardboard and became known to many generations of nurses and doctors as 'the Red Handbook'.[9] The book attempted to lay down standards for the work of the attendants and to provide guidelines for institutions intending to set up courses for them. The publication of the *Handbook* represented a significant shift from an oral culture of mental nursing, where the wisdom of one generation of nurses was passed down verbally to the next, to a written one with far greater power to pull together practice all over the country.

A national training scheme for attendants started under the aegis of the Medico-Psychological Association in May 1891. Those who successfully completed the course were awarded the MPA qualification and were permitted to use the Association's letters after their name. The MPA hoped that attendants trained by a particular asylum would have a greater sense of loyalty to it and be more inclined to continue to work within it. Reduced turnover of staff would help maximise the productivity of the asylum in terms of faster discharge of patients and continuity of supervision for ensuring that patients were fully and usefully employed. The MPA's agenda for training was not, however, stated in these or any other terms, but despite the absence of written aims and objectives, training was highly esteemed by attendants in the hope that it would help them to better themselves. These expectations were, unfortunately, completely unfounded, and attendants soon had to face the fact that successful completion of the MPA's training programme made no difference to their pay, their conditions of service or the kind of work they were expected to undertake. Suspicion of the motives of Medical Superintendents who introduced the training scheme into their asylums began to grow among attendants throughout the country, and suspicion soon turned into resentment and agitation. Attendants started to demand shorter working hours, better food, more time outside the hospital and the freedom to join a union. Superintendents became nervous, and many refused to allow attendants to hold meetings in their asylums. As relations between attendants and medical directorates deteriorated over the turn of the century, a series of strikes erupted nationwide, witnessing to the profound and widespread unrest within the asylum system.[6]

The Nurse's Registration Act of 1919 brought into being the General Nursing Council, which moved quickly to start to take control of attendants away from the medical profession. It set up a supplementary register for mental nurses and established its own training programme while agreeing, in May 1920, to make holders of the MPA certificate eligible for admission to the register. The GNC's bid for total control of the mental nurses was finally successful in 1948 when its own training scheme replaced the MPA's and the latter was stopped. For quarter of a century, two rival schemes of training for mental nurses had fought for supremacy, with the result that mental nursing found itself confused and divided at a critical time in the history of the nation's health care, culminating in the inauguration of the National Health Service in 1948.

THE IMPACT OF TWO WORLD WARS

The First World War was a critical period in the history of psychiatry. The mental hospitals were depleted of able-bodied staff called up for military service, while the patient population increased enormously. Health carers within psychiatry were expected to treat men suffering from 'shell-shock' and return them, cured, to the battlefield as quickly as possible. Shell-shock was an ill-defined but demonstrably 'real' condition which psychiatrists were considered able to address, and acknowledgement of their contribution to the war effort was made in 1926 when the Medico Psychological Association was awarded a Royal Charter and became the Royal Medico Psychological Association (RMPA). New honours, however, could not disguise the confusion which was widespread among doctors and Boards of Governors as to the role of the mental hospitals at a time when staffing levels had never been lower to cope with a never greater number of patients, while the country endured a raging economic depression which deprived health services of all resources.

In response to these pressures, psychiatry began, in the 1920s, to look to community care as a way of relieving the pressure on the hospitals. A new group of health professionals, the psychologists, and a small number of psychiatrists started to focus on preventive measures and child-rearing practices to reduce mental ill health among the population. Nurses played no part in this development, as their work was seen by government as self-evidently based in the institutions. The very early moves towards community care were consolidated in the Mental Treatment Act of 1930, which introduced the notion of voluntary treatment for the mentally ill. This represented a radical revision of the 1890 Lunacy Act which had legislated for every admission to a mental hospital to be certified, with the result that many individuals spent the rest of their lives in institutions. There was a spirit of optimism in psychiatry during the 1930s, born of the new Act and fostered by the building of more hospitals to relieve the chronic over-crowding in the Victorian asylums, the marketing of the drug cardiazol, and the introduction of shock treatment and insulin therapy. Optimism was, however, premature. By the end of the decade, another war had erupted causing intolerable strain on a system that was already seriously stressed. Little progress was made in the mental nursing profession during the 1930s and 1940s; the best that can be said is that it survived.

MENTAL HEALTH AND THE NATIONAL HEALTH SERVICE

The country was spiritually and economically drained by the two world wars. The creation of a National Health Service, free at the point of need to every citizen, represented the ultimate act of national altruism. It aimed to cushion people against poverty and to reassure industry that the health of the nation was of key importance to government in its efforts to create the best possible conditions for recapturing the economic status enjoyed by Great Britain during the nineteenth century.

The major restructuring of 1948 brought the former county asylums under the control of the new Regional Hospital Boards, while local authorities were charged with providing after-care facilities for patients. This division of responsibility for services for the mentally ill was to become the source of serious problems half a century later, when health policies would recommend that patients receive a 'seamless service'. The new arrangements did not diminish the role of the mental hospitals' Board of Control, which remained an important influence on management, and the hierarchy within the institutions went largely unchanged (see Chapter 15). Despite the advent of a nationwide health-service structure, the self-containment and remoteness of the mental hospitals, located as they often were in the countryside, meant that they were difficult to incorporate into the NHS and were able to continue with many of their traditional practices. In the late 1940s, the mental hospitals were self-supporting communities; nurses were provided with cheap housing and had access to an endless round of varied entertainments. It is small wonder that the staff were sometimes as intermarried as the Habsburgs.

When the NHS was inaugurated, 48 per cent of beds were in mental and mental deficiency hospitals, but by 1952 overcrowding was such that these hospitals were operating at 12.5 per cent above capacity, with every indication that the problem would get worse. Increased longevity, the rapid rate of social change, and a greater awareness of psychiatric illness were put forward as arguments to explain the rising number of in-hospital admissions. It was reported in the early 1950s that 1 in 12 people would experience a nervous illness during their lives, while 1 in 3 would seek medical advice for a complaint that was psychiatric in origin. The soaring incidence of mental health problems led some professionals to press for more links between mental and general nursing and a blurring of the boundaries between the two branches, so that general nurses could gain skills for coping with 'mild hysteria and the hint of suicide'.[10] At government level, a Royal Commission, under the chairmanship of Lord Percy of Newcastle, responded to the public concern about mental illness and set out: 'To examine the existing laws and administrative machinery governing people who are alleged to be suffering from mental illness or mental defect . . . and to make recommendations'. The Report of the Commission, published in 1957, became the basis of the Mental Health Act 1959. This Act dissolved the Board of Control and laid down new definitions of mental disorder. It relaxed the admission and discharge process by creating the category of 'informal' clients, so reducing the amount of time patients spent in hospital and aiming to improve the quality of community care. The Act was sadly flawed, however, because, while firmly placing responsibility on local authorities to look after patients not requiring the full range of hospital services, it only enabled them to provide accommodation for patients and nothing else. For their part, local authorities were reluctant to spend public money on problems that could be concealed within the hospital system.

Between 1954 and 1974, the number of psychiatric beds fell from 152,000 to 101,000, or 31 per cent of total hospital beds, although during the same period, admissions increased by 130 per cent.[11] In the space of 20 years, the hospital doorway changed from being an entrance to another world to a revolving door through which patients shuttled between the community and the hospital, belonging in neither place. The unsatisfactoriness of this state of affairs furthered moves towards wholesale community care, and in 1961 the Minister of Health, Enoch Powell, predicted that half the remaining psychiatric beds would be closed within 15 years.[12]

THE HOSPITAL PLAN

In 1962, Powell presented his Hospital Plan: 'The moment [has] come to take a comprehensive view of the hospital service as it is today and draw outlines for the service we would wish to create.'[13] The plan was based on estimates of need up to 1975 and beyond, and aimed to replace obsolete hospitals with District General Hospitals with 600–800 beds and serving a population of approximately 150,000. As for the Mental Health Services, the plan envisaged – incorrectly – a fall in demand, and proposed that 60 bedded Psychiatric Units for acute patients should be set within the District General Hospitals. The old mental hospitals were rightly alarmed by this as they saw themselves becoming the dumping ground for chronic and geriatric patients holding little clinical interest.

The Bonham Carter Report therefore suggested modifications to Powell's plan and advised that psychiatric and geriatric services should both be integrated into the District Hospitals which would thereby serve a larger area and have perhaps 1,000–1,750 beds. However, there was only lukewarm support for such a plan, which involved massive funding for extremely large hospitals, and, as a result, very few were built. The mentally ill remained largely in the Victorian institutions, with a small number being provided for in residential care, a small number at home and others swelling the ranks of the homeless.

ENQUIRIES INTO MENTAL AND MENTAL SUBNORMALITY HOSPITALS

As the National Health Service made mental institutions more visible to the public eye, an era of bad practice allegations commenced. In 1965, a letter to *The Times* signed by 10 distinguished persons drew attention to the fact that old people in mental and geriatric hospitals were often cruelly treated, denied the bare necessities of civilised life, and left to vegetate in loneliness and idleness.[14] The letter prompted a body calling itself 'Aid for the Elderly in Government Institutions' to make enquiries, which subsequently resulted in a book entitled *Sans Everything* and an uproar throughout the country.[15]

The Minister of Health, Kenneth Robinson, moved quickly to establish his own enquiry, reassuring Parliament that most of the allegations in *Sans Everything* were 'totally unfounded'. Many of those in public life and in the health professions were unconvinced by his rhetoric, and found their fears substantiated by the Committee established under Geoffrey Howe to investigate allegations of ill-treatment at Ely Hospital in Cardiff. Howe's committee found that it was virtually impossible for staff to make complaints about bad practice and negligence within mental hospitals. In the case of Ely, a member of staff, having tried all available official channels and receiving no satisfaction, approached the *News of the World*. Howe found that a quarter of the patients at Ely were unequipped to live outside the hospital even if there had been any accommodation to offer them, and suggested that a great deal more co-operation between different services with responsibility for the mentally ill was required before patients could be relocated.

The Ely enquiry was the first of 18 such public enquiries, all of which exposed neglect of patients, confused management, and doctors and nurses struggling to cope within a grossly under-resourced and apparently directionless system. A few nurses were praised for their devotion to duty in the face of appalling obstacles. The Payne Report, looking into the management of Whittingham Hospital near Preston, found two standards of care in operation, one for the acute wards and one for the long-stay wards. The latter, so-called 'back wards', were characterised by low levels of staffing and low morale, with much of the care being delivered by untrained people. This state of affairs was perpetuated by the General Nursing Council which insisted that certain wards, usually acute admission wards, be designated as training areas. Training wards received more resources and achieved reasonable standards of care at the expense of other wards. Back wards provided the focus for many of the hospital enquiries of the 1960s and 1970s.

SERVICES FOR PEOPLE WITH LEARNING DISABILITIES

The history of care for people with learning difficulties provides an interesting parallel to the development of community services for the mentally ill. In 1946, the National Health Act took back from local authorities the 'colonies' which provided services for clients then described as 'mentally subnormal', and renamed them Mental Deficiency Hospitals. By 1959 and the passing of the Mental Health Act, these hospitals had emerged as centres of 'clinical excellence'. Local authorities were invited to renew their interest in providing services for the mentally handicapped and in 1971, with the passing of the Education Act (Handicapped Children), the transfer of responsibility for the education of children with special needs resulted in the development of a range of special schools managed by local education authorities. In the same year, the Social Services Act introduced new arrangements for adult training centres and hostels, and the scene was set for a challenge to the franchise that the NHS had held on the provision of services to people with learning difficulties.

The White Paper *Better Services for the Mentally Handicapped* (1975) urged that moves towards community care be accelerated and during the 1980s, Government introduced a range of incentives to reduce the hospital population. Community mental handicap nurses were employed within multidisciplinary teams to support people with learning difficulties in their family homes and in local authority accommodation. Bridging finance was provided to develop new community housing schemes, and by the end of the 1980s there had been a 50 per cent reduction in in-patient beds and a vast increase in residential and day care provided by statutory, voluntary and private sector agencies.

Normalisation was the philosophy driving the changes towards community integration. In 1981, a further Education Act recommended that people with learning difficulties be included within ordinary schools. Progress to date has been slow on this front, but there has been a major change of attitude towards acknowledging the rights of this client group to ordinary patterns of living. The government, pleased with its community care programme, confirmed its commitment to transfer the major part of its programme for people with mental handicaps to local authorities through the legislation of the NHS and Community Care Act 1990. The Act differentiated between health and social care, and stated that only services for people with severely disturbed (or challenging) behaviour, with sensory deficits, mental health needs or severe health-related incapacity would remain within the province of the NHS. Others with learning difficulties would be supported in their own homes by community mental handicap nurses and other health-care staff. Although a few clients would still require long-term care in residential facilities for assessment, treatment and rehabilitation, the focus was to be on the community.

A CHANGING MENTAL HEALTH SERVICE

Disillusionment with institutional care for the mentally ill began to be voiced by critics of the system at the end of the 1950s and increased in vigour during the early 1960s. Overcrowding, the emphasis on conformity and the lack of individual treatment plans were identified as anti-therapeutic for patients, and the poverty of the working environment for staff, it was claimed, was evident from the difficulties in attracting and retaining appropriately trained medical and nursing personnel. So cogently presented was this criticism of hospital care that alternative approaches were eagerly and hastily sought. New drug treatments, most significantly the development of the phenothiazines in the early 1950s and of the anti-depressants a decade later, made it feasible to offer more care on an out- or day-patient basis. This encouraged the establishment of psychiatric out-patient departments within District General Hospitals, so reducing the numbers being admitted to the psychiatric hospitals. Community care which aimed to free patients from restrictive regimes, giving them back their independence and reuniting them with their family and friends, thus began to be realised as an alternative to institutional care.

Better Services for the Mentally Ill (1975) is regarded by social policy analysts as the first long-term strategy to provide locally based services for the mentally ill. The White Paper recognised that there would be a delay in fully implementing community care and stated that in the meantime, services were to remain centred on mental hospitals. It also recognised that the cultures of the two organisations involved in implementing community care – namely, the health services and the social services – were distinctly different, and that many changes would have to be made before the two systems could work harmoniously together to make community care effective.

After 1975, periodic statements from government reaffirmed or clarified the direction which services for patients should be taking, and regular exhortations issued from ministers and professional bodies urging that the best possible service be provided for all at the point of need. However, despite the changes already initiated, the most trenchant attack on the NHS was yet to come when, in 1979, the Royal Commission noted the enormous and unchecked expansion which had taken place in the health service since 1948, and decided that the NHS could no longer shelter from the country's chill economic climate.

By the beginning of the 1980s, political critics were accusing the health service of being too bureaucratic, too slow in decision-making and far too costly in respect of what it was delivering. In 1982, Area Health Authorities were abolished and competitive tendering was introduced in 1983. Hospitalisation came to be seen as a last resort. The cost of health care was reduced by closing long-stay hospitals or at least decreasing the number of patients in them, and justified on humanitarian grounds:

> The elderly, the mentally ill and the mentally handicapped were finally publicly noticed and the standards of care they received questioned. Was it really appropriate and cost-effective to keep people in the institutional environment of a hospital? The answer was clearly no, and the seeds of the policy of wholesale care in the community were sown – the full implications of which we are realising only now.[16]

In 1983, the Griffiths Report (1983) ushered in the new era of the general manager who was empowered to take decisions regarding the direction of health care in order to put it on a firmer financial footing. No longer were professionals permitted to determine their own destinies; henceforth they were subject to government policies and regional strategies, both of which were driven by financial considerations.

In the same year, the Mental Health Act was passed, which gave a new authority to nurses to exercise 'holding power', permitting them to detain patients for up to six hours until a doctor could take charge. It was not encouraging to mental health nurses that, despite their much-proclaimed emphasis on therapy for patients, communication and interaction, the government still appeared determined to see them only as controllers of patients and regulators of their lives.

In 1981, the General Nursing Council, in response to the climate of change, commissioned a new syllabus for mental nurses to update their training. The syllabus came out just before the Council itself was disbanded two years later in July 1983. The 'new' syllabus, as it was popularly and somewhat euphorically called, aimed to ensure the survival of mental nursing at a time when the structure of care for psychiatric patients was being radically rethought. The haste with which the syllabus was introduced was largely motivated by the Jay Report (1979) which had suggested that mental handicap nurses were inappropriately named and trained and that they would be better placed under the aegis of social services rather than the health service. The Report even proposed that a new profession should be devised to care for people with mental handicap. In order to prevent a similar fate befalling psychiatric nurses, the GNC moved quickly to change psychiatric nursing practice in line with the new ideas being advocated by health-care commentators and adopted by more innovative health professions. The new syllabus aimed to give nurses a sense of direction and professional identity which they had hitherto lacked.

It was, therefore, just less than a century after the introduction of the first training scheme for mental nurses in 1891 that the 'new' syllabus attempted to revolutionise mental health nursing in England. The 1891 scheme had appeared in the wake of government's strategy for institutional care; the 1982 syllabus appeared in the wake of an opposite strategy, which was based on the premise that psychiatric hospitals were self-evidently undesirable, an assumption often accompanied by an uncritical advocacy of 'community care'.[17] Despite its claim to be 'new', many of the ideas contained in the new syllabus were not, although the attempt was made to distance psychiatric nursing from mere role-modelling or rule-following, and to encourage nurses to see themselves as part of a self-directed and evolving profession.[18, 19] In order to confront the challenge of de-institutionalisation, the syllabus attempted to foster in nurses' skills appropriate to caring for people in the community.

THE IMPACT OF PROJECT 2000

Project 2000 (1986) represents the most far-reaching overhaul of training in the history of nursing. Hailed by some as revolutionary and by many as progressive, it was intended to be the means by which the nursing profession could take its place on equal terms with the other caring professions. It aimed to increase educational opportunities for nursing students, to establish links with institutions of higher education, to improve morale and to encourage the involvement of nurses in health promotion and disease prevention. This was the overt agenda for Project 2000; it has since become apparent that government had a hidden agenda which included shifting the burden of payment for nursing students from the National Health Service to the Department of Education and Science by introducing a grant system, reducing the number of trained nursing staff, and increasing the number of care attendants.

As far as mental health nurses were concerned, it seemed that the recommendations contained in Project 2000 would help raise academic standards and, by improving the status of the nursing profession in general, would boost their own alongside that of their colleagues from other branches of nursing. However, the driving force behind Project 2000 came from general nursing, and it is clear that general nurses had most to gain from it. In a climate where short-term planning has reigned supreme, general nurses are a far more attractive group to train and fund than mental nurses whose clients require extended care and therapy if lasting results are to be achieved. When Project 2000 courses got under way nationally, mental nursing was relegated to branch programme status and the amount of clinical experience offered to students drastically reduced. Critics have argued that the nature of the change in the training of mental health nurses embodies a serious, and perhaps intended, threat to the identity and very survival of mental health nursing in the United Kingdom.[20]

As the millennium approaches, it seems as if mental health nursing finds itself under serious threat as the part its nurses are to play in the challenging new world of health-care delivery remains undefined. The nursing profession cannot ignore the economic climate prevailing throughout the Western world, which has led to drastic cuts in public expenditure and, in particular, spending on the welfare services. Community care itself has been seen by some as merely a response to economic necessity: 'providing a service on the cheap in which large numbers of ordinary people are being exploited and attempts are being made to cut down considerably on the responsibility of the collective towards its more vulnerable members'.[21] If, in the future, purchasers seek to buy care as cheaply as possible, they may well prefer to opt for untrained assistants in preference to trained nurses. Already many patients are being provided for not by the health service but at centres run by untrained personnel.

The last government review of mental health nursing took place in 1968 and reported under the title 'Psychiatric nursing today and tomorrow'.[22] This review included evidence from the Joint Sub-committee of the Standing Mental Health and Standing Nursing Advisory Committees and declared that psychiatric nurse education was a substantive subject. It urged that separate training for psychiatric nurses was essential if a high standard of care for mental health patients was to be achieved. Twenty-five years will have gone by before the next enquiry into mental health nursing reports at the beginning of 1994, continuing a pattern whereby government interest in mental health care seems to be triggered only by crisis situations. The forthcoming report will look at how mental health nurses should be trained and in what ways they should practise as the year 2000 approaches.

In spite of government's repeated reassurance that it sees mental health nursing as providing an important service for mentally ill people, the signs are ominous that it is in decline. Nursing is, as a profession, attracting dwindling numbers into training, and this is especially true of mental health nursing. Indeed, some colleges of nursing are currently unable to run a viable mental health branch. As the number of nurses falls, the number of clients requiring care in the community rises. Strict budgetary control is likely to mean that a limited number of mental health nurses will be used to fulfil a supportive rather than a therapeutic role. A generic approach to health care may become the norm and specialism in nursing become an outdated fashion. The generic nurse, however, may be poorly equipped to cope with the complex and challenging problems of the long-term mentally ill. Should mental health nurses disappear, this may reflect a hardening in society's resolve to distance itself from the unsatisfactorily insoluble problems of people whose health problems do not make good media stories. If the nurses go, services for the mentally ill may be the next to follow.

REFERENCES

1 Salvage, J. (1985) *The Politics of Nursing*, London: Heinemann Nursing.
2 Walk, A. (1961) 'The history of mental nursing', *Journal of Mental Science*, 107: 1–17.
3 Adams, F. R. (1969) 'From Association to Union – a professional organisation for attendants 1869–1919', *British Journal of Psychiatry*, 20: 11–26.
4 Carpenter, M. (1985) *They Still Go Marching On – a Celebration of COHSE's First 75 Years*, London: COHSE Publication.
5 Digby, A. (1985) *Madness, Morality and Medicine – a Study of the York Retreat*, Cambridge: Cambridge University Press.
6 Nolan, P. (1993) *A History of Mental Health Nursing*, London: Chapman & Hall.
7 Connolly, M. J. (1992) 'The value of historical investigation', in J. I. Brooking, S. A. H. Ritter and B. L. Thomas (eds) *A Textbook of Psychiatric and Mental Health Nursing*, London: Churchill Livingstone.
8 Clarke, L. (1991) 'Ideological themes in mental health nursing', ch. 3 in P. J. Barker and S. Baldwin (eds) *Ethical Issues in Mental Health*, London: Chapman & Hall.
9 Rollin, H. R. (1986) 'The Red Handbook: an historic century', *Bulletin of the Royal College of Psychiatrists*, 10: 279.

10 Royal College of Nursing Conference (1952) *Mental Health Conference Proceedings*, London.
11 Office of Health Economics (1977) *Annual Report*.
12 Powell, J. E. (1961) Speech by the Minister of Health, the Rt Hon. Enoch Powell *Report of the Annual Conference of the Association for Mental Health*, London.
13 The Hospital Plan (1962) London: HMSO.
14 *The Times*, Letters section, 10 Nov. 1965.
15 Robb, B. (1967) *Sans Everything*, London: Nelson.
16 Clay, T. (1987) *Nurses – Power and Politics*, London: Heinemann, p. 14.
17 Weller, M. P. I. (1989) 'Mental illness – who cares?' *Nature*, 339: 249–52.
18 Bergman, R. (1983) 'Understanding the patient in all his human needs', *Journal of Advanced Nursing*, 8: 185–90.
19 Jolley, M. (1987) 'The weight of tradition: a historical examination of early educational and curriculum development', in P. Allan and M. Jolley (eds) *The Curriculum in Nursing*, London: Croom Helm.
20 White, E. (1990) 'The future of psychiatric nursing by the year 2000: a Delphi study', Department of Nursing Studies, University of Manchester.
21 Ramon, S. (1991) *Beyond Community Care*, London: Macmillan, in Association with MIND Publications, p. 7.
22 *Psychiatric Nursing Today and Tomorrow* (1968) *Report of the Joint Subcommittee of the Standing Mental Health and the Standing Nursing Advisory Committees*, London: HMSO.

FURTHER READING

Berrios, E. G. and Freeman, H. (eds) (1991) *150 Years of British Psychiatry 1841–1991*, London: Gaskell and Royal College of Psychiatrists.
Department of Health (1975) *Better Services for the Mentally Ill*, London: HMSO.
Griffiths Report (1983) *Recommendations on the Effective Use of Manpower and Related Resources*, London: HMSO.
Handy, J. (1991) 'Stress and contradiction in psychiatric nursing', *Human Relations*, 44: 39–52.
Martin, J. P. (1984) *Hospitals in Trouble*, London: Basil Blackwell.
Peplau, H. E. (1980) 'Future directions in psychiatric nursing from the perspective of history', *Journal of Psychosocial Nursing*, 27: 18–28.
Smith, L. D. (1988) 'Behind closed doors: lunatic asylum keepers 1800–1860', *Social History of Medicine*, 1(3): 301–28.
United Kingdom Central Council for Nursing, Midwifery and Health Visitors (1986) 'Project 2000: A new preparation for practice', London: United Kingdom Central Council.

Chapter 21

Health at work

Paul Lloyd
With Mavis Gordon

> Work may be a source of livelihood, or a significant part of one's inner
> life. It may be experienced as expiation, or as an exuberant expression
> of self; as a bounden duty, or as a development of man's universal
> nature. Neither love nor hatred of work is inherent in man, or inherent
> in any given line of work.
>
> C. W. Mills, *The White Collar – The American Middle Class* (1956)

Mills is delineating the ways in which some of man's basic needs are met
through work, and he rightly emphasises that love or hatred of work is not
the prerogative of any particular occupation and that it can be man's
apotheosis or his nadir.

One aspect of work that is unchanging is that it carries a variety of
hazards to health, for even wielding a pen can affect the posture and
milking cows carries some risk. The builders of the medieval cathedrals fell
off scaffolding. Roman slaves died in the silver mines, and labourers in
the feudal fields, as their bones testify, suffered from arthritis. Any
modest research into the admissions to hospitals in areas affected by the
early Industrial Revolution will detect a rise in the number of lacerations,
multiple fractures and burns, and the building of the railways sometimes
called for new hospitals to take the expected casualties.

As Marx pointed out, a change in the means of production is a most
powerful factor in social change; one reason why the health needs of
people altered in the early nineteenth century was that many changed the
way in which they earned their living. Before the Napoleonic Wars the
great majority were engaged in agriculture and fishing; by 1851 it was 22
per cent; and by 1911 only 8 per cent.[1] Instead of working on the land,
growing numbers were employed in factories and mines, where labour was
increasingly mechanised, with some industries giving rise to the hazards
described in Chapter 8. But apart from this there were psychological problems; in 1776 Adam Smith had demonstrated that the division of labour,
where each worker performed only a small part of the production, would
greatly increase productivity, and this made work more repetitive and

often boring. One of the problems of mechanisation was that there was a tendency to see the worker himself as a machine, and at the beginning of the twentieth century researchers like Frederick Taylor were trying to limit people to machine-like behaviour, and with a ruthless scientific approach, prescribe what movements they should make, the rests that were appropriate and the limitation of their contacts.[2] 'Taylorism' was not popular with the workforce but the 'man-as-a-machine' concept had an important bearing on the organisation of work in a number of industries and it left a legacy of hostility towards such things as time and motion study.

Since then the industrial psychologists have turned away from the mechanistic approach. The famous experiments carried out by Patricia Elton Mayo at the Hawthorne Works in Chicago in 1924 showed that the relationship between good physical conditions and psychological well-being is not as straightforward as was supposed. For although improvements in working conditions led to better productivity, the output remained high when the improvements were gradually withdrawn, the obvious conclusion being that people work better when they are aware that someone is taking an interest in what they are doing. This conclusion is substantiated by Maslow[3] who, in 1943, produced his hierarchy of needs (Figure 21.1) in which he pointed out that once the lower needs have been satisfied they lose their potency and are superseded by the needs on the next level. This model is in fact saying much the same and although it is an oversimplification, it is a reminder that occupational health is far from being a matter of physical hazard and accident.

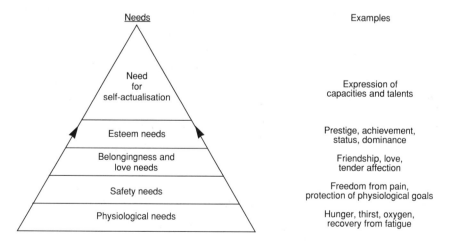

Figure 21.1 Maslow's hierarchy of needs

Through the twentieth century there have been a series of revolutions in the way people work and, consequently, of their occupational needs. Two world wars affected employment patterns; for example. the employment of women in heavy industry. By the 1970s, agriculture, fisheries and forestry employed 3 per cent of the working population. Thirty-eight per cent worked in manufacturing, leaving the rest employed in service industries such as finance, the professions, the sciences and public administration.

Further vast changes have occurred in the latter part of the century as large traditional industries declined (for mainly financial reasons) and smaller, often self-employed businesses emerged. Small companies were encouraged by the 1980s' political climate and the economy boomed. The type of work undertaken changed radically with the introduction of micro-electronics as fewer personnel were required to achieve the output of earlier manual operators.

By the 1990s, as a result of these changes, company privatisation policies and a deep economic recession, unemployment, redundancy and early retirement became commonplace. Employers struggled to maintain solvency as exports were reduced and cheaper products from overseas flooded the market. Workers were cut back in every sphere of occupation. It became increasingly common to find people working from home on a contract basis, the further development of micro-technology enabling communication by computer link and facsimile. Handy[4] states:

> Labour intensive manufacturing was traditionally managed with a large pool of relatively cheap labour, a lot of supervision and a hierarchical management structure. The result [of change] is not only a requirement for different people, but different organisations, organisations which recognise that they cannot do everything for themselves, that they need a central group of talented and energetic people, a lot of specialist help and ancillary agencies.

These changes have occurred over a comparatively short space of time and have resulted in the emergence of new occupational health problems. Fears of harm to the unborn baby from visual display unit operators arose. Repetitive strain injury became a common complaint from keyboard users and insecure employment prospects heralded dramatic increases in stress-related problems. As more people worked fewer hours, found themselves unemployed or retired early, the leisure and entertainment industry expanded.

DEVELOPMENT OF OCCUPATIONAL HEALTH SERVICES

Physicians like Ramazzini had written about the relationship of occupation and disease in the early eighteenth century but it was not until the Industrial Revolution that the subject was pursued in England. In 1775

Percivall Pott drew attention to the incidence of scrotal cancer in chimney sweeps, and in 1831 Charles Thackrah, in his *Effects of Arts, Trades and Professions and of Civic States and Habits of Living on Health and Longevity*, related life expectancy to a person's occupation and way of life, and, incidentally, pointed out the dangers of too much butcher's meat and high living. Later, as part of the Simon team, Edward Greenhow in 1860 made his pilgrimage through the factories and workshops of England examining the effects of industrialisation on pulmonary disease (see Chapter 8). Reformers in the nineteenth century were concerned with the effects of industrialisation on pulmonary disease (see Chapter 8). Reformers in the nineteenth century were concerned with the effects of industrialisation on two fronts. First, there were the actual hazards from new processes that gave rise to a variety of colourful complaints like 'grinder's colic', 'flaxman's bronchitis' and 'potter's rot', and the fact that some work like mining, grinding and cotton spinning seemed to shorten life and leave dependent widows. Second, there was a growing awareness that the long hours and conditions in the factories and workshops sapped the workers' vitality and destroyed them mentally and morally, and it was the fact that people could not be expected to lead Christian lives under such conditions – as Kay-Shuttleworth pointed out – that led the evangelical reformers like Ashley to take up the cause of factory reform.

The problem of intervention was that it was counter to the cherished theories of *laissez-faire* and the economic philosophies of Adam Smith and Ricardo; namely, that any distortion of the market forces by regulations would upset the natural economy. However, shocked at the treatment of the Poor Law apprentices sent to the factories, Sir Robert Peel (1750–1830), himself a manufacturer, persuaded William Pitt (1759–1806) to pass the Health and Morals of Apprentices Act in 1802, which was an unsuccessful attempt to limit the hours worked by pauper apprentices and to ensure that they had some schooling and religious instruction. Factory owners circumvented this simply by employing local children for whom no such embargo applied. In 1819, Robert Owen (1771–1858), the founder of the New Lanark Co-operative Villages, tried to persuade the government to forbid the employment of children under the age of 9 years in the mills and to limit the hours of those aged between 9 and 16 years, but in the emotional climate of Peterloo and post-war depression this was also doomed.

Then, after a decade, a fresh sense of purpose emerged, and the Reform Bill of 1832 enabled men like Richard Oastler (1789–1861) and Thomas Sadler (1780–1835), evangelical workers from Yorkshire, to press for legislation to control the work of children in factories. When Sadler, who stood as a Tory for Newark, lost his seat in the election of 1831, the leadership of the 'factory movement' passed to Lord Ashley, who, taking up the Sadler Report,[5] reintroduced the Bill prepared by Sadler for a 10-hour day. After much delay this was lost, but Althorp, the Chancellor, produced his own Bill which became law and limited the hours of children between 9 and 13 years to an eight-hour day and forbade the employment of children under 9 altogether. Two hours were set aside for education, work at night was forbidden for all persons under 18, and above all, four Factory Commissioners were appointed. Although the Act only applied to certain factories Althorp's Factory Act of 1833 was a milestone in social legislation. The Chief Factory Commissioner was Leonard Horner (1785–1864), who had been the head of the new London University, and who served the cause of factory reform with distinction for the next 15 years with reports that eventually shocked the conscience of Victorian England and led to further legislation.

In 1844 a further Act required that 'certifying surgeons' be employed to certify that the children employed in the textile mills had the ordinary strength and appearance of a child of 9 years, a necessity that tells its own story. Then, under the provisions of the 1867 Act, the surgeons were required to examine young persons under 16 years as to their fitness for work. Meanwhile, the Factory Inspectorate continued under the aegis of the Home Department, and as the work increased they appointed 'super-intendents' to deal with particular branches of the work. In 1898 the first medical inspector was appointed, Thomas Legge (1863–1932) – later Sir Thomas – who was himself a distinguished contributor to the body of knowledge on occupational disease and hazard.

Few employers in the nineteenth century provided any medical services for their workers, and those who did, like Colmans, were motivated by parental benevolence rather than prevention, and social welfare rather than illness arising through work. However, in 1897 the Workman's Compensation Act gave an impetus to the idea of a 'works' doctor', and some firms found it worthwhile to employ a doctor to help them protect themselves against claims for compensation.

The growth of what was known as 'industrial health services' in the twentieth century owes much to the stimulus of the two world wars. During the First World War the Ministry of Munitions had a medical department to advise on hygiene and, because of the increase in the number of women workers, more attention was paid to health and welfare (see Chapter 10). As a result of the war-time experience and the efforts of bodies like the Industrial Welfare Society and enlightened employers, in the inter-war period more doctors and nurses were appointed to work as industrial health practitioners and, as they built up a body of knowledge, so 'occupational health' became an important post-basic study. The Second World War again increased the interest in a health service for aspects of work, but it was the coming of the National Health Service that raised questions about its future and relevance.

Occupational health nursing

Most branches of nursing were nascent before the nineteenth century, the exception being occupational health nursing, which reflects the social changes and attitudes of the second half of the Industrial Revolution; inasmuch as it is concerned with prevention and education, it is a twentieth-century medical concept. The First World War demonstrated the value of trained nurses to industry as a positive force for the improvement of standards. In the 1916 Annual Report of the Chief Factory Inspector it stated, 'Even before the formation of the Welfare Department at the Ministry of Munitions some manufacturers were employing trained nurses, lady superintendents and providing improved cloakrooms, rest rooms and washing conveniences.' The Report goes on to comment on how these measures have improved the whole standard of life in the factory, and since this part of the Report is about the value of women workers, adds a gentle suffragette plug, 'women have been kept back too much', and goes on to hope that the better standard of hygiene and the employment of qualified nurses would continue.[6]

After the war, with the return of men, most women workers returned to their homes, but a number of nurses remained in industry. In 1928 the Industrial Welfare Society called a national conference in London in which the need for a special training was discussed, and in 1934, partly as the result of these deliberations, the Education Department of the College of Nursing produced a syllabus and a course of training that was the forerunner of the present Occupational Health Nursing Certificate. Between 1939 and 1945 there was again an expansion of the health services in industry, mainly due to the various requirements of the Emergency Orders; then after the war a number of firms continued to employ doctors and nurses and, because of the greater understanding of the relationship of work to health, universities and other institutions started to offer courses for a Diploma in Industrial Health.

Over the years, education for nurses in the field of occupational health developed to a higher academic level, keeping pace with changes in general nursing education. Until 1988 the Royal College of Nursing was the central body for Occupational Health Nursing Certificate course validation across the United Kingdom. Responsibility for occupational health nurse education passed to the national boards for England, Scotland, Wales and Northern Ireland, in 1988. At that time institutions started to develop diploma and degree level courses in occupational health nursing, the Institute of Advanced Nursing Education leading the way in 1990. At this time it also became necessary for all nurses, midwives and health visitors to re-register with the United Kingdom Central Council-on a three-yearly basis. It is proposed that evidence of approved post-basic educational enhancement will be required for registration in the future.

The National Health Service, however, was short of both nurses and doctors. Complaints were voiced to the government that industry, and particularly the new nationalised industries, were duplicating services and diverting doctors and nurses who would be better employed in the National Health Service. In 1949 the Prime Minister, Clement Attlee, set up a committee under the chairmanship of Judge Edgar Dale,[7] to examine the relationship between the preventive and curative health services provided for the population at large and the industrial health services which call upon manpower, and to consider what measures should be taken to ensure that manpower was used to the best advantage.

The Committee on Industrial Health Services had 2 nurse members out of a committee of 12, and was, to this extent, a measure of the improved status of the occupational health nurse. Reporting in 1951, the Committee stated that there was no appreciable overlapping with the National Health Service, that the industrial health services were performing a necessary and separate function, and that 'there should eventually be some comprehensive provision for occupational health covering not only industrial establishments but non-industrial occupations'. To this end the Committee urged further research, pointing out that the Gowers Committee of 1949 had already commented on the needs of non-industrial undertakings. Both enquiries pointed to the wide range of services being offered, the largest being that organised by the National Coal Board, but the Report stressed that the majority of workers were employed in small establishments whose owners could not possibly afford a health service. The Dale Report showed that out of 243,769 factories, 202,868 had fewer than 26 workers – a typically British situation, and only 4,884 had more than 250 employees. Few of the smaller factories offered any medical service, and the services provided by many of the larger firms were not much more than first aid.[8] To overcome the difficulties of providing services to smaller undertakings a number of experiments were tried, the oldest being the Slough Industrial Health Service established in 1947 with a grant from the Nuffield Trust; since then a number of experimental schemes to provide services have been set up, especially in the 'new towns', but while voluntary endeavour produced some results it obviously did not provide full cover and the question remained: should there be a service in some way linked to the National Health Service?

The Safety and Health at Work Committee under the chairmanship of Lord Robens took a more cautious view and reiterated the danger of duplicating the facilities provided by the National Health Service. For this reason, and for other political and economic considerations (see Chapter 25), the Act providing for the reorganisation of the Health Service, when it did come, contained no proposals for linkage with the occupational health services.

In spite of the uncertainties about the future of the occupational health services and whether or not they should be more closely associated with the health service, there has been a slow if unspectacular provision of occupational health services.

Organisation of occupational health

The growth of occupational health services in Great Britain in the 1990s has not been dramatic, despite the volume of EEC directives and domestic health and safety legislation. Only about 30 per cent of the workforce has any occupational health provision, and there is no legislation requiring employers to establish or have access to occupational health services.

The use of health professionals was surveyed[9] by the Health and Safety Executive in 1976 and again in 1993. The 1976 survey[10] revealed that in the sectors surveyed some 5.5 per cent of private sector employers employing 52 per cent of the workforce employed medical and or nursing staff.

The 1993 survey revealed that employees in the private sector, covering 15.9 million workers, had 'any health professional' in 36 per cent of cases, or a nurse (full- or part-time) in 14 per cent of cases. In the public sector the figures were much better, being 98 per cent or 86 per cent respectively for 5.8 million workers. This can be seen clearly in Table 21.1; along with analysis of doctor availability.

Table 21.1 The use of health professionals, 1993

	Total employees (21.7m) (%)	Private sector (15.9m) (%)	Public sector (5.8m) (%)
Any health professional	53	36	86
Nurse (full or p/t)	35	14	86
Doctor (full or p/t)	34	20	72

The survey also revealed that the roles of health professionals (nurses) had broadened from carrying out treatment of sickness or accidents to:

- monitoring health and safety procedures (66 per cent of private-sector establishments);
- advice on preventive measures (43 per cent);
- regular health checks (39 per cent);
- control of substances hazardous to health assessments (28 per cent);
- health and safety management (26 per cent);
- implementation of health and safety procedures (25 per cent);
- monitoring of sickness absence records (22 per cent);
- treatment was carried out in 4 per cent of establishments (40 per cent in large establishments).

Factors which have influenced these developments include legislation pressures, risk assessments, and HSE/Employment Medical Advisory Service activity.

Occupational health services have developed in the service sectors such as local government, the police and the fire services.

Aims and functions of occupational health service

In 1959 a joint committee of the International Labour Organisation and the World Health Organisation on occupational health defined the aims of the service as the highest degree of physical, mental and social well-being of workers in all occupations. The same year the International Labour Organisation's Recommendation No. 112 (later endorsed by the European Economic Community in 1962 and the Council of Ministers in 1972) defined the purposes of an occupational health service as:

1 protecting the workers against any health hazard which may arise out of their work or the conditions in which it is carried on;
2 contributing towards the workers' physical and mental adjustment, in particular by the adaptation of their work and assignments to the jobs for which they are suited;
3 contributing to the establishment and maintenance of the highest possible degree of physical and mental well-being of the workers.[11]

Later, in 1985 the ILO produced two further instruments; namely, Convention 161 and Recommendation 171 on the Organisation of Occupational Health Services. The British government adopted the Recommendation but had not ratified the Convention by 1993. The Convention defines

> occupational health services as meaning services entrusted with essentially preventive functions and responsible for advising the employer, the workers, and their representatives on the requirements to establish and maintain a safe and healthy environment which will facilitate optimal mental and physical health in relation to work, and the adaptation of work to the capabilities of those performing it in the light of their state of physical and mental health.

The situation with regard to the European Community Law is quite different because the UK government has no option but to implement the EC Directives concerning health and safety arrangements in member states. A Draft Directive is sent to member states for consultation. Agreement is then reached as far as this is possible, and the European Parliament then implements the Directives requiring all member states without exception to enact or modify domestic legislation to comply with the intent of the Directive within a specified time scale.

Directives have been issued on:

1 The Management of Health and Safety at Work Regulations, 1992;
2 Manual Handling Operations Regulations, 1992;
3 Personal Protective Equipment Regulations, 1992;
4 Workplace (Health Safety and Welfare) Regulations, 1992;
5 Provision and use of Work Equipment Regulations, 1992, and other regulations covering Substances Hazardous to Health Regulations, Biological Agents Regulations and many others.

Role and function of the Health and Safety Executive

The government enforcement and national advisory agency is the Health and Safety Executive (HSE). This consists of a national field force of Health and Safety Inspectors, qualified occupational health doctors and nurses, scientists and other specialists. Their function is to undertake routine inspections of workplaces and offer advice, and in certain cases inspectors can impose improvement or prohibition notices on employers where the risks of injury or disease to workers is unacceptable.

This field force also carry out surveys and conduct research, publish advisory documents and collect data on occupational accidents and diseases reported to the agency under the statutory reporting arrangements imposed on employers, general practitioners, or appointed doctors carrying out health surveillance on behalf of the HSE.

The means of reporting are through the Reporting of Injuries, Diseases and Dangerous Occurrences Regulations 1985 (RIDDOR). Steps are being taken to expand these reporting arrangements and to harmonise these with a European schedule of occupational diseases.

The House of Lords Select Committee on the Future of Occupational Health and Hygiene Services reported in 1984, and could only agree that occupational health should be provided on a voluntary basis by employers. Enforcement through legislation was not considered at that stage to be appropriate. Therefore, the task fell to the HSE to persuade employers of the value of occupational health services by offering advice and information about the occupational health implications of their workplace activities.

The RCN recommend that qualified occupational health nurses should be based in health centres to give advice on the occupational health aspects of patient referrals. This recommendation was accepted by the Select Committee.

In 1990 the government wanted to extend the development of National Vocational Qualifications (NVQs) into the health and safety sector. For the first time both doctors and nurses working in the specified field of occupational health had to produce their competencies on paper, a task which was beset with many problems.

The organisational pattern and structure of Occupational Health Services has undergone a radical change since the mid-seventies, with the wholesale demise of the large industries such as coal mining and steel manufacture. Further dramatic changes have been wrought by the introduction of auto-mative processes robotics, mechanisation and new technologies, which have tended to make the more dangerous industries like glass manufacturing or chemicals cleaner and safer.

This has resulted in a dramatic reduction in the numbers of occupational health nurses required to work a 24-hour shift system who provide emergency and continuing first aid and ongoing treatment for injured workers.

There has been and continues to be a gradual decline in the manufacturing base in the United Kingdom due to the opening up of world markets and the development of the EEC. One of the purposes of the EEC is to allow the free passage of goods and services between member states.

Due to the decline in manufacturing and the improvement in manufacturing methods, there is an increased awareness of the health risks and better inspection and enforcement arrangements by the government's Health and Safety Inspectorate.

An occupational health service for the NHS staff

As long ago as 1943 the King Edward Hospital Fund issued a memorandum on the Supervision of Nurses' Health. In 1949 the Horder Report urged a new approach to the care of staff in hospitals, and the Dale Report recommended occupational health services 'for non-industrial occupations'. During the next 15 years there was an upsurge of interest, and services, like the one at Slough, increased their coverage by sixfold – an interest not shared by the NHS. In 1964, prompted by the Occupational Health Section, the Royal College of Nursing published a booklet, *A Hospital Occupational Health Service*, which set out the objectives and functions of such a service and the staffing and accommodation necessary. As a result of this and the fact that the Ministry had issued a multiplicity of circulars on the subject that remained unheeded, a committee was set up in 1965 under the chairmanship of Sir Ronald Tunbridge, 'to examine the standards and the scope of the health services provided for hospital staffs of all grades.' The Tunbridge Committee reported in November 1967, with the main recommendation that 'Hospital authorities should aim at setting up an occupational health service for all their employees.[12] The Report contained guidance about the functions of such a service and its relationship with other departments of the hospital. However, most Hospital Management Committees were slow to consider its implementation, and the nursing profession itself was not always enthusiastic. First, the hospital ethos was antipathetic to a service whose aims were not curative, and as most staff saw the service in terms of diagnosis and treatment, they considered that this was provided by the present arrangements. The other obstacle was confidentiality: hospitals were used to being employer and medical adviser; indeed, the two functions could be combined in one person, and they were sometimes confused. The idea of senior nursing and medical staff not having access to the medical records of the staff was revolutionary, and an indication of the need for change. As more staff became non-resident and the hospital bureaucracy more remote, these problems tended to dissolve, but there remained the question of finance, and the health care of staff still had a low priority in the NHS compared with the best industry. The Royal College of Nursing in its evidence to the Royal Commission on the Health Service said, 'in spite of notable experiment and advance, for the most part not only are the cobbler's children badly shod, in many cases they have no shoes'.

However, by the 1990s most hospital staff had access to occupational health units, but each has developed independently and there are wide variations in services provided. Nurses tend to manage the NHS units, but more hospitals are now employing occupational health consultants to lead the service.

A wide spread of occupational health problems are faced by NHS staff, most commonly back injury in nurses and ancillary workers. The risk of exposure to chemical and biological hazard is high, and a programme of protection against hepatitis B for health-care workers has been implemented. The lifting of 'Crown Immunity' from hospital premises and the introduction of the Control of Substances Hazardous to Health Regulations (1988) raised awareness and action for health and safety. Pressure on NHS staff from increased workloads and cutback led to stress-related problems.

Health authorities are currently moving into the purchase/provider concept as trust status is sought, leading to the most enormous changes to be faced by hospital services since the inception of the NHS. All these changes are inevitably affecting occupational health services, some staff becoming an 'essential' component of the organisation as they 'sell' occupational health services to outside agencies, thus generating income. In contract, however, some units are being cut back or closed, as managers have a poor perception of the occupational health function and potential. A publication from the Health Services Advisory Committee (1993) provides guidance to health service managers on the provision of occupational health services for their staff.

REFERENCES

1 Parker, S. R. *et al.* (1972) *The Sociology of Industry*, London: Allen & Unwin, p. 24.
2 Brown, J. A. C. (1954) *The Social Psychology of Industry*, London: Penguin Books, pp. 12 ff.

3 Maslow, A. H. (1943) 'A theory of human motivation, *Psychological Review*, 50: 370–96.

4 Handy, C. (1990) *The Age of Unreason*, London: Arrow Books.

5 *Report of the Select Committee on Factory Children's Labour* (the Sadler Report) (1831), London: HMSO; see Fraser, D. (1973) *The Evolution of the Welfare State*, London: Macmillan, p. 234.

6 *Annual Report of the Chief Factory Inspector for 1915*, Parliamentary Papers (1916), Cmnd 8276, London: HMSO.

7 *Report of the Committee of Inquiry on Industrial Health Services* (Dale Report), (1957) Cmnd. 8170, London: HMSO.

8 Ibid., Appendix E, Table A.

9 Bunt, K. (1993) *Occupational Health Provision at Work,* HSE Contract Research Report No 57/1993, London: HMSO.

10 *Occupational Health Services*, (1977) London: HMSO, Health and Safety Commission, pp. 20, 21.

11 *Report of the 43rd Session, International Labour Organisation Conference* (1959) London: HMSO, Geneva.

12 *The Care of the Health of Hospital Staff*, (Tunbridge Report) (1986) Scottish Home and Health Department, London: HMSO.

FURTHER READING

Fraser, D. (1973) *The Evolution of the British Welfare State*, London: Macmillan.

The Control of Substances Hazardous to Health Regulations (1988) SI 1988/1657, London: HMSO.

The Management of Occupational Health Services for Health Care Staff (1993), London: HMSO.

Chapter 22

Nurses as managers

June Clark

> How few men, or even women, understand either in great or in little things what it is the being 'in charge' – I mean how to carry out a 'charge'. From the most colossal calamities down to the most trifling accidents, results are often traced (or rather not traced) to such want of someone 'in charge' or of his knowing how to be 'in charge'.
>
> Florence Nightingale, *Notes on Nursing*, 1859

> In short, if Florence Nightingale was carrying her lamp through the corridors of the NHS today she would almost certainly be searching for the people in charge.
>
> Sir Roy Griffiths, *NHS Management Enquiry*, 1983

Miss Nightingale, having considered various alternatives, and realising the problems of basing a system of nursing on a religious movement, especially in the acute religious sectarian strife of the nineteenth century, decided to base her reforms of the pattern of the voluntary general hospitals, where, in spite of the over-blown claims of the reformers, there were already nurses of standing. Miss Nightingale grafted on to the system new and important principles: first, all nurses should be trained, and promotion should depend on nursing and leadership merit, and second, in matters affecting nursing the matron should be supreme. The matron now became head of nursing service and nurse training while retaining much of her old responsibility for the hospital housekeeping. The hospital steward, now often called the secretary, had overall responsibility for the general administration of what was becoming a complex institution, while the doctors, who were usually honorary and worked through committees, were responsible for purely medical matters. Thus began the tripartite system of control that characterised voluntary hospital administration and later became the accepted pattern for the National Health Service.

The new municipal hospitals, which had evolved from the Poor Law infirmaries built after the Metropolitan Poor Law Act of 1867, developed along different lines and presented the framers of the National Health Service Act with a second type of administration. Once medical care, rather than Poor Law relief, was established as the reason for the institution, the doctors wrested the ultimate power from the Master and established a hierarchical administration under a Medical Superintendent to whom both the nursing matron and the lay administration were subordinate. Until the late nineteenth century, when hospital administration was comparatively simple, both systems were uncomplicated; but as at the beginning of the nineteenth century when medical advance had imposed tasks upon nurses for which they were neither recruited nor trained, so, in the twentieth century, further advance and the new expectations of patients placed new strains on nursing administration for which it was not prepared. The matron could no longer cope single-handed with her three-fold task as head of nursing service, nursing education and general housekeeper, and assistants had to be brought in. Tutors were needed for nurse training, and assistants were required to help with the increasingly complex side of nursing service: some had special tasks like the supervision of the nurses' home; others merely assisted over a wide range of tasks, some of which had little to do with nursing.

As the hospitals developed, new groups of workers came into being, each carving out its own empire. Often these groups did not provide a 24-hour service, but nurses had often done these tasks, such as taking X-rays, before the new groups came, and because nurses were adaptable the range of tasks they encompassed, especially at weekends, tended to be wide. The para-medical groups such as physiotherapists, radiographers, dieticians and occupational therapists often had their own training departments within the hospital, and for some of these the matron had no responsibility, while for others she had a nominal responsibility but no authority. On the housekeeping side, simple quartering of patients gave way to a sophisticated hotel service with caterers, laundry firms, domestic supervisors and even contract cleaners, who were accountable to the hospital secretary although the matron might be expected to take some responsibility for deficiencies in the service.

As was shown in Chapter 16, the tripartite pattern of administration from the voluntary system did not fit comfortably into the hierarchical structure of the health service with its three tiers of management and its crucial decision making at Group Management level where there was no nursing voice. The recommendations of the Bradbeer Committee (see Chapter 16) were too equivocal to produce any real improvement, and the growing disenchantment with nursing administration meant that it was difficult to fill posts. In 1961 the Royal College of Nursing carried out an enquiry into the fate of all nursing administration posts advertised in the *Nursing Times* between October 1959 and March 1960; the results showed that one-fifth of the posts remained vacant, over one-third attracted only one candidate or were left unfilled and rather more than a third were filled by internal promotion. The number of candidates who had done a course in administration was negligible, and most candidates were over 40 years old and had no qualification other than State registration.

As the result of the survey and pressure from its membership, in 1964 the Royal College of Nursing issued *Administering the Hospital Nursing Services – a Review*, which examined the current problems in the three main areas: administration, education and clinical nursing. The Report showed that in administration nurses compared unfavourably with other hospital administrators; their duties were manifold and often included responsibility for non-nursing areas, hours were long and difficult, and residence was often a condition of employment which fostered an unfavourable image. Similar pressures had altered the situation of the tutor, who often felt restricted, lacking in academic freedom and the chance of a more heuristic approach to education, and whose discontent was both vociferous and manifest in shortages. The post of ward sister which should have represented the apex of clinical nursing had also suffered a sea change. The ward sister was often placed in a cruel dilemma: changes in surgery and medicine and the increased pace of patient turnover meant that the physical strain was greater than many could bear until retirement day, and the only escape was into administration or teaching; moreover, it was only by going into administration that the clinical nurse could improve her salary, and consequently her pension prospects. In this, nursing was in direct contrast to medicine, where clinical consultancy was the pinnacle for the profession; a contrast that threw some doubt on the claim of nursing to be a profession, since the actual practice of nursing seemed to be lowly regarded from the point of view of salary and, apparently, prestige only came through the practice of some other skill like administration or teaching.

The Report, which was intended to be read in conjunction with the Platt Report on education (see Chapter 23), set out proposals which it was hoped would offer a career pattern to the well-qualified candidate in clinical nursing, in education or in nursing administration – three equally regarded ladders. The proposed pattern of nursing administration was based on the concept of the District General Hospital within the current framework of the health service; the nursing head of the group would be the group nursing officer who would not have day-to-day responsibility for a particular hospital as 'senior nursing officers' would have charge of individual hospitals in the Group – in other words, they would fulfil the old role of matron, but now they would look to a nursing rather than a lay head of the service. Then, instead of using 'deputy matrons' and 'assistants' the hospitals would be divided into clinical areas under the control of a nursing officer, who would be able to offer clinical advice to the less experienced sisters who were being appointed at an ever earlier age. This type of post would offer the ward sister promotion while retaining her clinical skill. The College, now a champion for sex equality in nursing, wished to drop the title 'matron' as it implied that the head of nursing service was expected to be a woman.

THE COMMITTEE ON SENIOR NURSING STAFF (THE SALMON REPORT)

The outcome of pressure from the Royal College of Nursing and the Association of Hospital Matrons was that in 1963 the Minister of Health, Kenneth Robinson, invited Mr Brian Salmon (later Sir Brian) to chair a committee of management experts and nurses to 'advise on the structure of senior staff in hospitals and the methods of preparing staff for those posts'. The Committee, after two years of research, reported in December 1965 with radical recommendations which represented an attempt to come to terms with modern management in the structure of the health service *as it then was*. The Committee was not asked to address itself to the problem of whether the basic structure of the health service was sound.

On the whole, the Report was welcomed by the nursing profession because it restored nursing to the decision-making process, and although this meant sacrificing the notion that each hospital and its staff were a separate identity, many people already realised that because of the haphazard growth of the hospitals in the historical past, this rationalisation was inevitable. To get over the confusion of the 16 administrative grades where the so-called 'assistant' matrons often deputised and the 'deputy' matrons assisted, and where structural authority might be through triadic, or even dual triadic, control, it was necessary to establish a simple logical system of line authority with each nursing post responsible to the one above. The Committee, having examined the administrative and management skills required of nurses, came to the conclusion that there were three distinct areas of management in nursing, each of which required a different type of preparation: the 16 grades could be condensed into six with two grades for each type of management. For convenience's sake, and unfortunately, the management grades were numbered from five to ten – unfortunately, because the new job titles were quickly replaced in common parlance by the grade numbers, a habit which merely strengthened the criticisms of the Report's opponents.

First-line management

This group included staff nurses, senior enrolled nurses and ward sisters; these were the people who ordered and co-ordinated others caring for the patient. The administrative task of the ward sister was essentially organisational because she allocated tasks to the team; on the one hand, she was under the structural authority of the matron, while on the other she acted under the direction of the doctor, but she herself, by virtue of her own clinical experience, exercised some authority, which the Committee described as 'sapiential authority'. This grade, the Committee pointed out, was now marrying earlier and had continually to be replaced. Other posts in first-line management were certain posts at that time designated as 'departmental' or 'clinical' manager.

Middle management

By analogy with the computer, the Committee grouped the tasks of 'programming' into middle management; that is, the planning and providing of resources for first-line management to execute. For example, it might be agreed that the whole group would change to central sterilisation; middle management would withdraw old equipment, see that the staff were instructed in the new techniques, and in consultation with those who were to run the programme, plan the operation of the new service. However, the most important recommendation for this group was the misunderstood and hotly debated concept of the 'nursing officer' – significantly called by the Committee 'matron', but in common parlance 'the number 7'. This post was intended to deal with the rapid turnover of young ward sisters. By promoting the experienced clinical practitioner as an adviser on nursing practice, as indeed happened in the armed services, it was hoped that the young and inexperienced would be supported, and that those with clinical skill and judgement would not waste it by going into administration. However, if Miss Nightingale had instilled the idea that the matron was supreme and no other nurse had authority over her, the idea had spread downwards, and it was soon clear that there would be opposition to the idea of any other nurse advising a ward sister on clinical matters.

Top management

Traditionally nursing policy was formulated by the General Nursing Council, the Nursing Division of the Ministry of Health and the professional nursing organisations, but under the system before 1966 there was no way in which nursing policy could be presented to a Hospital Management Committee. In order to overcome this lacuna the Committee recommended that the policy-forming function should be undertaken by nurses in top management – men and women suitably selected and prepared for such posts, with a chief nursing officer (the 'number 10') now acting as the spokesman for nursing. The hospital groups would be organised in 'divisions' and, for example, a group of 2,000 beds might have a division for general nursing, maternity services, psychiatry and a teaching division. Each division would be controlled by a principal nursing officer (the 'number 9'), who would be responsible to the chief nursing officer, who might have control over all the divisions, or, depending on the size and variety, have control over some but a co-ordinating function for the others.

Preparation and selection

In order to organise courses of preparation and to provide assessors for the new posts, the Committee recommended the setting up of National and Regional Nursing Staff Committees which, it was suggested, might co-operate with the Royal Colleges of Nursing and Midwifery to institute advanced courses and qualifications. The Committee, in Appendix 9 of the Report, made specific proposals about the length and content of the various courses. In other appendices the Committee set out a number of specimen organisational plans and job descriptions for the different grades in the various types of group. The Report was comprehensive and offered a blue print for implementation.

The implementation of the Report

The Report was accepted by the Ministry of Health and a National Nursing Staff Committee was appointed. The nursing division, in consultation with regional hospital boards, selected suitable management groups as pilot schemes. The criteria for such schemes were that the management committee concerned and the associated medical and administrative staff had to be willing to accept the principles of the Report; the group should have reasonable stability and there should be an expectation of obtaining staff in the quantity and of the quality required. One problem was that the scheme had implications for the Whitley Council and the negotiations were likely to be protracted. Did 'parity of esteem' mean parity of salary? If not, why not? But if 'top' nurses were lifted out of the traditional low pay for nurses, how long would it be before there was a new set of differentials and the whole nursing budget raised? The year 1966 saw a sterling crisis and an attempt at 'severe restraint deflation'; the situation was complicated by the well-known and oft-repeated proviso, 'the report is accepted in principle but there can be no extra money for its implementation'. But money was what successful implementation needed. It was imperative that the pilot groups be given the best possible education so that they might train others, but this was not forthcoming and there was no money for extra staff while the staff were away being trained – which did not endear the scheme to those left behind. The pilot schemes also had the difficulty of being unable to send staff to suitable courses in advance, and there were the inevitable difficulties about the salaries that were paid on an *ad hoc* basis which in no way reflected the new responsibilities and which provoked the editor of the *Nursing Times* into the terse comment that 'Salmon was being had at cod prices'.[1]

Although the report was welcomed as being rational and logical there were serious criticisms The Royal College of Nursing, still annoyed about the non-acceptance of 'A reform of nursing education', pointed out that a reform of nursing administration should have been a concomitant of a different approach to nursing education, and they feared that unless nurses were prepared with a more liberal education they would not be able to make the best contribution to the new system. The College was critical of the way nursing education had been dovetailed into the management structure and of the criteria the Committee had used in estimating the number of tutors required and their grades. Many people argued that the most urgent need was for *nurses to be better prepared as nurses*. At the same time there was disappointment, and some conflict, about the standard of the course proposed for top managers; the College always hoped there would be a Diploma of the University of London for nursing administration to take its place alongside the Diploma offered for tutors and the Diploma in Nursing for those in clinical practice. In fairness to the Committee, nursing education was not part of their brief and they had to deal with the situation as it was, and when it came to planning courses for management it was a question of the art of the possible, and they did say that they hoped such posts and courses would attract candidates holding degrees.

Apart from the serious criticisms there were many emotional attacks, with perhaps the most rancorous coming from the medical profession. All institutions are conservative, and in the face of change they exhibit what Dr Schon once described as 'dynamic conservatism'; that is they fight to preserve the stable state.[2] For the doctors the stable state was the Nightingale system although a hundred years earlier they had bitterly opposed its implementation. Not only did doctors dislike the idea of nursing administrators in the upper echelons, as their predecessors had disliked the idea of the 'new matrons' with control over nursing – they were also concerned that at ward level there would be interference by the new type of nursing officer in the clinical judgement of 'their' ward sister, and in some vicarious way, with their own clinical freedom. As it happened, for better or for worse, the fear was unfounded and the post rarely developed as a clinical adviser. In these criticisms by the doctors there was a tendency to compare nursing with medicine where advancement (and higher salary) came with the advancement of skill in practice. In some ways the comparison was refreshing – though it is doubtful if the critics were prepared to see this through to the logical conclusion, and it led to useful discussion about the possibility of using nurses with particular nursing skills and expertise as advisers to others.

As the pilot schemes were being organised in 1967, the current pay scales, awarded by the Whitley Council two years earlier, came up for revision. However, at the beginning of 1966 the Wilson administration had announced a six months' pay and prices freeze and had set up a National

Board for Prices and Incomes to deal with the period of restraint that followed. Accordingly, the Board examined the pay claim by nurses and in 1968 issued *Report No. 60 on the Pay of Nurses and Midwives*. This Report was important because a number of consequences flowed from it, for it not only made recommendations about pay, but as the result of research and analysis, also made a number of general comments. It was highly critical of the uneven standard of entry into nursing, a criticism that had been made by reports and investigations since 1937, and urged that in the long term 'large group training schools be set up'. However, the severest criticism was reserved for the structure of the health service itself, which it saw as the source of many problems. The Report stated, 'we think there is a diffusion of authority and a fragmented system of management which makes it difficult to increase efficiency in the hospital. We suggest that in the long term the present system might give way *to a simple tier system** in which authority and management functions would be concentrated in a small number of Area Health Boards or similar bodies.'[3]

As a corollary of this recommendation, the Board stated that the senior nursing management structure recommended by the Salmon Committee should be brought into operation as soon as possible because this was seen as a pattern that would fit into a reorganised rationalised health service. To this end the Board made recommendations about salaries for key posts in the so-called 'Salmon grades' which, although not comparable with the salaries paid in general administration, which is what the staff were asking, were a considerable improvement.[4]

As the result of *Report No. 60* there was a Gadarene rush into the new system. Now, in the desire to see the report of the Committee on Senior Nursing Staff Structure implemented as quickly as possible, few had a chance of full preparation, and the lessons of the pilot schemes were not absorbed; indeed, some senior staff did not have the opportunity for preparation until after they were in post, and even then it was not of the standard and length suggested by the Committee. Moreover, in spite of a spate of conferences all over the country, it was clear that not everyone understood the goals of the new system. Therefore, in a number of cases it was not a question of 'Salmon' having been tried and failed; it was never tried as it was intended.

SALMON IN RETROSPECT

In spite of the early enthusiasm, the Report subsequently tended to have a bad press. While some of the criticism was justified, much of it has was emotional and displayed an elliptical regard for the truth. The Report showed that demographic change was such that ward sisters would marry

---

* Author's italics

and stay in post a shorter time. This came true, but the Salmon Report, like Cassandra, was destined to tell the truth and not be believed; when the event foretold was palpably true it was the prophet who was blamed.[5] But although the turnover of staff was greater because of social mobility, it is untrue to say that the implementation of the Report increased the number of nursing administrators at the expense of the wards. If anything, the reverse is true. The British Medical Association promoted the myth and their evidence to the Royal Commission on the Health Service stated (on the subject of 'Salmon'), 'an army of the best and most capable nurses upon whom he (the consultant) depended have been removed from a clinical sphere to an administrative one'.[6] In fact, a report issued by the Department of Health in 1972 had shown that out of a sample of 20 schemes, all but three had a higher ratio of ward sisters and staff nurses to the numbers in nursing administration than there had been in 1966.[7] This conclusion was substantiated by the Royal Commission itself,[8] and by the Department of Health statistics.[9]

In several important respects the philosophy of the report was not put into practice. The post of nursing officer has never been developed as was intended. There are many reasons for this; first, there was the problem of fitting into the new system numbers of nurses who in the past had been translated to the matron's office and, through no fault of their own, were out of touch with clinical matters. Second, ward sisters, often supported by their consultants, looked askance at what might be interpreted as clinical interference. Ward sisters were used to looking above for administrative advice, but if they wanted help in clinical matters they looked horizontally to nursing and medical colleagues. Ward sisters were well used to tapping other people's sapiential authority. A more potent reason for the non-development of the nursing officer as a clinical grade was that clinical changes were taking place so rapidly that a nurse with no specialist practice of her own could soon be out of date on matters of detail. Moreover, hospitals did not divide into neat parcels; the chances were that a unit would be heterogeneous, and even if the nursing officer was a specialist in one field, say orthopaedics, she would have no particular expertise to offer the other wards in her unit. In the last analysis the reason why the nursing officer post did not develop as intended was that the numbers of nursing *administrative staff did not increase*, but the burden of paperwork, reporting, staff problems, labour relations work, legislation and the number of committees did.

Since the nursing officer was forced into administrative rather than clinical work people began to argue in favour of using the nurse who had developed special nursing skills in a different way. In the past ten years new attention has been given to the problem of providing care. It is now accepted, in a way that was not possible in 1966, that some nurses, by study and research, can develop special skills in aspects of nursing – for example, terminal care, stoma care and oncology – and that such nurses may be used to advise their colleagues both in hospital and the community and to play a part in teaching other disciplines. This development of the nurse specialist, arising as it has done from the clinical situation itself, is proving more fruitful than the solution proposed as part of a management structure. In essence, the perceived failure of the Salmon proposals was due not to the proposals themselves but to the circumstances of their implementation. In particular, the speed at which the proposals were implemented following the Prices and Incomes Board Report exacerbated misunderstandings about the underlying principles and led to the over-hasty use of inappropriate training models based on industrial models, which nurses believed were of limited relevance to their work. Most critical, however, was the absence of parallel proposals (which were outside the remit of the Salmon Committee) for the development of a clinical structure, because this meant that a move into nursing management became not just one option, but in practice the only possible career advancement for the nurse who had excelled in the clinical practitioners role.

The real success of the Salmon reforms, however, was the preparation which they afforded nurse managers for their new roles following the 1974 reorganisation.

NURSING MANAGEMENT IN THE REORGANISED HEALTH SERVICE

Five years of Salmon-style structure and training meant that by 1993 nursing was better prepared than almost any other group to take advantage of the new management arrangements introduced by the 1974 reorganisation of the NHS.

The management arrangements to support the new NHS structures of Regional Health Authorities, Area Health Authorities and Districts (see Chapter 25) were prescribed explicitly and in great detail in what became known as 'the Grey Book'.[10] At each level a management team was established consisting of a doctor, a nurse, an administrator and a finance officer. Further reorganisation of the NHS in 1982 removed the Area 'tier', but the management principles remained intact. There were two key principles:

1 *Functional management.* Each discipline managed its own business, its own budget and its own staff: the chief nursing officer managed nursing, the nursing budget and all nursing staff.
2 *Consensus management.* At each level the management team operated as a team of equals, making decisions by consensus: the team was usually chaired, but was not controlled, by the administrator, and in the event of disagreement, any one member of the team could impose a veto.

These arrangements gave nursing powers which were unprecedented in the history of nursing. For the first time nurses not only sat at the policy table at every level of decision-making, but sat as equals alongside doctors, administrators and finance directors. The fact that they were paid less than the other members of the team provoked a review (the Speakman Review) which justified the nursing claim to equal status and partially rectified the financial unfairness. But the nurse's key source of power was the size of the nursing workforce which was reflected in the size of her budget. The chief nurse was able to assemble around her a team of nurses in staff posts to help her with the responsibilities associated with the management of such an important function and so large a workforce (for example, her own personnel staff and direct management of nursing education), and the power of the nursing team within the management team was in many places formidable. It was perhaps inevitable, and certainly not unique to nursing, that some exercised their power wisely and well and others did not; those who did not provided ammunition for future use by others who still saw nursing as a subordinate occupation and resented the power it was acquiring.

Meanwhile, the concept of consensus management was seen to be incompatible with the developing Thatcherite ideologies of the market – efficiency and managerialism – and was denigrated as slow, inefficient, cumbersome, bureaucratic, and leading to 'lowest common denominator decisions'.

THE INTRODUCTION OF GENERAL MANAGEMENT

The change came, in October 1983, in the form of a letter to the Secretary of State, Norman Fowler, from Roy Griffiths, the managing director of Sainsbury's plc, who had been appointed, with a small group of three other people, 'to give advice on the effective use and management of manpower and related resources in the NHS'. The letter pointed out that 'All our recommendations are designed to be implemented without delay; none of them calls for legislation nor for additional staff overall.' The proposals were specifically presented, in a massive government 'promotion' which included leaflets, a video, meetings and conferences and a prepared 'question and answer brief for speakers, as 'not another reorganisation'.[11] After a minimal period of formal consultation (during which almost the only opposition came from the Royal College of Nursing), the recommendations were rapidly implemented.

The main recommendations of the 'Griffiths Report' were:

1. At DHSS level the Secretary of State should:

establish within the DHSS, a Health Services Supervisory Board and a full-time NHS Management Board.

The role of the Supervisory Board was 'to be concerned with:

a) determination of purpose, objectives and direction for the Health Service;
b) approval of the overall budget and resource allocations;
c) strategic directions;
d) receiving reports on performance and other evaluations from within the Health Service'[12]

The Supervisory Board would be chaired by the Secretary of State, and would include the Permanent Secretary, the chief medical officer, the chairman of the management board and two or three non-executive members. The chief nursing officer was not included, but was subsequently reinstated following intensive lobbying by the Royal College of Nursing.

2 At Health Authority (RHA and DHA) level, Regional and District Chairmen should:

a) identify a general manager (regardless of discipline) at authority level, charged with the general management function and overall responsibility for management's performance in achieving the objectives set by the authority;
b) review and reduce the need for functional management structures at all levels from unit level to authority level, and ensure that the primary reporting relationship of functional managers is to the general manager;
c) initiate major cost-improvement programmes for implementation by general managers.

3 At unit level, District Chairmen should:

a) Clarify the general management function and identify a general manager (regardless of discipline) for every unit of management;
b) ensure that each unit of management has a budget and develops management budgets which involve clinicians (i.e. doctors) and relate work load and service objectives to financial and manpower allocations.

The measures which were subsequently implemented 'in the name of' the Griffiths Report in fact considerably exceeded its actual recommendations. For example, the Report itself made no recommendations for the replacement of functional management by general management below the unit level, and specifically stated: 'This is not intended to weaken the professional responsibilities of the other Chief officers, especially in relation to decision taking on matters within their own spheres of responsibility.'

As in the case of the Salmon Report almost two decades earlier, the manner of implementation produced considerable trauma for many people and dysfunctional consequences which were never intended by the originators of the proposals. In the event, far from being 'not another reorganisation', the restructuring which followed the Griffiths Report produced huge and irrevocable change which had much more impact on service delivery and on the vast majority of staff than any of the formal 'reorganisations' which had taken place since the NHS was established in 1948.

In marked contrast with the 1974 and 1982 reorganisations, local structures and the manner of implementation were seen as issues to be determined locally and not a subject for DHSS guidance. The result was great variation across the country. In particular, different kinds of hybrid posts were created, especially for nurses, whose previous influence and span of control were dramatically reduced.

THE SIGNIFICANCE OF THE GRIFFITHS REPORT FOR NURSING

Just a few weeks after the Report was published, Roy Griffiths commented: 'The proposals don't threaten nurses at all. The nurses are doing a good job, and the changes that are being talked about aren't designed to affect them, except beneficially.' While the sincerity of the remark may be unquestionable, its naïvety is breathtaking. If, as many commentators have suggested, the target of the Griffiths reforms was medicine (see below), nursing was the discipline and nurses were the staff group which was most seriously and most immediately affected. At a stroke the 1984 reorganisation removed nursing from nursing's own control and placed it firmly under the new general managers, very few of whom in the event turned out to be nurses.

At national level, the chief nursing officer was not included in the new Supervisory Board (nor in its successor the NHS Policy Board). At Regional and District level, the chief nurse no longer held the nursing budget nor managed the nursing workforce but became merely an 'Adviser' to the authority. Chief nurses became increasingly marginalised and excluded from the policy-making machinery at all levels. Many senior nurses were 'eased out', and there was evidence of 'settling old scores'. Within units new management structures were created which took the general management principle down to the level of the ward sister in hospitals, and first-line 'locality' management in community nursing services.

There were also significant implications for nursing in the recommendation that the Secretary of State should appoint, as a member of the NHS Management Board, a personnel director, whose responsibilities would include 'carrying forward the DHSS work ... in determining optimum nurse manpower levels in various types of Unit ... so that Regional and district Chairmen can re-examine fundamentally each Unit's nursing levels'. The establishment of a strong Directorate of Personnel at national level, mirrored in local management structures, and coupled with the loss of the chief nursing officer's responsibility for the nursing budget and nursing workforce, also removed the determination of nursing numbers and skill mix from nursing control. Even more significantly, the linkage between manpower and training needs, and the inclusion of training among the personnel director's responsibilities, paved the way for a similar transfer of responsibility for nursing education.

THE NEW MANAGERIALISM

The Griffiths Report was a major milestone in a dramatic change in the organisational culture of the NHS which culminated in the NHS reforms some seven years later. The introduction of general management meant the end not only of consensus management but also of professional management (namely the management of health professionals by one of their own kind), and the rise of the 'professional' manager. This concept included the notion that management was essentially the same whether the organisation sold groceries, made cars or provided health care. It followed that people who had managed private-sector commercial enterprises or military organisations could manage the NHS, and many such people were appointed to the new management posts. Professional goals and values were replaced by commercial goals and values, such as customer satisfaction and cost-improvement programmes. The new values were reflected in the new language: sisters became ward managers, directors of nursing services became directors of operations.

As this 'wind of change' swept away a large part of the older generation of nurse managers, a new generation and a new breed of nurse managers began to emerge. One aspect of the business orientation promoted by Griffiths was an emphasis on quality of service and 'putting the customer first', and nurses, who already had an established track record in quality assurance (based on the work on nursing standards which had developed in many countries through the 1970s and 1980s), began to develop new roles in this field. A distinction began to be made between 'managing nurses' (the focus of concern of the 'old' nurse managers) and 'managing nursing' (the focus of the 'new' breed).

THE RESOURCE MANAGEMENT INITIATIVE AND CLINICAL DIRECTORATES

It had long been recognised that one of the problems of managing the NHS was that most of its expenditure was determined not by finance officers or even by general managers, but by the clinical decisions of doctors; and yet doctors were not involved in the management process, were not held financially accountable, and indeed often protested that costs were 'not their business'. The Resource Management Initiative, introduced on a pilot basis in 1986, attempted to tackle this problem through a costing system based on three key components: developing a clinical database, establishing a case-mix management system for recording patient treatment resource usage and costs, and implementing effective computerised systems for deploying nursing staff (Nursing Management Systems).

The information-based costing system became the core of a new decentralised management structure, initially for acute general hospitals, which was modelled on the system developed in the Johns Hopkins Hospital, Baltimore.[13] The system involved the division of hospital activity according to broad clinical specialities (usually a surgical directorate, a medical directorate and so on). Each directorate is headed by a clinical director (almost universally a medical consultant) who controls the budget and all the staff, including the nurses. The clinical director is typically assisted by a business manager and a nurse. Initially nursing concern about the model was focused on the consequent loss of authority of the hospital's director of nursing services or the loss of the post altogether (a UK deviation from the original model), and on the fear that, under financial pressure, directors would seek to contain their budgets by reducing or diluting their nursing workforce, ignoring the advice of nurse 'advisers'. The requirement that NHS trusts include a nurse executive director on the board has to some extent relieved the first concern, and there is increasing evidence that many of the 'new breed' nurse managers are rising to the challenge of new roles within directorates and are achieving authority on the basis of their expertise (which Salmon described as sapiential authority) in spite of their relatively weak structural position.

OPPORTUNITY 2000

Nursing management is also beginning to benefit from recent initiatives to raise the number of women in key appointments in the NHS. The appointment of a female Secretary of State for Health (Mrs Virginia Bottomley) undoubtedly influenced the decision by the Department of Health to be the first government department to join the Opportunity 2000 Campaign, a national business-led campaign to improve the quality of the participation of women in the workforce. One part of this initiative is the establishment of a register of senior women managers. All women on the register are offered access to a properly funded positive action programme to help equip them for career development. The current reality, however, is that there are still very few women, and even fewer nurses among the ranks of NHS chief executives or clinical directors.

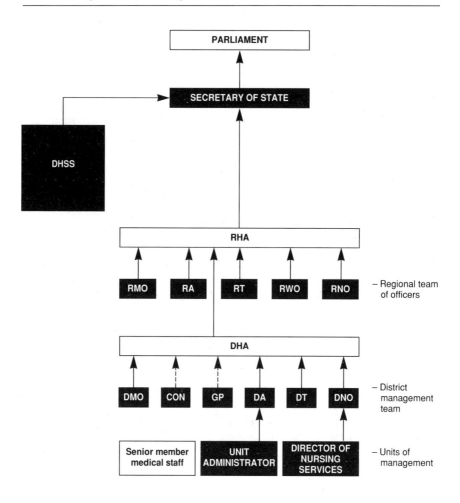

Key

RMO	Regional Medical Officer	DA	District Aministrator
DMO	District Medical Officer	DT	District Treasurer
CON	Consultant	RNO	Regional Nursing Officer
GP	General Practitioner	DNO	District Nursing Officier
RA	Regional Administrator	RGM	Regional General Manager
RT	Regional Treasurer	DGM	District General Manager
RWO	Regional Works Officer	UGM	Unit General Manager

Figure 22.1 Health authority management – before Griffiths
This is a simplified representation of the main present management relationships
in health authorities and their links with DHSS, the Secretary of State for Social
Services and Parliament.

MANAGEMENT AND LEADERSHIP

The power and influence of nursing was devastated by the introduction in the 1980s of the new managerialism, and a generation of nurse leaders was lost. One of the lessons which nursing learned from the trauma, however, was that management is not synonymous with leadership, and there are hopeful signs that the 1990s may see the emergence of new models of clinical leadership which may contribute far more to nursing's influence

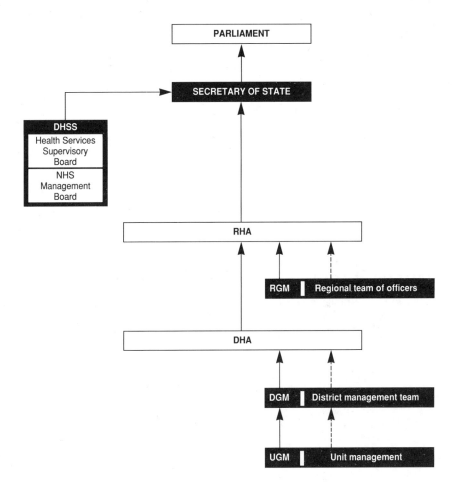

Figure 22.2 Health authority management – after Griffiths
This is a simplified representation of the key future management relationships in Health Authorities and DHSS, how they link to each other, to the Secretary of State for Social Services and to Parliament.
These management developments will all take place within the existing account-ability arrangements and statutory framework.

on health care than was possible for nurse managers in the traditional management hierarchies of the 1960s and 1970s.

REFERENCES

1 *Nursing Times*, 3 May, col. 64, no. 18.
2 Schon, D. (1970) *Beyond the Stable State*, Reith Lectures, London: BBC Publications.
3 *Pay of Nurses and Midwives in the National Health Service* (1968) Report No. 60, Cmnd. 3585, London: HMSO, paras. 157 ff.
4 Ibid, para 138. Recommended scales (CNO £2,180–2,950).
5 *Evidence to the Royal Commission on the Health Service* (1977) Royal College of Nursing, para 64.
6 *Evidence to the Royal Commission on the Health Service* (1977) *British Medical Journal* ch. 8, AN 7, p. 322, 29 Jan.
7 *Report on the Progress on Salmon* (1977), DHSS.
8 *Royal Commission on the National Health Service* (1979) London: HMSO, para 4.12; *also* Table 4.1.
9 Nursing and Midwifery Staff, England & Wales, Statistics Division, Table 1, Sheet 1 (1976) DHSS.
10 *Management Arrangements in the Reorganised Health Service* (the Grey Book) (1972), London: HMSO.
11 HMSO (1979) *Review of Top Posts in the National Health Service* (the Speakman Review).
12 *NHS Management Enquiry*, DA(83)38 (1983) DHSS.
13 Heysell, R. M. *et al.* (1984) 'Decentralised management in a teaching hopsital', *New England Journal of Medicine*, 310 (22); 1477–80.

FURTHER READING

Strong, P. and Robinson, J. (1990) *The NHS Under New Management*, Milton Keynes: Open University Press.

Chapter 23

Nursing education – 'Reports are not self-executive'

Margaret Green

In 1963 the Committee on Higher Education published its report, and in its outline on procedure dismissed nursing with these words:

> We received evidence about training for nursing and some of the occupations associated with medicine. Since this does not form part of higher education as we defined it, we have not specially considered this wide opportunity for girls. But we are aware that at certain points contacts with universities and colleges are now being established.

Why was nursing not considered higher education, and how did the Committee define it? In the next chapter, on the aims and principles of higher education, there is a paragraph that is significant:

> While emphasising that there is no betrayal of values when institutions of higher education teach what will be of some practical use, we must postulate that what is taught should be taught in such a way as to promote the general powers of the mind. The aim should not be to produce mere specialists but rather cultivated men and women. And it is a distinguishing characteristic of healthy higher education that, even when it is concerned with the practical techniques, it imparts them on a plane of generality that makes possible their application to many problems – to find one in the many – the general in the collection of particulars.[1]

Judged by these criteria, nursing in 1963 was not higher education. Nursing at that time taught what would be of practical use on the plane of practicality rather than generality; its aim was to produce safe practitioners rather than cultivated men and women, and its concern was with the particular rather than the general characteristic in a collection of particulars. Because nursing evolved from a simple pupillage to a long apprenticeship where the apprentices became the main labour force, nursing had not been able to use accepted educational methods, such as reasoning from first principles and working from the known to the unknown. Techniques had to be performed and jobs done by the person on hand to do them, and if there was time to show 'how' there was seldom time to explain 'why'.

The service needs took precedence over the educational needs of the student.

The fact that nursing developed this way was an accident of history. On the Continent, nursing remained based on religious orders which were in many cases a product of the Counter-Reformation and on a 'mother house' system which was emulated by the Protestant deaconesses in Germany. In America, nursing developed along another path due to a different hospital tradition and the more democratic educational system to which nursing was often linked. In England, it so happened that 'reformed nursing' preceded the Education Acts at the end of the century and the foundation of colleges of higher education for women; however, the colleges for women, the entry of women into professions and 'reformed nursing' must all be seen as part of the movement to free women from 'ideas that were used to validate social disapproval of intellectual and professional attainments in women based on the preconceived ideas about the psychology of women'.[2]

NURSING EDUCATION AFTER REGISTRATION

Registration came not through the profession but through a new statutory body set up by Act of Parliament (see Chapter 12). The new Ministry of Health was responsible for the health of the community as well as the registration of nurses, and, as the country was under-nursed, it is not surprising that the Ministry was persuaded that specialist hospitals should be training schools and that the probationers when 'trained' placed on a supplementary register. Leaders of the nursing profession who wished to see nursing develop parallel to medicine argued against this and in favour of one basic training with specialisation to follow. In fact, the rigidity of registration itself increased the disunity and barriers between the branches of nursing. If a nurse qualified in one branch and wished to pursue study in another, she had to undertake two or more years' training even though there was a common core of knowledge in all branches. Hospitals not only had a vested interest in a long training; they also had a financial stake in the fragmentation of training. Gaining 'a wide experience' meant being a poorly paid probationer for years. Ironically, even administrative posts in purely specialist hospitals usually went to the candidate with the most certificates.

THE COLLEGE OF NURSING

Education has been one of the important activities of the College since its inception. The first full-time educational activity, an international course in hospital administration, training school administration, methods of teaching and the history of nursing, was established in 1924. In the same year a part-time education officer was employed. In 1930, an Education

Department was established, and Miss H. C. Parsons was appointed Director of Education.

In the hospital service the first nurse tutor to be appointed was Miss Agnes Gullan at St Thomas's Hospital in 1914. The first training for those who wanted to teach was through the Diploma in Nursing of the University of London, approved in 1926 and first examined in 1927, with an optional paper in methods of teaching and elements of educational psychology.

The College of Nursing played a significant part in the development of the diploma, which continued as the route for training teachers of nursing until 1950, while the Sister Tutor Diploma commenced in 1947, at first as a one-year course and subsequently as a two year course in 1952. This Sister Tutor Diploma course was organised by the College of Nursing, Queen Elizabeth College and Battersea Polytechnic, now the University of Surrey, and subsequently by the South Bank Polytechnic. It was discontinued in 1981, being replaced by a one-year Diploma in Nursing Education for those nurses who already held a Diploma in Nursing or other qualification of similar standing.

In 1944 a one-year, full-time course in nursing administration was established at the College for potential hospital matrons. This was a popular course attended by a significant number of nurses. However, nurses had increasing difficulty in obtaining funding to attend this course, despite generous funding by the Hospital Saving Association in the form of scholarships.

Although health visitors had been receiving training since 1890, their position was anomalous, and often it did not prepare them to meet the demands of new legislation. Recommendations were made to the Ministry of Health, and in 1925 regulations were issued defining the training required and the Royal Sanitary Institute was approved as the examining body for the Health Visitors Certificate. The College of Nursing and other colleges of further education were approved to run courses and prepare candidates. By the time the College received its charter in 1928, there were nearly 6,000 trained nurses a year attending the special courses, seminars and lectures it organised. In 1934, in response to nurses working in industry, the College organised a six-month course in Industrial Nursing and granted a certificate (see Chapter 21).

As the Education Department undertook more work it became known as the Educational Division, and was classified as a major establishment of further education. In 1970 the Division was renamed the Institute of Advanced Nursing Education, with centres in London, Birmingham, Scotland and Northern Ireland.

The 1990s saw another significant development in the educational work of the Royal College of Nursing. The Institute became recognised as an institution of higher education and was approved by the Department of Education to run degree courses. It is an accredited college of the

University of Manchester, and the majority of their degree courses and some diploma courses are validated by that University. The Institute now offers a wide range of basic degree courses on a modular basis, and from 1993 will commence offering a postgraduate modular scheme with six Master's degrees.[3] The Institute continues to offer a variety of short courses.

Associated with the Institute is the Library of Nursing, which was established in 1923 and now has over 50,000 volumes and is a reference and research centre for all bona fide enquirers. The Library also has a research collection, including the Steinberg Collection, which has over 700 volumes at Master's and Ph.D. levels.

OTHER POST-REGISTRATION TRAINING AND EDUCATION

Apart from the College of Nursing, there were a variety of hospital-based trainings for clinically based studies. A number of these were nationally recognised courses, such as those organised by the British Tuberculosis Association (BTA), founded in the mid 1920s, subsequently to become the British Thoracic and Tuberculosis Association (BTTA), the Ophthalmic Nursing Board, the Midland Institute of Otology, and a Joint Examination Board set up in 1935 for the award of the Orthopaedic Certificate.

Other courses were not recognised, and in 1970, arising from discussions following the *Reform of Nursing Education* (the Platt Report), a Joint Board of Clinical Studies was set up which brought some order into the many earning and learning schemes.

The Board was an excellent example of co-operation between the medical and nursing professions. The Board was composed of representatives from the Royal Medical, Nursing and Midwifery Colleges, and it worked through a series of specialist panels of doctors and nurses, set up to devise outline curricula in their specialities. These were in turn approved by the Board. Hospitals applied to them for approval. The hospital was then visited by a small team of doctors and nurses with a member of staff, and the Board would then approve the course.

Working in this way, the Board was able to develop and maintain standards of training in a wide range of clinical courses and institute the award of nationally recognised certificates to successful course members.

Not all post-registration training was hospital-based. District nurses had for many years been trained and examined by the Oueen's Institute of District Nursing, which offered its own special courses in further education; these functions have now passed to the Panel of Assessors for District Nurse Training (see Chapter 19). Since 1902 midwives, on the other hand, have been licensed by the Central Midwives Board, but Teachers of Midwives had a course arranged, and the certificate granted, by the Royal College of Midwives. There are therefore a number of separate bodies dealing with different aspects of post-registration training. Although the Nurses, Midwives and Health Visitors Act of 1979 was designed as an enabling Act so that the philosophy of nursing education outlined by the Briggs Committee could be introduced, it has brought some semblance of order into the multiplicity of training, examining and certificate-granting bodies that confuse the public and the profession.

DIPLOMA IN NURSING

In 1924 the Royal College of Nursing, in conjunction with the University of London, discussed the introduction of the Diploma in Nursing. This was established in 1926. The University of Leeds also established a Diploma in Nursing, followed by Hull. The object of the Diploma was to enable suitable candidates to fit themselves for further responsibilities, and a syllabus was prepared for an examination to be taken in two parts – Part A dealing with the general sciences, the development of nursing and ethics, and Part B covering the particular aspect of nursing offered by the candidate – with the final examination including a written paper and a viva. For those teaching, or wishing to teach, this could be offered as an optional extra. In 1980 the university undertook a complete revision of the Diploma in Nursing, and the new diploma commenced in 1982. This diploma was approved by a university validation panel, and could only be organised through a combined centre of a higher education establishment and a college of nursing.

The new diploma was organised in units taken on a day-release basis, with parts of the course taking place in higher education and the others in the college of nursing. Units 1 and 2 concentrated on the human and social organisation and social change; units 3 and 4 covered the application of care and the emergence of modern nursing, while unit 5 looked at research in nursing and unit 6 was devoted to nursing and the search for excellence in nursing. Students successfully completing this course were subsequently able to take a full-time year at King's College, University of London, to obtain a degree in nursing. Later, a part-time mode was established at the Royal College of Nursing.

PRE-REGISTRATION NURSE TRAINING – EMPLOYEE OR STUDENT?

Both the Athlone (1937) and the Lancet (1932) Reports had commented upon the equivocal position of the student nurse, and foresaw the time when this type of training would be out of step with modern thinking. This conclusion did not have the wholehearted support of the nursing profession, many of whom 'regarded the element of apprenticeship as a more important part of nurse training than [their] theoretical studies'.[4] This attitude was not surprising, since the apprenticeship system itself, with its emphasis on obedience, discipline, and copying precept and example, militated against an enquiring attitude. But by the time of the Horder (1941) reports there was a new attitude among many nursing leaders; study of the systems in other countries made people realise that it should be possible to select tasks that would fulfil the educational needs of the student rather than merely the service needs of the hospital, but to do this it would be necessary to provide sufficient ancillary staff to relieve the student of non-nursing tasks.

The next major report was the Report of the Working Party on the Recruitment and Training of Nurses (1947),[5] under the chairmanship of Sir Robert Wood. This working party was established by the Ministry of Health, the Department of Health for Scotland and the Ministry of Labour and National Service. Sir Robert had four other members: Miss Daisy Bridges and Miss Elizabeth Cockayne (later Dame Elizabeth), both nurses, and Dr Cohen from the Cabinet Office and Mr Inch from the Department of Health in Scotland. Their remit was to review the whole nursing service and its problems. Their recommendations were revolutionary and included a two-year training with full student status, a shortened working day, a five-day training week of 40 hours and six weeks' holiday. The first 18 months of training would be devoted to the fundamentals common to all fields, including midwifery, followed by six months in a chosen field, after which there would be a year's supervised practice. There would be one common register. Another significant recommendation was for the establishment of Regional Nurse Training Committees. The working party also suggested that there should be research units established. They also recommended the development of experimental training schemes, and a review of the General Nursing Council.

The reception to the Wood Report was very mixed and in the main was negative, but it was largely overshadowed by the advent of the National Health Service. However, pressure for reform continued, which led to the Nurses Act 1949. This Act provided for the establishment of Area Nurse Training Committees and included provision for experimental training schemes to be submitted to the Secretary of State for permission to proceed. The Area Nurse Training Committees were given limited powers under the 1949 Act, mainly acting as a channel for the distribution of moneys from the General Nursing Council for England and Wales to the training schools for staff salaries, equipment and travelling expenses. They were in no way given freedom to function as the Wood Report envisaged.

The National Health Service, when it came, left the student nurse legally as an employee, and students continued to supply most of the service needs of the hospital, many of which did little to enhance their education or their understanding of the patients. The view that 'nursing was falling into disfavour' with young people and those who advised them' (see Chapter 13) seemed to be true. Lack of agreed educational requirements for entry led to a wide range of ability and was frustrating to tutors; the increasing ratio of untrained to trained meant there was insufficient supervision and ward teaching, and the student was confused by what happened on the ward and what was taught in the classroom, and this contributed to the high wastage rate, which in turn created further shortage and gave a poor image of the profession. In the light of what appeared to be a worsening situation, in 1961 the Royal College of Nursing decided to set up another enquiry into nurse training.

A REFORM OF NURSING EDUCATION (THE PLATT REPORT)

This committee first met under the chairmanship of Sir Harry Platt in 1961 and reported in 1964. The Report was divided into three sections: 'The case for reform', 'The means of reform and achieving reform'. The nub of the case was that 'all who wished to nurse and were prepared to be persistent in seeking admission to general training were likely to be accepted'.[6] This meant that there was no chance of candidates coming forward for enrolment in any numbers, and a second level was vital to the balance of the team. Therefore, the Committee recommended that the standard of entry for the Register be raised and the number of training schools be reduced from the current 987 to about 200, and that Regional Councils be set up. The student should receive a training grant and have an entry standard of five subjects at Ordinary level and should pursue a course of controlled clinical experience for two years, with a third under supervision as a paid member of the team. The enrolled nurse, who would also receive a training grant, would also train under the aegis of the school and there should be a clearer distinction between the Register and the Roll.

The Report was debated widely and, while the profession reacted favourably, the reactions of administrators and doctors were depressingly reactionary: they feared that nurses with five Ordinary levels would be too academic. This complaint was expressed by doctors when the standard of entry to medical schools was being pushed ever higher. The General Nursing Council stated that it did not think such reform was necessary or desirable and it urged evolution rather than revolution.[7]

Evolution proceeded slowly. In 1962 there was a new syllabus, which gave way to a revised syllabus in 1969, in which students were required to have more experience in controlled situations, but, since the student was the main labour force, this led to greater conflict. However, no report is ever lost; each acts as a catalyst and a basis for the next push forward. Those who at the time 'perished for Platt' did not do so in vain, for the result was a new impetus to experimental schemes which attracted the more academic candidate who might have otherwise been lost.

EXPERIMENTAL SCHEMES IN PRE- AND POST-REGISTRATION NURSE EDUCATION

In Scotland as early as 1956 a Department of Nursing Studies had been set up under the Faculty of Arts within the University of Edinburgh, with entry through the Universities Central Council on Admissions, and this admitted candidates who satisfied the university requirements and the nursing officer of the associated hospital. The course lasted four years and six months and led to a degree, BSc (Social Science–Nursing).

In England, the first integrated course was approved and commenced in 1957 and was organised between St Thomas's Hospital, London, and Southampton University. It enabled the students to become SRNs and obtain the Health Visitors Certificate (HV Cert), together with Part I of the Central Midwives Board Examination. In 1958 further integrated schemes were developed, and in 1959 one that had particular significance was between Manchester University and Crumpsall Hospital, Manchester, where the students obtained an SRN, HVCert and the National District Nursing Certificate, and included midwifery experience. In 1969 this course was granted degree status, and Manchester became the first university to award degrees in nursing.

In 1966 the first course leading to a degree in human biology and a nursing option was proposed between the University of Surrey and St George's Hospital. A number of other courses developed, commencing in 1968, in conjunction with other universities, leading to a nursing qualification and a variety of different degrees in economics, sociology, social science and life sciences.

In 1969 the first proposal for a degree in nursing was accepted at the Welsh National School of Medicine. A number of other degrees in nursing were introduced at various universities during the 1970s. The polytechnics were not far behind in this development, with the Council for National Academic Awards enabling nursing degrees to be set up in 1974 in Leeds, Newcastle and the South Bank. Others followed. Although degree courses in nursing continued to develop, they remained a relatively small percentage of registration courses. Another important trend at this time was the development of post-registration degrees. The first course was developed at the Welsh National School of Medicine in 1979 and was a full-time, three-year course. In 1980, Leeds Polytechnic commenced a part-time course spread over four years. A number of other courses have developed, some, as already indicated, based on a diploma in nursing or professional studies. A small number of Masters' degrees in nursing have also been established.

Experimental courses ceased to be classified as such in 1964: some continued until 1980; others were phased out because of the difficulty in meeting the requirements of the EEC directives, in which students of nursing must have experience in specified clinical areas and have a specified balance of theory and practice.

Another imaginative mode of education that might be applied to aspects of post-basic nursing education comes from the Open University, where there are already courses in the social sciences that are applicable to nursing studies. There is no detailed breakdown of the occupation of students taking degrees with the Open University, but it was calculated that in 1977 some 800 nurses were involved in degree courses.[8] Although many of these students were senior nurses, especially tutors and health visitors, some were nurses in training trying to fill the intellectual gap that yawned after leaving the sixth form.

TOWARDS THE COMMITTEE ON NURSING

Out of the rejection of Platt came an increase in the range of experimental courses, and a greater flexibility in existing courses, but the student remained an employee, a pair of hands, and service demands continued to make priority over training. Tutors remained concerned about their difficulties in presenting an educational programme, and the students became increasingly discontented. Following a letter from the then General Secretary of the Royal College of Nursing, Catherine Hall, to the Deputy Secretary of the then Ministry of Health, two meetings were held between representatives of the Ministry and the RCN. At the second of these meetings it was agreed that a working party be set up. The terms of reference were: 'To identify the current and foreseeable education and training needs of student and pupil nurses and the role of teaching staff in meeting these needs and to examine the resultant staffing pattern.'[9]

It was agreed that the General Nursing Council for England and Wales join the Ministry of Health and the RCN on the working party, which became the Nurse Tutor Working Party under the chairmanship of Dame Kathleen Raven, Chief Nursing Officer of the Ministry of Health. Although the Nurse Tutor Working Party was largely overtaken by the establishment of the Committee on Nursing, it did publish an interim report in 1970.[10] One of its main recommendations was for a modular system of training. Further recommendations concentrated on the need to increase the number of teachers and to facilitate their work. The Raven Report received little recognition, but it did alter the thinking in a number of schools, and four modular schemes were established.

Nurses, however, continued to feel dissatisfied with the existing system, considering that a radical review was required throughout the United Kingdom. Following a meeting of the RCN Representative Body, the General Secretary wrote to the then Secretary of State, Richard Crossman, requesting a meeting because of the increasing difficulty in providing an adequate standard of care for patients. A further matter of concern was that of the status of nurse learners and the degree of responsibility that students were expected to undertake, for which the students knew themselves to be inadequately equipped. The concern was not only for the students but also for the patients who were exposed to this situation.

At the meeting that was arranged with the Secretary of State in February 1970 there was extensive discussion on standards of care, on the increase in the demands on the service, on the lack of trained staff to supervise care and the need to reform the system of training. At the same time as the RCN was making representations, the Association of Hospital Matrons were also expressing concern at a meeting with the Minister of State, Baroness Serota.

THE COMMITTEE ON NURSING (BRIGGS)[11]

On 2 March 1970, the Secretary of State for Social Services announced to the House of Commons that he, together with the Secretary of State for Scotland and the Welsh Secretary, had decided that a Committee on Nursing was to be established under the chairmanship of Professor (now Lord) Asa Briggs. Briggs' terms of reference for his independent committee were: 'To review the role of the nurse and the midwife in the hospital and the community and the education required for that role so that the best use is made of available manpower to meet present needs, and the needs of an integrated health service.'

The Committee was composed of 20 individuals, the majority of whom were nurses, plus three doctors and six others. They were well supported by a team of research staff. They received evidence from 581 individuals and organisations.

The Committee recommended that all candidates start on the same course, a common portal of entry (entry age being 17 years) to an 18-month foundation course leading to a certificate in nursing practice. A further 18 months for the more able student would lead to registration. This could include or be followed by a higher certificate, non-statutory, in a particular branch of nursing or midwifery. They proposed a new grade of worker in the community, a family health sister, who would have a higher certificate in community preventive nursing.

The central recommendation of the report was that there should be one statutory body concerned with basic and post-basic training in Great Britain, with an Advisory Board for Scotland.

It took one and a half years before the Secretary of State responded to the report. It had not been helped by the fact that the Secretary of State who set up the Committee was Richard Crossman, the one receiving the report was Keith Joseph, and finally it was Barbara Castle who responded in the House in May 1974.

The Report was received with qualified approval. There was concern that the position of the student nurse had not been clarified. The common portal of entry was not popular, and the notion of a new governing body was very unpopular with the health visitors and midwives, who previously had had separate governing bodies. In 1975 the government issued a statutory framework making provision for delegated powers in the case of midwives. Once this had happened, other groups, such as district nurses, asked for similar concessions. As the debate widened, comparisons were made with 1919, when sectarian squabbles within the profession handed control to government.

In 1977 action was initiated by the Department of Health, setting up the Briggs Co-ordinating Committee under the chairmanship of the Minister of State, Roland Moyle, but the delay continued, with competing claims of various specialist groups wanting statutory recognition. Finally, it was accepted that there should be a United Kingdom Central Council for Nursing, Midwifery and Health Visiting, with provision for a statutory committee for midwifery, with four National Boards all with their midwifery committees. To this was added a Joint Committee for Health Visiting and, at the last moment, a Joint Committee for District Nursing.

On 13 November 1978 the Nurse Midwives and Health Visitors Bill had its second reading and, as Parliament was about to be prorogued in April 1979, it became law. The first Chairman of the United Kingdom Central Council (UKCC), Catherine Hall, later Dame Catherine Hall, was appointed in August 1979, and the Council and Board members were appointed and met for the first time in shadow form in 1980. The first elections to the National Boards took place in 1983.

TOWARDS PROJECT 2000

The next attempt at reform was by the UKCC. They set up a number of working groups to look at elements of their work in order to produce consultation papers for the profession's consideration. Working Group 3 produced Consultation Paper 1 on the Development of Nurse Education. They proposed a single route to registration, with ample opportunities for conversion. They rejected student status and went for controlled learning situations. The professions were very critical of the report, and the report was shelved by the Council to await the elected bodies in 1983.

When the newly elected bodies took office, one of the early matters on the agenda was reform of nursing education. In late 1984 there was much discussion among the five bodies about who should take the lead. Finally it was agreed that the UKCC should take the initiative and, further, that the Education Policy Advisory Committee should be responsible for the work, and it was subsequently agreed that the whole committee should form the Project Group under the chairmanship of Margaret Green. There were 20 members representing Boards and Council. The membership included all disciplines plus four educationists. A project officer, Dr Celia Davies, was appointed to assist the Committee, who were given a target date for completion in the autumn of 1986. The project became known as Project 2000.

The terms of reference for Project 2000 were: 'To determine the education and training required in preparation for the professional practice of nursing, midwifery and health visiting in relation to the projected health care needs in the 1990s and beyond, and to make recommendations.

In 1984 the Royal College of Nursing, concerned about the delay in reforming education and the apparent lack of action by the statutory bodies, set up its own Education Commission under the chairmanship of Dr Harry Judge.[12] In April 1985 the Judge Report, *The Education of Nurses: a New Dispensation*, was published. The Judge Commission had travelled widely throughout the United Kingdom to meet a range of members and others, and received considerable evidence. They also commissioned two pieces of research. The main recommendations were threefold:

1 transfer of nursing education to the higher education sector;
2 student status;
3 A three-year course commencing with a one-year foundation course, a second year in adult nursing and a third year in a speciality.

The English National Board's (ENB) strategy was published in May 1985.[13] They produced concepts and not recommendations. These included a common core initial programme leading to qualifications in each speciality; direct entry to district nursing, midwifery and health visiting; student status for two years; and collaborative links with higher and further education.

The RCN's report was received by the project group, together with research that they had commissioned from the Institute of Manpower and the Centre for Health Economics at the University of York. The ENB's document was also received, together with the results of the consultation exercise as material to be taken into consideration in the production of the project group's final report. The direct result of the publication of these reports on Project 2000 was a request from Council to report ahead of schedule. The project group had already decided to work in an open way and produce a series of discussion documents, including a detailed analysis of projected health needs, and to hold meetings throughout the United Kingdom to meet with the professions and listen to their comments. The papers were widely circulated, and the nursing press gave generous cover to the documents. A wide range of comments was received by the project office at the UKCC, and these informed the final report, which was published on 13 May 1986.

PROJECT 2000: A NEW PREPARATION FOR PRACTICE[14]

The main recommendations of the Report were:

1 A three-year programme with a common foundation programme of two years and one year in a branch, the total programme to lead to a Diploma in Higher Education;
2 branches to include midwifery, adult nursing, children's nursing, nursing the mentally ill and mentally handicapped;
3 second-level training to be phased out;
4 full student status, no contribution to rostered service;
5 improved educational facilities and the development of links with the higher education sector.

Included in the Report was information on the changing pattern of health needs.

The Report went out for professional consultation, and 1,200 comments were received. The final recommendations went to the Minister of Health, Tony Newton, in January 1987 and took into consideration a cost-benefit exercise that had been conducted. The final proposals were amended to allow a 20 per cent student contribution to service because of the high cost of full student status. The midwives did not want to be part of Project 2000, so direct entry was proposed; the mental illness branch was changed to mental health; and the common foundation programme reduced to 18 months.

The Minister agreed to circulate health authorities in March 1987, but it was not until May 1988 that Tony Newton met with the UKCC, accepting in principle the recommendations, and Council agreed that further work was required. Three days later the Secretary of State, John Moore, made an announcement to the RCN Congress. The further work was completed and in May 1988 the Secretary of State, Kenneth Clarke, announced 13 demonstration districts in England that were to commence Project 2000 in 1988/89. Project 2000 was launched, but it was not until 1993 that all colleges of nursing and midwifery had changed to the new Project 2000 programmes, with the links with higher education fully established.

POST-REGISTRATION EDUCATION AND PRACTICE

One of the recommendations of Project 2000 was that there should be a coherent, comprehensive, cost-effective framework beyond registration. In 1989 the second elected and appointed Council launched a new project, 'The Post Registration Education and Practice Project' (PREPP).[15] Again the Education Policy Advisory Committee, under the chairmanship of Margaret Green, took the lead role, but with the addition of 12 extra National Board members.

As with Project 2000, the project took shape within the context of the future health needs of the population and the professional practice required to meet those needs. The group again worked in an open manner, producing a discussion paper that was widely circulated and undertaking a series of meetings throughout the United Kingdom in which the professions were asked their views. A questionnaire was also included in a copy of the Register, which went to every practitioner. There was a total of 35,999 responses.

The PREPP Report envisaged practice as a continuum on which to build a structure that would maintain and enhance professional standards. After registration, each practitioner was to receive support from a preceptor. This recommendation came into practice in March 1992. The remainder of the recommendations required legislative change, and in September 1993 had not yet been implemented.

PREPP required that all nurses must demonstrate that they had maintained and developed their professional knowledge and competence, and they were to record their development in a professional profile. A minimum of five days' study leave was to be undertaken every three years, prior to periodic registration. It was also recommended that after a break of five years, every practitioner wishing to return to practice should undertake a return to practice programme.

The PREPP proposals received wide acceptance and produced a way forward for the professions. Further work was needed on community education and practice and a sub-group was set up in 1991, under the chairmanship of Kay Rodgers,[16] and it reported in 1992. A new community health-care nurse was recommended, which would include all nurses working in the community including those who were engaged in direct care, disease prevention and health promotion as employees of the NHS health authorities or trusts, nurses employed by general medical practices, those engaged in occupational health nursing, those employed by private agencies and those practising independently. A modular preparation was envisaged for the community care nurses, with shared learning across what had previously been different professional groups.

The Report of the Post Registration Education and Practice Project (PREPP) and those of the Community Education and Practice group were agreed by the professions, and became UKCC policy. Further work was then needed to establish the required standards for post-registration education and practice. This work was completed in March 1993 prior to the end of the second Council's term of office. The proposals for the standard kind and content of post-registration education[17] were, in September 1993, the subject of consultation.

The final proposals for post-registration education and practice establish a new model for nursing practice, which include primary, specialist and advanced practice, and for midwifery practice, which include primary, enhanced and advanced practice. They also include standards for education and standards for teaching. The teachers of the future must be graduates with an advanced nursing or midwifery qualification and must have an appropriate teaching qualification. All teachers must have relevant and up-to-date clinical knowledge and subject expertise. The Council has also agreed to use a system of credit accumulation and transfer which will acknowledge not only academic worth but also professional experience. This will then enable registered nurses and midwives to build on their qualification at registration. The system will take account of previous knowledge and experience at registration and future qualification at higher diploma level, nursing education being seen as a continuum from registration until retirement. The PREPP proposals have been accepted in principle by the government. The response on the proposed legislative changes is first required from the profession and then from the Secretary of State.

CONCLUSION

The long and difficult path to the reform of nursing education/training has taken over 50 years, but during those years the various reports did lead to change, albeit gradual change. Thirty years after the Committee on Higher Education published its Report, nursing can be said to be higher education, with nurses being taught on the plane of generality even though it is concerned with practical techniques. Students of nursing have become true students, receiving on completion of their course a higher diploma that has academic credit enabling them to register with the statutory body.

A framework has been created for education and practice which is responsive and relevant to the needs of patients and clients wherever they are nursed, which will improve the quality of care. This framework provides for a more effective match between education and practice throughout a professional life. Nurse training has at last become nursing education.

REFERENCES

1 *The Report of the Committee on Higher Education* (1963) ch. 2, para 26, Cmnd 2154, London: HMSO.
2 Duffin, L. (n.d.) 'Women and medicine in the nineteenth century', *Medical Historical Association Bulletin*, 21.
3 *Institute of Advanced Nursing Education: Prospectus* (1993) London: Royal College of Nursing.
4 *The Report of the Commission on Nursing* (Lancet Report) (1932) London: HMSO.
5 *The Report of the Working Party on the Recruitment and Training of Nurses* (1947) Chairman, Sir Robert Wood, London: HMSO.
6 *A Reform of Nursing Education* (1964) p. 6, para 17, London: Royal College of Nursing.

7 GNC (1965) Comment on a Reform of Nursing Education, *Nursing Times*, 1 Oct. 1965.
8 *Evidence to the Royal Commission on the NHS* (1977) p. 47, Royal College of Nursing (quotes information from the Bursar of the Open University to Baly).
9 Ministry of Health Central Health Services Council, (1966) *The Post-Certificate Training and Education of Nurses*, London: HMSO.
10 *The Report of the Nurse Tutor Working Party* (1970) Chairman, Dame Kathleen Raven, London: Department of Health and Social Services.
11 *The Report of the Committee on Nursing* (1972) Chairman, Professor Asa Briggs, Cmnd 5115, London: HMSO.
12 *The Education of Nurses: a New Dispensation* (1985) Commission on Nursing, Chairman, Dr Harry Judge, London: Royal College of Nursing.
13 *Professional Education/Training Courses* (1985) Consultation Paper, English National Board for Nursing, Midwifery and Health Visiting.
14 *Project 2000: a New Preparation for Practice* (1986), London: United Kingdom Central Council for Nursing, Midwifery and Health Visiting.
15 *The Report of the Post Registration Education and Practice Project* (1990), London: United Kingdom Central Council for Nursing, Midwifery and Health Visiting.
16 *Report on Proposals for the Future of Community Education and Practice* (1991), London: United Kingdom Central Council for Nursing, Midwifery and Health Visiting.
17 *The Council's Proposed Standards for Post Registration Education* (1993), London: United Kingdom Central Council for Nursing, Midwifery and Health Visiting.

FURTHER READING

Allan, P. and Jolley, M. (1982) *Nursing, Midwifery and Health Visiting since 1900*, London: Faber & Faber.
Burnard, P. and Chapman, C. (1990) *Nurse Education: the Way Forward*, London: Scutari Press.
Clay, T. (1987) *Nurses' Power and Politics*, London: Heinemann.
Evidence to Committee on Nursing (1971), London: Royal College of Nursing.

Chapter 24

Nursing research

June Clark

Nursing must become a research-based profession.
Report of the Committee on Nursing, 1972

In 1948 Dr Cohen dissented from certain parts of the report on the *Recruitment and Training of Nurses* and wrote his own minority report because he maintained that the majority report had failed to examine the key problems of the future demand for health services and the changing role of the hospitals. Until these problems were examined it was impossible to decide on the function of the nurse; Dr Cohen therefore urged further research (see Chapter 15).

In spite of the fact that Miss Nightingale herself had based her reforms on investigation and was a member of the Statistical Society, to which she presented a paper on 'Uniform Hospital Statistics',[1] her initiative was not followed up, and the lack of such statistics and particularly those relating to nursing manpower is a common complaint from all investigators, from the Lancet Commission to the evidence to the Royal Commission on the National Health Service in 1977. Although there had been a few attempts at surveys such as the questionnaire circulated by the College of Nursing in 1919 seeking information about nurses' pay and conditions of service, for the most part it was assumed that problems on nursing could be solved by distinguished men and women exchanging views in committee supplemented by written evidence. 'Such methods', wrote Dr Cohen with restrained understatement, 'had not been altogether successful.' It was the Minority Report rather than the Majority that was in the end to have the most effect on nursing, because after 1948 a number of people both inside and outside the profession applied research techniques to problems connected with nursing.

The Minority Report itself attempted to use scientific methods; Dr Cohen had intended to deal with the whole problem of planning health services in relation to the total manpower and other resources of the country, but unfortunately Geoffrey Pike, Dr Cohen's distinguished colleague, died, and the work remained unfinished. The Report did, however, introduce nurses to the idea of relating good nursing care with the length of the patient's stay and his recovery rate and to such methods as job analysis.

In the past a number of facts have militated against the nursing profession becoming research-minded. The main concern of the early reformed nursing had been to 'carve itself an empire' and to propagate the Nightingale system – not to question it. The discipline of the apprenticeship system itself demanded obedience without query, and enquiry is the life blood of research. As a contributor to the *Nursing Record* wrote in 1888, the nurse soon learned 'never to ask "why" and as rarely as possible, "how"'. Furthermore, before 1918 the position of women in general, and the relationship of nurses to doctors especially in hospital, gave little opportunity for effective questioning, and during the inter-war years, with most hospitals in debt, there were more pressing problems than those arising from the nurses' questioning of why they did certain tasks.

The first response to Dr Cohen's plea was the setting up of an Advisory Panel by the Nuffield Provincial Hospitals Trust in 1948, the outcome of which was the *Work of Nurses in Hospital Wards* which reported in 1953 (see Chapter 17). This report, which was in places received with marked hostility, was widely debated and at least introduced nurses to the mysteries of research techniques, time-and-motion studies, direct observation and interview techniques. The attitude to research would never be the same again

THE EARLY DEVELOPMENT OF NURSING RESEARCH

In 1990 a group of nurse scholars met as a Task Force on International Nursing Research at the headquarters of the International Council of Nurses in Geneva. They represented nine different countries across all five continents. They reported the rapid growth of nursing research, albeit from a relatively late start in the 1920s, but with great unevenness between countries. In 1990 in some countries there was still no such thing as nursing research, in others (notably the United States) nursing research was well established alongside research in other disciplines, well respected and reasonably resourced. On two major principles agreement was universal:

1 the need to develop scientific knowledge to under-gird nursing practice, and

2 the need to bridge the gap between practice and research so that research findings are incorporated into practice and topics of research needed are channelled from practitioners to researchers.[2]

Although the United Kingdom would have been seen as among the countries where nursing research was most developed, it was not until the 1950s that the first tentative research activity by nurses began in the United Kingdom. The starting point, well-described by Marjorie Simpson[3]

(who could herself be described as the midwife of nursing research in the United Kingdom) was a focus on nurses as an occupational group rather than on nursing itself; studies of the recruitment and selection of nurses[4] and of nurses' work[5] undertaken by social scientists in the 1940s and 1950s established an orientation and a methodological approach which has dominated nursing research in the United Kingdom ever since – a pragmatic, atheoretical approach, utilising survey methods and quantitative forms of analysis, based in service settings such as hospitals and health authority offices rather than in the academic setting of the universities. Most of the early studies by nurses used the same approach, including the pioneering studies of recently qualified nurses,[6] staff nurses[7] and enrolled nurses[8] undertaken by Gertrude Ramsden and Muriel Skeet for the Dan Mason Nursing Research Committee, and the studies of district nurses undertaken by Lisbeth Hockey for the Queen's Institute of District Nursing.[9, 10]

The first studies of nursing practice were also relatively simple surveys, but their exposure of the inadequacies of current nursing practice provided a foundation for later, more sophisticated work. A Nuffield study of 'Present sterilising practice in six hospitals'[11] in 1958, reinforced by Lisbeth Hockey's study of district nurses' sterilising practices,[12] were instrumental in replacing the ward 'fish-kettle' and the district nurse's 'biscuit tin' with sterile dressing packs. Meanwhile, the first truly clinical research was being pioneered by Doreen Norton in her seminal work on pressure sores,[13] and the first of what later became fashionable as 'patient satisfaction surveys' were being undertaken by Muriel Skeet ('Home from hospital', 1970[14]) and Winifred Raphael[15] who, although not herself a nurse, was a core figure in this early nursing research community.

These pioneers of nursing research – Norton, Raphael, Ramsden, Skeet, Hockey, and a small number of others – were the founder members of a Research Discussion Group (RDG), which was established in 1959 under the auspices of the Royal College of Nursing. The RDG subsequently became the RCN Research Society, and over the next 30 years became a significant focus point and educational resource for the next generation of nurse researchers. But the most influential figure of all in the long term, although she was not herself an active researcher but saw her role as primarily to facilitate others, was Marjorie Simpson, who, after a distinguished first career in occupational health nursing, was appointed as Research Officer first to the Royal College of Nursing and then, in 1963, to the (then) Ministry of Health. In this position Marjorie Simpson established a policy framework and a developmental programme for nursing research based on three key elements:[16]

1 preparing nursing to undertake research;
2 the development of research centres;
3 the dissemination of research fundings.

The programme included:[17]

- a research fellowship scheme, started in 1967, which enabled experienced nurses to obtain research training while undertaking a higher degree;
- the appointment of regional nursing research liaison officers, whose role was to advise services and individual nurses about nursing research;
- the establishment of nursing research units – at the Royal College of Nursing to develop method for measuring the quality of nursing care (see below); at the General Nursing Council for England and Wales to evaluate experimental programmes of nursing education, at Chelsea College London; and at Northwick Park Hospital (later transferred to the University of Surrey); in addition, the Scottish Home and Health Department supported a Nursing Research Unit at the University of Edinburgh.
- the establishment in 1976 of an Index of Nursing Research, followed two years later by a quarterly journal, *Nursing Research Abstracts*;
- underwriting a series of research monographs published in association with the Royal College of Nursing.

THE STUDY OF NURSING CARE PROJECT

Probably the most influential initiative was the Study of Nursing Care project, which was conceived by Marjorie Simpson, who persuaded the Ministry of Health to fund a project to be carried out by the Royal College of Nursing in order to try to develop measures of the quality of nursing care. Under the leadership of Jean McFarlane, the project took the form of 12 studies, introduced by an initial monograph by Jean McFarlane herself and aptly entitled *The Proper Study of the Nurse*,[18] and with a concluding monograph by her successor, entitled *Towards a Theory of Nursing Care*[19] and published in 1975. The projects explored such basic issues as patients' bowel habits,[20] pre-operative starvation[21] and pain.[22] The significance of the project was far greater than the impact of its individual studies. For example, the project was the basis of the very influential work on standards of care which the RCN began in the late 1970s and which was later developed in the 1980s and 1990s under the leadership of Alison Kitson; and several of the individual research assistants went on to become the first generation of professors of nursing and heads of the newly developing academic departments of nursing in British universities. Some 25 years after its conception, Jean McFarlane (by now Baroness McFarlane of Llandaff, Emeritus Professor of Nursing of the University of Manchester) reflected on the project in the Tenth Winifred Raphael Memorial Lecture[23] as follows:

Limited as the Project was by virtue of its place at the beginnings of nursing research in this country, I suggest that it has had a profound effect on subsequent developments in stating for all time that the study of the practice of nursing care is the central concern of nursing research; that there is a need for all nurses to be educated in appreciation of research applicable to their practice; and for some to be skilled researchers; that the methods used in nursing research may well be adopted from other disciplines but other methods may evolve which are more specific to nursing problems; that the analysis of theories and models of nursing practice which had their beginnings in the Project are an important part of any continuing study of nursing care; and that the issue of quality assurance and standard setting whilst conceptually complex is still a central concern to the profession.

NURSING RESEARCH AND HIGHER EDUCATION

Unusually, when compared with other countries and other disciplines, nursing research in the United Kingdom was not rooted in higher education. In the United Kingdom nursing as an academic subject (and therefore a discipline deriving its knowledge base from research) took a long time to penetrate higher education (see Chapter 23), and the important role which universities play in research in any discipline came to nursing research comparatively late. Few of the pioneers were university graduates, although many of them later achieved distinguished academic careers based on their research activities, and in 1970 in the United Kingdom there were very few nurses with higher degrees.

The Report of the Committee on Nursing (the Briggs Report), published in 1972, marked a new milestone in the development of nursing research, because it brought the issue of research in nursing to the attention of the profession as a whole, and its much-quoted sentiment that 'nursing must become a research based profession' became something of a slogan or rallying cry for the development of nursing research through the 1970s and into the 1980s. Research appreciation courses for practising nurses began to proliferate, and a few universities (such as the University of Surrey) began to make more serious research methods courses at Master's level available to non-graduate nurses. Meanwhile, the rapidly expanding pre-registration undergraduate programmes were beginning to produce a new generation of nurses whose basic qualification not only gave them unquestioned access to university Master's and doctoral-level programmes, but also established in them from the very beginning the critical and analytical approach to nursing which is a prerequisite for undertaking research. The nursing research of the 1970s and 1980s was mainly, although not entirely, in the form of studies undertaken in pursuit of higher degrees; by 1990 the Steinberg Collection of Nursing theses held at the Royal College of

Nursing, which had been started in 1974 with a small collection of master's-level dissertations, contained over 700 doctoral theses. The intellectual environment of the academic nursing departments also encouraged a more theoretical approach to nursing research, and the development of new methodological approaches which many considered were more appropriate and relevant for understanding nursing than the positivistic survey and experimental methods drawn from medicine and traditional social sciences. Qualitative approaches and grounded theory became not only more popular as methods of investigating nursing and nursing problems, but, thanks to the careful work of nurse researchers such as Kratz,[24] Melia[25] and others, increasingly more credible.

Academic departments of nursing in British universities still face an up-hill struggle. The system of funding of universities is increasingly based on research productivity, yet nursing still lacks the educational infrastructure of other disciplines – for example, there is still a shortage of nurses able to supervise other nurses undertaking doctoral studies, and because of the professional requirements of nursing education, the teaching responsibilities of academic staff in nursing are usually much heavier than academics in other disciplines. In 1980 the Universities Funding Council undertook an exercise in which all academic departments were required to detail their research activity and funding for purposes of grading on a five-point scale, the topmost of which (grade 5) indicated 'research quality which equates to attainable levels of international excellence in some sub-areas of activity and to attainable levels of national excellence in virtually all others'. No UK nursing department achieved the top grade; three (King's College, London, the universities of Surrey and Manchester) achieved grade 4; but overall, nursing came bottom of the list of 17 subject areas reviewed.

RESEARCH FOR HEALTH: A RESEARCH AND DEVELOPMENT STRATEGY FOR THE NHS

The cry for 'effectiveness and efficiency' which dominated so many health-service developments through the 1980s also included research activity. From the beginning, most nursing research (unlike most other disciplines) has been directly funded through the government health departments. Following the publication of the Rothschild Report in 1971, which advocated that all government-funded research should have a designated 'customer', a Nursing Research Liaison Group was established within the Department of Health to commission research in nursing and to advise the government's Chief Scientist (the head of the governmental research programmes) on the development and allocation of research resources. A House of Lords Select Committee on Science and Technology report on Priorities in Medical Research in 1988 reinforced the need for 'customer' orientation, and in April 1991 a Research and Development Strategy for the NHS was launched.[26] Two nurses, Dr Deborah Hennessey and Professor Karen Luker, were appointed as members of the Central Research and Development Committee, and the committees which were established at regional level also included nurses.

The main report was followed a year later by the Report of a Taskforce on the Strategy for Research in Nursing, Midwifery and Health Visiting.[27] Separate but parallel strategies were prepared for Scotland and Wales. The Report recognised the need for investment in nursing research, but specifically rejected the case for ring-fenced resources and the suggestion that, because of its disadvantaged position compared with medical research, nursing should be treated as a 'special case'. Instead, they recommended that 'research in nursing should be fully integrated within health services research and that the nursing profession should be enabled to make their proper contribution to this endeavour'. Their 37 recommendations ranged across four areas: structure and organisation, research education and training, funding for research, and integrating research development and practice.

INTEGRATION OF RESEARCH WITH NURSING PRACTICE

The purpose of nursing research has to be the improvement of nursing practice.[28] But this goal cannot be achieved unless its findings are used by clinical practitioners and incorporated into the knowledge base which underpins nursing practice. In 1981 Hunt suggested five reasons why research fundings are not properly utilised by practitioners: that nurses do not know about research findings, do not understand them, do not believe them, do not know how to apply them, or are not allowed to do so.[29] Six years later, a recently qualified graduate nurse was still able to claim that 'academic research findings are being ignored by practising nurses because they are too often unavailable, irrelevant, incomprehensible and impractical'.[30] As Hunt later concluded, on the basis of a study of the process of translating research findings into practice,[31] the process requires educational changes and changes in the organisational systems within which nursing care is delivered, as well as the knowledge and willingness of the individual nurse.

RETROSPECT AND PROSPECT

It will undoubtedly take some time before the Briggs Committee's challenge, which was quoted at the beginning of this chapter, is achieved, but given the shortness of the history of nursing research compared with the history of nursing described in this book, progress towards it has been considerable. In the first edition of this book, this chapter consisted mainly of a summary of some key research studies together with an overview of the methodological approaches then in use. At that time, the extent of research in nursing was such that it might have been possible to detail all work in progress and to know of all nurses who were involved in research. The amount of nursing research at the time of the preparation of this third edition is such that it is now impossible even to attempt to list or to summarise individual studies, and it would be almost as difficult to pick out a small number of special significance. Perhaps the best summary would be to quote from the United Kingdom's annual report to the Workgroup of European Nurse Researchers presented at the meeting held in Prague in August 1993 by Dr Alison Tierney, Chair of the RCN's Research Advisory Group.[32] On the positive side she reported:

- in addition to the Index of Nursing Research (which is accessible to on-line computer users and in a quarterly publication of *Nursing Research Abstracts* which for the year 1992 contained almost 500 entries), nurses in the United Kingdom have access to research reports in a wide range of generalist and specialist nursing journals as well as at least three scholarly journals;
- nurse researchers regularly present papers at national and international nursing conferences and at multidisciplinary research meetings;
- research training in the form of supervised postgraduate study leading to a master's or PhD degree is now available at many academic nursing departments, the number of which has now increased to over 30;
- the recently reformed system of nursing education (Project 2000) should produce a new generation of nurses who are more research aware and better prepared to function in the reformed NHS in which there is a growing commitment to research-based practice;
- The Royal College of Nursing has established a Research Committee as one of the standing committees which advise Council on major policy matters.

On the negative side she reported:

- much of the research undertaken is small-scale, project-type work; by accepted definitions of research, the volume and range of nursing research in the United Kingdom is limited;
- of the government-funded nursing research units only one (at King's College, London) remains;
- although government funding for nursing research has increased over the years it remains small in relation to the need for research investment in nursing and the cost of nursing services. . . . For funding from other sources the problem is not one of lack of available funding, but rather a lack of grantsmanship expertise within the nursing profession.

REFERENCES

1 Woodham-Smith, C. (1960) *Florence Nightingale*, London: Constable, p. 335.
2 International Council of Nurses (1990) *Nursing Research Worldwide: Current Dimensions and Future Directions*, Geneva: ICN.
3 Simpson, M. (1971) 'Research in nursing – the first steps', 13th *Nursing Mirror* Lecture, *Nursing Mirror* (12 March).
4 Houlistor, M. (1946) 'Selection tests for nurse applicants', *Nursing Times* 42: 808.
5 Goddard, H. (1953) *The Work of Nurses in Hospital Wards*, Oxford: Nuffield Provincial Hospitals Trust.
6 Dan Mason Nursing Research Committee (1966) *The Work, Responsibilities and Status of Recently Qualified Nurses*, London: DMNRC.
7 Dan Mason Nursing Research Committee (1966) *The Work, Responsibilities and Status of Staff Nurses*, London: DMNRC.
8 Dan Mason Nursing Research Committee (1962) *The Work, Responsibilities and Status of the Enrolled Nurses*, London: DMNRC.
9 Hockey, L. (1966) *Feeling the Pulse*, London: Queen's Institute of District Nursing.
10 Hockey, L. (1968) *Care in the Balance*, London: Queen's Institute of Nursing Research.
11 Nuffield Provincial Hospitals Trust (1958) *Present Sterilising Practice in Six Hospitals*, Oxford: NPHT.
12 Queen's Institute of District Nursing (1965) *Safer Sterilising of Equipment*, London: QIDN.
13 Norton, D., McLarent R. and Exton-Smith, A. N. (1962) *An Investigation of Geriatric Nursing Problems in Hospital*, re-issued 1975, Edinburgh: Churchill Livingstone.
14 Skeet, M. (1970) 'Home from Hospital', London: Dan Mason Nursing Research Committee.
15 Raphael, W. (1969) *Patients and their Hospitals*, London: King Edward's Hospital Fund for London.
16 Simpson, M. (1973) 'Research in nursing' (ch. 14), in Nuffield Provincial Hospitals Trust (1973) *Portfolio for Health 2: the Developing Programme of the DHSS in Health Services Research*, London: Oxford University Press.
17 Lelean, S. (1980) 'Research in nursing: an overview of DHSS initiatives in developing research in nursing', *Nursing Times Occasional Papers*, 76(2): 5–8, and 76(3): 9–12.
18 McFarlane, J. K. (1970) *The Proper Study of the Nurse*, London: Royal College of Nursing.
19 Inman, U. (1975) *Towards a Theory of Nursing Care*, London: Royal College of Nursing.
20 Wright, L. (1974) *Bowel Function in Hospital Patients,* London: Royal College of Nursing.
21 Hamilton-Smith, S. (1972) *Nil by Mouth*, London: Royal College of Nursing.
22 Hayward, J. (1975) *Information: a Prescription against Pain*, London: Royal College of Nursing.
23 McFarlane, J. K. (1990) 'The study of nursing care: the Tenth Winifred Raphael Memorial Lecture', in P. Denton (ed.)(1992) *They Speak for Themselves: the Winifred Raphael Memorial Lectures 1981–1990*, London: Royal College of Nursing.
24 Kratz, C. (1978) *Care of the Long-term Sick in the Community*, Edinburgh: Churchill Livingstone.

25 Melia, K. (1982) 'Tell it as it is – qualitative method and nursing research', *Journal of Advanced Nursing*, 7(4): 327–36.
26 Department of Health (1991) *Research for Health: a Research and Development Strategy for the NHS*, London: Department of Health.
27 Department of Health (1992) *Report of the Taskforce on the Strategy for Research in Nursing, Midwifery and Health Visiting* London: Department of Health.
28 Royal College of Nursing (1993) *The Research Role of the RCN*, London: Royal College of Nursing (in press).
29 Hunt, J. (1981) 'Indications for practice: the use of research findings', *Journal of Advanced Nursing*, 6: 189–94.
30 Chellell, A. (1987) 'Learned practice', *Nursing Times*, 83(21): 64.
31 Hunt, J. (1987) 'The process of translating research findings into nursing practice', *Journal of Advanced Nursing*, 6: 189–94.
32 Royal College of Nursing (1993) Workgroup of European Nurse Researchers, 16th Annual Meeting, held in Prague (23–25 Aug.) Annual Report from the United Kingdom, Royal College of Nursing, unpublished Report.

Chapter 25

The road to reorganisation

Monica E. Baly and June Clark

We trained hard but it seemed that every time we were beginning to form up into teams we would be reorganised. I was to learn later in life that we tend to meet any new situation by reorganising, and a wonderful method it can be for creating the illusion of progress, while producing inefficiency and demoralisation.

Gaius Petronius, AD 66

The years since the inauguration of the National Health Service have seen a social change as great as that experienced between 1780 and 1820, when industrialisation transformed so many lives. The so-called affluent fifties gave way to the swinging sixties and the problems of inflation in the seventies, and then to the recession of the late eighties and early nineties. The western world is facing an energy crisis, the problems of pollution, global warming and endemic unemployment. As in the past, rapid social change produces new health needs, which challenge existing institutions and attitudes to health care.

The most important of these challenges comes from the changed population profile (Chapter 18). At present the birth rate is 13.8 per thousand and the death rate 11.2 (Chapter 1). The population figure is 57,561, of which 3 per cent are other nationals which is less than the figure for other EEC countries. Demographic forecasting is an inexact science, but it looks as if the population will continue to grow slowly and reach 59 million by the end if the century (see Figure 25.1).

The main change since 1960 is that the population is older. There are 10.6 million pensioners, a rise of 16 per cent since 1971, and by 2031 there will be 14 million.[1] This increased longevity has come about because life expectancy at birth has increased. By the turn of the century women will have a life expectancy of 80 years, and this means there will be an increase in the number of the very old living alone. More than one-quarter of all households are one-person households, which is double the number in 1961, and of these 16 per cent are pensioners.[2] This is an enormous challenge to the health and social services and to the community care services (Chapter 19).

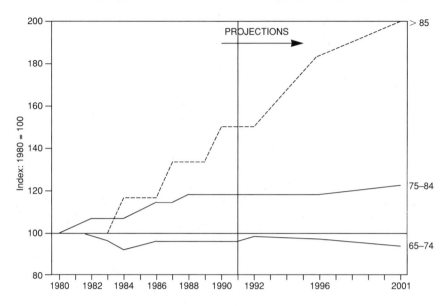

Figure 25.1 Population projections to the turn of the century, UK: the elderly
Source: NAHAT (1993) *NHS Handbook 1993–4*

Perhaps more than any other group the elderly have been the victims of the fact that during the past 20 years 'the rich have got richer and the poor poorer'. In the 12 years up to 1991 only those with a present-day pre-tax income of £38,000 saw an increase in the amount that they could spend. Those in the lowest categories found that their disposable income had almost halved. For those relying on savings, the pound of 1951 was worth 7 pence in 1992. A special survey of the poorest households shows that 70 per cent of their income comes from social security benefits.[3] Although inflation has fallen to 2.6 per cent, the poorest, who often include the elderly, are disproportionately affected by rises in VAT. Inability to heat homes adequately will have an effect on health.

Another social change that affects health is the rise in unemployment, which in 1993 rose to just below 3 million, though this is by no means the highest figure in Europe. One in three of the poorest group is unemployed, but, apart from poverty, unemployment is often the harbinger of chronic ill health and disruption and discord in family life. Among other social changes that have a bearing on health has been the change in housing. Rising land values, cuts in the bank rate and the property boom of the late 1960s and early 1970s saw an acceleration of changes begun in the inner cities. Offices replaced houses and housing accommodation tended to be in high-rise blocks. As in the nineteenth century, when railways replaced homes, so now motorways and offices replaced cheap living accommodation and people moved out and had to travel further to work, the cost of which was soon to be increased by rising fares and the oil crisis. At the same time, cheap rented accommodation fell in availability; 1.4 million council houses were sold off and the number of owner-occupiers doubled between 1961 and 1991. However, mortgage repayments and rents have remained above the rate of inflation, and in 1991 over 75,000 properties were repossessed, a fivefold increase in two years.[4] Shortage of low-priced accommodation, especially in the rented sector, has meant an increase in homelessness, and there are now 160,000 people in priority need with all the attendant problems of malnutrition and infection (Chapter 19).

On the other hand, expectations rose. More children stayed at school longer, more under-5s were attending school and large classes are becoming a thing of the past. In 1992, 22 per cent of all girls and 20 per cent of boys obtained two or more A levels, and 82 per thousand are in full-time education; nevertheless, we have the lowest rate in Europe and the western world for the number of children progressing to higher education.[5] While there are still opportunities for the brightest for those who design the programmes for the micro-electronic era, the future for those displaced by the new equipment does not look so good. On these grounds recruitment to nursing should be easier, especially recruitment to Project 2000, which is educationally more demanding. However, the question that now arises is not how many students we need but how many we can afford, and colleges of nursing have reduced their student intake. The health service budget is fixed, and any salary increase for staff has to come out of 'efficiency savings' and, because of their high proportion of the labour costs, this often means reducing the nursing staff.

THE HEALTH NEEDS OF THE 1990s

The first need is that increased survival means survival of the frail and more people suffering more episodes of ill health – people whose needs are not so much cure as *care*. Recorded morbidity has risen, but this may be due to better diagnosing and the fact that some social groups seek advice earlier. The number of general practitioners has risen by one third since 1960. The more effective the service, the greater the number of clients. More than ever, the health service has to do with degenerative changes that are complicated and difficult to treat, with the patient requiring the whole gamut of the health and welfare services. Because people live longer, the genetic component is more likely to play a part in disease, and these factors, about which little can be done, may determine the way of death.

The other important consideration stems from the way people behave. Apart from this there is the question of the environment; for example, the effect of petrol fumes on respiratory diseases and asthma. Medicine cannot stand aside from the debate about motorways versus public transport. The White Paper, 'The health of the nation: a strategy for health in England' and parallel documents for the other three countries of the United Kingdom, identified the major causes of premature death and initiated a major programme of action to tackle them. The five key areas selected were:

- coronary heart disease and stroke,
- cancers,
- mental illness,
- HIV/AIDS and sexual health,
- accidents.

Although the strategy acknowledges the importance of inter-sectoral collaboration (which it calls 'healthy alliances'), it does not include any consideration of the underlying problem of poverty and it specifically eschews fiscal measures such as the tax structure and the banning of tobacco advertising. In her introduction to the Strategy, the Secretary of State wrote:

> We must be clear about where responsibilities lie. We must get the balance right between what the government, and the government alone can do, what other organisations and agencies need to do, and finally, what individuals and families themselves must contribute if the strategy is to succeed.

In spite of the propaganda and health education, a quarter of a million children are regular smokers, more likely in families where the adults smoke, and more alarming is the fact that in the age group 20–24 years smoking is actually increasing. Another cause for alarm is that there are nearly ten times as many drug addicts reported in 1991 as in 1973, with the vast majority addicted to heroin, while there has been an increase in the number addicted to methadone, and deaths from solvent abuse are on the increase (Chapter 19). The question posed in the 1979 Royal Commission to those giving evidence, 'To what extent are people responsible for their own health?', is still relevant.

MEETING THE HEALTH NEEDS: THE REORGANISATIONS OF THE 1970s

The main services meeting these needs in the early 1970s were the health and welfare services provided by the local authorities, the hospital services provided by the Regional Hospital Boards and the family practitioner services: the tripartite National Health Service together with an assortment of voluntary services.

The local authority services

In 1871 the Local Government Board gathered together most of the services given through municipal authorities (see Figure 8.2). In 1888 and 1894 Local Government Acts provided machinery for elected authorities through which these services could be administered. In 1919 the new Ministry of Health took over the multifarious tasks of the Board, some of which were clarified by the Local Government Act of 1929, with the local authorities continuing to administer what were now municipal hospitals, and the personal health and welfare services. In 1948 the municipal hospitals were taken over by the Regional Hospital Boards. The division was now between the curative and the preventive services, with the family practitioner services semi-independent. This tripartite structure failed to meet the needs of the community. The fragmentation of the services had practical and human consequences; co-ordination was difficult because of the number of agencies to be co-ordinated, there was waste of resource through overlap, many patients were in hospital who could have lived out had there been support in the community, but local authorities were not responsible for the health service and were unlikely to use ratepayers' money for accommodation to relieve the pressure. Other disadvantages were obvious; the bewildering variety of agencies confused the public and the diversity of advice was at best complicated and, at worst, dangerous. Medical and nursing education was targeted, not on the health needs of the population, but on a close-up picture of a limited hospital population. Both the local government health services and the social services had grown up empirically, and, in isolation, both were considering plans for reform.

The personal social services – the link in the chain

The social services had developed from the chequered history of the Poor Law and the voluntary services. In the nineteenth century services for the relief of poverty and the care of ill health were often interdependent. The Poor Law medical officer, the parish nurse, the relieving officer and the visitors from many voluntary societies dealt with the same users, usually 'the perishing classes'. Later this interdependence extended, the school medical service dealt with physically and mentally handicapped children who were probably the concern of the Poor Law and possibly, one of the voluntary services like the Society for the Prevention of Cruelty to Children. On the other hand, some social services developed as off-shoots of other local authority services. School attendance and housing officers encountered families in distress, so various services developed a welfare function. As with the local authority services, there was lack of co-ordination.

In 1966 a Committee under the chairmanship of Sir Frederic Seebohm was set up 'to review the organisation and responsibilities of the local authority personal social services in England and Wales and to consider what changes are necessary to secure and effective family service'. The Seebohm Report was published in 1968 and made a detailed review of the growth of the social services; it looked at future trends and analysed present difficulties. The Committee came to the conclusion that there were difficulties in both the range and quality of the service, that they were poorly co-ordinated, difficult of access and lacked adaptability. A number of solutions were examined, but in the end the Committee came to the conclusion that the only solution was an independent Social Services Department in each authority under the control of a director of social services who would have the responsibility for the social services of the authority.

Behind this solution the report conveys the sense of frustration on the part of the social workers ,who were tired of being an appendage of medicine. However, the Seebohm solution, coming as it did when chronic illness had taken the place of episodic disease, was ironic. Never since the nineteenth century had the two services been so interdependent. Although there were strong advocates for the report in the Lords, the health organisations advised against its acceptance. The unification of the health service would be a Pyrrhic victory if it were gained at the expense of the divorce of health and welfare. Advice from the health service was overruled, and the Local Authority Social Services Act gained assent in May 1970. The division between health and welfare had begun. Attempts to minimise that division now dictated much of the planning in the health services. That is why Seebohm is the link in the reorganisation chain.

Reform of local government

As the public health medical services had grown up under the local authorities (Figure 8.2), it was accepted that the reforms of the health services would be bound up with reforms in local government. However, in 1960 the structure of local government was still what it had been in 1888 when the population was 28 million. In 1951 the local authority functions of the Ministry of Health were transferred to the Ministry of Housing and Local Government (to become the Department of the Environment in 1970), and in 1963 the Greater London Council (since disbanded) replaced the old London County Council.

In 1966 a Royal Commission under the chairmanship of Lord Redcliffe-Maude was set up to consider the structure of local government outside London. The Committee, which sat for three years and took monumental evidence, came to the conclusion that the local authority areas did not fit the life and work of the people of England, that there was an unreal division between town and country and that the fragmentation into 124 major authorities and 1,086 County District Councils was wasteful of resource. The Commission recommended new boundaries for local government based on the 'city region'; these unitary authorities would be large enough to assume responsibility for all local governing services. The Commission looked at the need for a unified health service and suggested that the unitary authorities would be a suitable basis for health authorities and would have the merit of keeping the social services closely related to health. This concept influenced the proposals put forward for a reform of the health services by the Rt Hon. K. Robinson in 1968.

The Report of the Commission was debated in 1969 and the recommendations accepted by the Labour Government, but the findings were not universally popular; not all those connected with local government thought that fewer meant better. The health professions, particularly the doctors, were against local authorities being in any way responsible for health. In 1969 the Secretary of State, the Rt Hon. R. Crossman, at the new Department of Health and Social Services, was faced with a commitment to unify the health services but with little room to manoeuvre; he rejected the Redcliffe-Maude proposals on the grounds that the resources of the local authorities would not be sufficient to take over a service now costing £14,000 million.[6] The Department concluded that the only way round the dilemma of keeping health and welfare linked was to revert to the idea of independent 'health authorities' which operated within the same boundaries as the local authorities. At this point there was a general election, and the Labour government went out of office.

A compromise solution for local government reform

The incoming government rejected the findings of the Royal Commission and the new Secretary of State for the Department of the Environment, the Rt Hon. Peter Walker, produced his own White Paper. Although accepting some of the philosophy of Redcliffe-Maude, it produced a different solution. The major authorities were to be the counties, and several new ones were created, with special arrangements for the metropolitan areas. Outside London there were 44 county councils, which were responsible for the planning and administration of the major services such as education, transport and the social services. However, within these major authorities the existing 900 councils were organised into district councils and given responsibility and resource for housing, land acquisition and what were termed 'purely local services'. In due course the White Paper became the Local Government Act, which set up new authorities in April 1974.

There is now another Commission on Local Government which is considering the possiblity of unitary authorities.

THE NATIONAL HEALTH SERVICES REORGANISATION, 1974

The new legislation had consequences for the health service. The major authorities would have no responsibility for either the preventive or curative health services, but they would have responsibility for the social services. On the other hand, some matters that impinged on health remained with the District Councils. If the growing dichotomy between health and welfare were not to worsen, liaison between the services must be strengthened; those whom usage had joined together the planners had put asunder. The Secretary of State at the Department of Health, the Rt Hon. Sir Keith Joseph, consulted the Brunel Institute whose thinking was set out in Hospital Organisation[7] and whose advice was reflected in the Management Arrangements for the Reorganised National Health Service. The legislation came into force in 1974 to coincide with the reorganisation of local government. The Brunel Institute advised that hospital organisation be understood in terms of 'areas of consensus'. The philosophy was translated into practice by placing heavy emphasis on line management with maximum decentralisation and delegation of decision-making, within the policies laid down by the Regional and Area Boards and that 'delegation downward be matched by accountability upwards'.[8]

The structure of the reorganised health service

The Regional Hospital Boards became Regional Health Authorities, whose jurisdiction covered the same areas. Below the region there was a second management tier, the Area Health Authority, based on 38 non-metropolitan and six metropolitan areas outside London, with special arrangements for London. The Area Health Authorities were coterminous with the major local authorities, with which they set up liaison committees. To meet the needs of medical teaching, certain areas were designated teaching AHA(T). Each authority set up a Family Practitioner Committee to administer the contracts of the general practitioners, who were adamant that it was a 'contract for service', not 'of service'.

During the debate on the Bill there was considerable criticism that the service was governed by members appointed by the Secretary of State. To meet this criticism a section was added to the Act which provided for the setting up of Community Health Councils . The Community Councils had no executive power, but they had the right to inspect hospitals and were expected to produce a report. In spite of efforts to strengthen their position, evidence to the Royal Commission on the National Health Service shows that these councils made little impact and did not make the service more democratic.

As the areas were too large for the day-to-day execution of policy, the areas were sub-divided into into districts covering populations of up to 500,000. Some areas had only one or two districts, others had four or five. The District Management Team was in a staff relationship to the Area Health Authority and was responsible for providing an integrated health service within its District. Regional Health Authorities were responsible for planning health services, allocating resources and monitoring the performance of the Area Authorities in their Region, including the personal health services and the family practitioner services, and for contact with outside agencies.

As far as nursing was concerned, integration was achieved by the fusion of the 'Salmon' and 'Mayston' structures and by selecting the staff according to elaborate algorithms set out by the National Staff Committee. Not all the plans achieved the objective of integration. Putting district nurses, health visitors and medical officers of health on the pay-roll of an AHA did not in itself produce integration. True totality of care will only come when all health professionals are educated to have this as their aim.

Resource Allocation Working Party (RAWP)

One of the difficulties in providing continuing care is the fact that resources are unevenly distributed between geographical areas and branches of medicine. The cost of keeping a patient in a mental hospital was less than a third of that for an acute hospital, and hospital services still account for two-thirds of all expenditure. The National Health Service has done little to redistribute health care. Each area builds on its historical past. Liverpool has a high rate of hospital beds, and Merseyside has the lowest hospital waiting list but is a low spender on community care.

A start was made on the redistribution of resources by the Working Party, but it admitted that as yet there were no tools available to measure health care deprivation and there is an urgent need to develop measurement skills. The common measuring rods are the peri-natal rate, the infant mortality rate, the standard mortality rate for various age groups and the number of days lost from work for such things as the suicide rate. Then there are morbidity rates from selected scourges like infectious diseases, bronchitis and rheumatism; but most of these yardsticks are not measures of the quality of the service but more often the failures of the social system. Some, like the infant mortality rate, are a reflection of the social and economic life of the community. All this endorses the fact that positive health is largely promoted by factors outside the health services. To paraphrase Miss Nightingale: 'There are many reasons why chronic sickness and days lost from work are higher in the north than in the south, but lack of provision of hospital beds is not one of them.' (See Table 25.1, 'Health-care expenditure in 24 OECD countries' and Table 25.2, 'Selected health status measures.)

Criticism of the 1974 reorganisation

Although there was agreement on the need to unify the health services there was by no means universal endorsement of the proposed methods. Those

Table 25.1 Health-care expenditure in 24 OECD countries: percentage of gross domestic product spent on health, 1989

	%		%
USA	11.8	Luxembourg	7.4
Sweden	8.8	Ireland	7.3
Canada	8.7	Belgium	7.2
France	8.7	Finland	7.1
Iceland	8.6	New Zealand	7.1
Netherlands	8.3	Japan	6.7
Austria	8.2	Denmark	6.3
Germany	8.2	Portugal	6.3
Switzerland	7.8	Spain	6.3
Australia	7.6	UK	5.8
Italy	7.6	Greece	5.1
Norway	7.6	Turkey	3.9

concerned with preventive medicine were critical of the barriers between health and welfare and were unhappy about the new status of the Medical Officer of Health. The Royal College of Nursing made a strong protest about the number of 'tiers of management' which would elongate the management chain, be expensive of resource and delay decision-making, and the *Nursing Times* was forthright about the massive superstructure that seemed to be an end in itself. Many organisations were critical of the proposals to set up a separate statutory body for family practitioners, pointing out that unless those who gave care were truly members of the team, the service would remain divided and failures in communication would still occur.

THE ROYAL COMMISSION ON THE NATIONAL HEALTH SERVICE

In 1976, the government having changed again, the Wilson administration appointed a Royal Commission whose job it was to consider the interests of both the patient and those who worked in the National Health Service and the best use and management of the financial and manpower resources. The Commission, which took wide-ranging evidence, reported in July 1979 and found much that was good in the National Health Service; not all its faults could be laid at the door of reorganisation. Like all reports since that of the Webbs in 1909, it saw the logical organisation of the health services as being in some way connected with local government, but this was a possiblity for the future. For the present, it suggested a simplification of the structure with a single tier below the Regional Health Authority and the abolition of the Family Practitioner Committees with their functions absorbed in the health authorities. The Report made a number of recommendations, some of which could be implemented without an enactment,

Table 25.2 Selected health status measures

	Male life expectancy at birth	Female life expectancy at birth	Male life expectancy at 40	Female life expectancy at 40	Infant mortality	Peri-natal mortality
France	72.0	80.3	34.3*	41.4*	0.76	1.12**
Germany	71.8*	78.4*	34.0*	39.9*	0.83	0.73
Netherlands	73.5	80.1	35.8	41.9	0.64*	0.92
Sweden	74.5	80.2	36.1	41.1	0.61	0.71
UK	71.9	77.6	34.0	39.1	0.91	0.88
USA	71.5	78.3	34.7	40.3	1.00	1.00

Note: All figures relate to 1987 unless stated otherwise
* 1986 figures
** 1984 figures
Source: OECD, Paris

but others would require legislation. The Labour government fell from office in 1979, and the incoming administration rejected most of the Commission's proposals.

MEETING HEALTH NEEDS: THE REORGANISATIONS OF THE 1980s

The structural deficiencies of the 1974 reorganisation were not the only problem: the real problem was that the post-war period of economic growth was over. The rise in oil prices of 1973, and the onset of a recession, which was combined, unusually, with inflation, forced the Treasury in 1976 (under a Labour government) to introduce cash limits on public expenditure, including health care; only the General Practitioner service escaped. The planning system which the Department of Health had introduced in 1976 as an attempt to implement national priorities, including the plans for financial redistribution, came under increasing pressure.

The change of government in 1979 (the first Thatcher government) heralded the onset of a new political ideology – Thatcherism – which included a totally new approach to public services, including the NHS. The new approach emphasised managerial efficiency, cost considerations as the basis for decisions, cost containment, and commercial goals such as efficiency savings and income generation, competitive contracting and the development of the private sector. Out went ideas such as consensus, consultation and collaboration – represented by committees such as the Royal Commission and 'representative' health authorities; in came individual advisers (drawn mainly from the business world), management consultants, and 'enquiries' or 'reviews' undertaken by small teams of people directly appointed and selected more for their political and commercial orientation than for their experience of health care or as 'representatives' of particular interest groups. The first example – and with hindsight the catalyst for the new approach – was the NHS Management Enquiry undertaken by Roy Griffiths (see Chapter 22).

The first reorganisation of the 1980s, however, was that which had been recommended by the Royal Commission – the reduction of the number of 'layers' of the NHS by the removal of the area tier. The 90 area health authorities and the area teams of officers disappeared; the district management teams were strengthened and supported by the creation of approximately 200 district health authorities. The new authorities and their officers were given greater devolved responsibilities and greater freedom to plan their services. Below the level of the district, services were divided into units, each with a unit management team.

With hindsight, however, the wrong tier was removed. The geographical definition of the area had been linked with the boundaries of the local authorities which were responsible for the provision of social services and education (both of which interface closely with health services) and also formed the boundaries of the Family Practitioner Committees which managed the contracts of general practitioners and the other family practitioner services. The loss of this co-terminosity meant that either multiple management links and arrangements for collaboration had to be established or the different services would 'go their own way'. The developing philosophy of replacing central planning and central direction with devolution and local freedom ensured that it was the latter tendency which prevailed.

The 1980s saw a sequence of changes which were introduced as 'efficiency improvements' but which in their effects constituted structural and cultural changes as significant as the 'formal' reorganisations of 1974 and 1982. The most important, which was specifically described as 'not another reorganisation' was the introduction of general management as a result of the Griffiths Report in 1983, but the presentation of other developments in list form gives some indication of the range and extent of the changes:

1982   Dissolution of AHAs, creation of DHAs and units of management;
       Raynor scrutinies of services such as the provision of staff accommodation;
       system of annual accountability reviews started.
1983   Annual accountability reviews extended to Unit level;
       comparative performance indicators introduced;
       value for money audit programme introduced;
       manpower planning systems revised;
       competitive tendering introduced;
       NHS Training Authority established;
       Griffiths Report published;
       Health Services Supervisory Board established.
1984   Directives on implementation of Griffiths Report, appointment of new chief executives (district general managers);
       Chief nursing officers and directors of nursing services become 'advisers';
       cash limits, manpower targets and service developments brought together;
       cost-improvement programmes established;
       NHS Management Board created.
1985   Quality assurance programmes introduced;
       Cumberlege Report on community nursing services in England published, followed by similar reviews in other UK countries.
1986   Publication of 'Project 2000' Report;
       introduction (in some areas) of 'neighbourhood nursing' and locality management of community health services

1988   Restructuring of nurses' salary structures through the introduction
        of clinical grading.

THE 1990 REFORMS: THE 'NEW' NATIONAL HEALTH SERVICE

But it was not enough. The government remained unhappy about the NHS, and was particularly sensitive about public criticisms of cuts in services so soon after a general election (in 1987), in which the future of the NHS had been a major issue and Mrs Thatcher had claimed it to be 'safe in our hands.' By the autumn of 1987 it was clear that the NHS was in yet another financial crisis. In December the British Medical Association issued a statement claiming that the funding of hospital services was seriously inadequate and a major injection of resources was needed, and the presidents of all the Royal Colleges, in an unprecedented show of unity, issued a joint statement claiming that the NHS had reached breaking point.

The funding crisis was undoubtedly the result of cumulative under-funding over a long period of time, exacerbated – paradoxically – by the improved efficiency of the service (unlike manufacturing or commercial enterprises, an increase in productivity in health care increases total costs), but the trigger for action came in the form of the heart-rending stories of two little boys whose badly needed heart operations were repeatedly cancelled and delayed because the Birmingham Children's Hospital could not afford to employ enough specialist nurses. The form of the response was equally bizarre: in an interview on the BBC television programme 'Panorama' on 25 January 1988, the Prime Minister announced that she had decided to initiate a fundamental review of the NHS, the results of which would be published within a year.

In fact, neither the ideological shifts of the 1980s nor the problem of cost-containment in health care, which came together to produce the 1990 NHS reforms, was unique to the United Kingdom. Similar changes were made in the health-care systems of New Zealand, Australia, and most countries of western Europe, while in the United States the 'health-care crisis' came to a head in the 1992 presidential elections. For countries such as the United Kingdom which already had a nationalised, tax-funded health care system, the key change was the replacement of the traditional public service model by the introduction of the concept of the 'internal market' – an idea which is usually attributed to the American economist Alain Enthoven, who in 1985 published a monograph entitled 'Reflections on the Management of the NHS.'[9]

The review which led to the reforms of 1990 was very different from those which had preceded earlier reorganisations. The Prime Minister established a small committee of senior ministers chaired by herself to undertake the review, supported by a group of civil servants and political advisers. There were no 'Green Papers', and the review was conducted in private. However, a number of institutions and individuals, including the Royal College of Nursing,[10] tried to influence the outcome by publishing their own proposals; among the most influential were the right-wing policy think-tanks such as the Adam Smith Institute and the Centre for Policy Studies, whose director at the time was David Willets, a former member of the No. 10 Policy Unit.

The results came in the form of the White Paper 'Working for Patients', which was published in January 1989. The White Paper reaffirmed the key principles of the NHS established in 1948; namely, that the service would continue to be available to all and would be funded mainly out of taxation. The principle that the service should be free at the point of contact had long been breached by the introduction of prescription and other charges, but no new charges were introduced at this time. The key change was the introduction of the internal market in the form of the 'purchaser/provider split': instead of being responsible for the provision of services as in the past, health authorities would use their money to 'purchase' services for their resident population from the hospitals and other health facilities which would now become 'independent' provider units to be called 'NHS Trusts'. General practitioners, subject to eligibility criteria based on the size of practice, would similarly be able, as 'GP fundholders', to purchase certain services for their patients. The purpose of this introduction of 'purchasers' and 'providers' within a 'health-care market' was to create the 'competition' between providers which would, it was claimed, improve quality and force down costs.

There were more structural changes and new management arrangements. In the new Department of Health, the Supervisory Board and the Management Board were to be replaced by a Policy Board and a Management Executive. In health authorities (RHAs and DHAs), the old 'committee' format was to be replaced by a Board of Directors. Family Practitioner Committees were to be replaced by Family Health Service Authorities which would be directly accountable to Regional Health Authorities and would thus, for the first time, achieve some accountability and budgetary control over the general practitioner services. The new powers given to the health authorities and the new NHS Trusts represented a major increase in managerial control at all levels.

The main focus of *Working for Patients*, and of the debate around the reforms, was the acute hospital services. Proposals for the development of primary health care (namely, general practitioner services) had already been published in 1987 in the White Paper 'Promoting Better Health'. Proposals for community care – which covered both the community health services provided by the NHS and the health-related services for elderly, mentally ill and disabled people provided by local authorities, were contained in the White Paper 'Caring for People'.

The proposals contained in the three White Papers were incorporated into the NHS and Community Care Bill which was published in November 1989 and received the Royal Assent as the NHS and Community Care Act in June 1990 – just 18 months from the Prime Minister's 'Panorama' interview.

Detailed analysis of this most radical reorganisation of the NHS since its inception in 1948, and of the events since, are outside the scope of this book. Most readers of this book will themselves be part of the history of its implementation, whether as providers or as users of 'the new NHS'. Whether these latest reforms represent, as suggested by the government, a further step in the improvement of the NHS, or, as others have suggested, the beginning of the end of the NHS, only time will tell.

REFERENCES

1 *Social Trends* (1992) London: HMSO.
2 *General Household Survey* (1992) London: Office of Population Census and Surveys.
3 *The Times*, 27 Jan. 1994.
4 *Social Trends* (1992).
5 Ibid.
6 Department of Health and Social Security (1970) 'The future structure of the NHS' (Green Paper), London: HMSO.
7 Jacques, E., Rowbottom, R. *et al.* (1972) *Hospital Organisation*, Brunel Institute; see also *Management Arrangements in the Reorganised Health Service* (The Grey Book – DHSS).
8 Ibid.
9 Enthoven, A. (1985) *Reflections on the Management of the NHS*, Oxford: Nuffield Provincial Hospitals Trust.
10 Royal College of Nursing (1992) *The Health Challenge*, London: RCN.

FURTHER READING

Ham, C. (1992) *Health Policy in Britain: the Politics and Organisation of the National Health Service*, London: Macmillan.
Social Trends (1992) London: HMSO.
Webster, C. (ed.) *Caring for Health: History and Diversity* (1992) Health and Disease Series, Book 6, ch. 7, Milton Keynes: Open University Press.

Chapter 26

Nursing, economic change and industrial relations

Val Cowie

And when they came they that were hired received every man a penny. But they that came first supposed that they should have received more ... and when they had received it they murmured against the goodman of the house saying, 'these last have wrought but one hour and thou hast made them equal to us which hath borne the heat and burden of the day'.

Matthew 20: 9–14

Since time immemorial men have argued about differentials and threatened action against unfair treatment. But the labourers in the vineyard had no case; they had agreed a contract and they had been paid the rate for the job. What struck them as unfair was that someone else got the same for doing less and they were using that time-honoured negotiating ploy of pointing to an anomaly to push up the basic rate. But life and reward are not fair; Mozart lies in an unmarked, poor citizen's grave.

The more complicated society the more difficult it is to find yardsticks by which to measure the value of labour. Karl Marx (1818–83), when he inveighed against the capitalist system, produced his theory of values,[1] and since then many non-Marxist economists have developed other theories to calculate the value of work – but they remain theories. Under the system of *laissez-faire* the value of work was simply what the market would bear, but even in the heyday of Adam Smith (1723–90) and David Ricardo (1772–1823), the market was never the sole determinant of wages; justices fixed minimum rates and the state intervened on behalf of children. At the other end of the economic spectrum there are the collectivist societies where there is no profit motive and the state controls prices and wages. However, most western industrial societies are pluralistic – that is to say that both systems operate in varying ratios, and the state, no matter the political complexion of the government, is forced to play a greater role, while in spite of 'cuts in spending' the public sector becomes larger.[2] In pluralistic societies, wages are often a pragmatic, and at times uneasy, amalgam of market forces in the private sector, and, related to this, what taxation will bear for the public sector. The problem of pay in the private sector depends on the constraints of the market, but in the public sector on the willingness of the government to provide funds; therefore, no matter how the government tries to wash its hands of pay, disputes in the public sector become political.

Doctors and lawyers maintained their financial superiority because the pace-setters came from the private sector where they charged the fees the market would bear, and in the nineteenth century that was a considerable amount. Moreover, the learned professions controlled their standard of entry and the numbers of their intake; thus they had both intellectual and social cachet and a scarcity value. Nurses were seldom private practitioners and, even after registration, thanks to internecine squabbles, the profession did not control its entry standard, its numbers, nor yet its basic training. But these factors are nugatory compared with the fact that most nurses were women. The overriding reason for low pay in nursing is not, as has been suggested, because nurses emanated from the Nightingale ladies – who were a minority group – but because they were not men.

The depressed economic position of women in the nineteenth century was the launching pad for twentieth-century woman. First, there was the sheer preponderance of women and the fact that in 1840 there were more unmarried women than at any time before or since. Second, women were confined to the skills they exercised in the pre-industrial era: the making of textiles, laundry work, catering, the teaching of small children and nursing the sick. Third, in the early years of the Industrial Revolution, the cheap labour of women was seen as a threat to the living standards of men and for the first time women and men were in economic competition. After the collapse of Chartism in 1848, and as industry changed from the family business to the joint stock company, so unionism changed from the craft and skilled work organisations to embrace the unskilled where new national unions organised on industrial lines with rules, regulations and paid officials, a world from which working women were largely excluded. Women did produce leaders like Annie Besant (1847–1933) but when they organised it was in separate women's organisations. In 1891 fewer than one in 200 women were in unions, compared with one in five men.[3]

Apart from the rapidly expanding workforce receiving surplus women into its mechanical arms there was another outlet for their traditional skills. With increasing wealth the expanding middle classes moved from their shops or the vicinity of the factory to the new suburbs now swathing the cities, where Victorian gentility, large families and the needs of larger houses increased the demand for servants, nannies and governesses, who, being plentiful, were poorly paid. There was also opportunity for employment in the houses of the landed gentry where the servant class 'were a group withdrawn from the mass of common people, and, committed to life-long service, were decisively influenced only by the ability to pay them'.[4]

Some were exploited, but within the expectations of the times, many found companionship, shelter and a satisfactory and often interesting life in someone else's home. The hierarchy of those who gave service in a large house had much in common with those who gave service in a voluntary hospital which, in the early days, was run on much the same lines. The 'servant class', often referred to disparagingly by the new, reformed nurses, were in fact often well-trained and knowledgeable.

On the other hand, by the late nineteenth century, some of the daughters of the employing class, frustrated by what Miss Nightingale called 'busy idleness', burst their bonds, but when they escaped it was into the traditional pastures of social work, teaching and nursing, or later as secretaries, inevitably subordinate to men who ensured that their pay was also suitably subordinate. Although historians should be wary of examples from literature, the pen portrait of the woman pupil-teacher in *The Rainbow*[5] is a reminder that women teachers were as exploited as nurses and men as tyrannical masters as the abused matrons.

The other reason for the poverty of women was that until the Married Women's Property Acts of 1870, 1882 and 1893, married women had no property rights. As Virginia Woolf points out, men left their money, and their wife's, to male colleges and institutions which became wealthy – women's colleges came from bazaars and fêtes organised by the dedicated few. The men drank wine, the women drank water.[6] The quintessential characteristic of women's emancipation was the background of comparative poverty. Spinster sisters did not earn the same as their bachelor brothers.

THE ECONOMIC POSITION OF THE NURSE SINCE 1948

As pointed out previously, comparison with nursing before 1948 is invidious because the contents of the nurse's emoluments package was so variable and it is impossible to be sure of comparing like with like. Prices had doubled in the war, so the Whitley Award did little more than put gross salaries back to where they were. Pay in the public sector was linked with the post-war economic situation. The government increased its intervention in employment policies and adopted the economic policies of Lord Keynes (1883–1946) which, together with the needs of the Cold War, ensured full employment, which pleased the unions, who thus negotiated from strength. From this there developed the 'post-war consensus', with the government tacitly pledged to full employment and the unions to reducing the areas of conflict.

One effect of this consensus was that Sir Stafford Cripps, with the co-operation of the unions, was able to freeze all wages, and it was against this background that negotiations on nurses' pay took place. With no hope of a fundamental restructure it was the mixture as before, but at least there was almost no inflation.

The Conservative government of 1951 was helped by the post-war commodity boom and with the prospect of ever-continuing growth, wages were allowed to rise; this, however, precipitated a sterling crisis which, together with the Suez episode, produced further instability and a cut-back in the expansion of public services. Every crisis was felt in the public sector, where the government was the paymaster; moreover, 'cutting public spending' had an immediate election appeal.

Although modest gains had been made, the pay of nurses was still low and this had a number of consequences. Recruitment was difficult and in some areas non-selective; since career prospects were poor, retention after training was low and poor pay of itself led to an exaggerated concern with small differentials and special payments, so that the salary scales were confused, cumbersome and riddled with anomalies. In 1958, at the worst stage of the recession, the Conservative government took a firm stand against pay increases and, having won the busmen's strike in 1961, introduced a 'pay pause'. The dockers threatened strike action and were awarded 9 per cent: the nurses, who did not, were held to 2½ per cent. Many nurses were earning less than office cleaners, and in 1962 professional nurses for the first time canvassed public support. Led by a group from Manchester and subsequently backed by the Royal College of Nursing, they held lobbies of the House of Commons and a mass meeting at the Royal Albert Hall involving speakers from the three main political parties. The campaign attracted considerable attention; the government lost four by-elections mainly on the issue of pay, and the new MP for Orpington, Mr Lubbock (later Lord Avebury), made his maiden speech on the subject of nurses' pay. The pay pause faded and nurses were given a special award of 9 per cent.

The election in 1964 brought a change of government, and the Wilson administration started with a policy of a return to free collective bargaining, but with a sterling crisis and a damaging seamen's strike they were soon pushed into asking for 'voluntary restraint', then direct intervention through the medium of the Prices and Incomes Board now invested with the power to investigate and make recommendations in special cases. For nurses, PIB Report No. 60 charted scales and differentials for the new Salmon grades and broke the deadlock. In 1969 rising unemployment and union unrest caused the government to abandon controls, wages rose by 16 per cent and nurses were left behind again.

THE 'RAISE THE ROOF' CAMPAIGN

Organised by the Royal College of Nursing, this campaign started in the autumn of 1969 with public meetings and culminated in lobbies in the House of Commons for four weeks in January 1970. A debate on nurses' pay in the House on the last day of the lobbies brought major concessions and an award of 22 per cent, then considered astronomical.

Shortly after this breakthrough all controls were abandoned and prices started to rise. An election brought a change of government, wages accelerated and unemployment rose to 3½ per cent registered unemployed. The government clamped down on the public sector, for which it adopted the 'n – 1' policy – each settlement had to be 1 per cent less than the last. After the postmen's strike the Heath government introduced statutory wage controls, to operate in three phases – a freeze, followed by limited rises, with special arrangements for those in lowly-paid or unpleasant work. Meanwhile, world commodity prices continued to rise, sending the RPI up by 15 points. The miners went on strike, the country went on a three day working week and the government called an election, which proved inconclusive.

The gains achieved by nurses in 1970 had, by 1974, been whittled away and unions and professional organisations both faced angry members. In May 1974 the Royal College of Nursing submitted evidence to the Secretary of State, the Rt Hon. Barbara Castle, calling for an independent enquiry into nurses' pay. The submission showed that the volume of work had risen without an appreciable increase in the number of registered nurse hours and nurses' salaries had fallen behind those of secretaries and shorthand typists, while the earnings for male nurses were as much as £20 a week below those of a primary school teacher.

THE HALSBURY REPORT

As a result of this and other submissions and delegations, the new Labour government set up a Committee of Enquiry under the chairmanship of the Rt Hon. the Earl of Halsbury, FRS. The Committee, which reported in September 1974, had two main aims: to re-evaluate the professions of nursing and midwifery, taking into account the intention to implement the recommendations of the Briggs Committee in full; and, second, to simplify the pay structure which had grown in a 'haphazard and opportunistic way'. The Report set out detailed recommendations on pay which represented an overall increase of 30 per cent, but with a return to free collective bargaining other groups obtained similar increases, so in relative terms nurses were no better off.

Further economic problems in the years which followed led to another sterling crisis, and the government, at the behest of the International Monetary Fund, was forced to cut its public spending and have its future budgets cleared by the Fund. This had an immediate effect on the health service, where workers were not replaced, recruitment was halted and wages were held down – the back-cloth to the winter of discontent in 1979. The submission by the Staff Side of the Nurses and Midwives Council in the spring of 1979 bore a distinct resemblance to that produced for the Halsbury Committee; the figures needed up-dating but they showed the same falling behind, bearing out the theory that those without industrial power tend to gain during incomes policies and lose during free collective bargaining. The years 1980 and 1981 brought no real improvement in the pay of nurses, and expressions of anger and betrayal were being voiced ever more widely.

THE REVIEW BODY FOR NURSING STAFF, MIDWIVES AND HEALTH VISITORS

The annual pay negotiations for 1982 departed dramatically from the practice of previous years, and instead of a settlement being reached before or only shortly after the operative date for the new salaries of 1 April, negotiations within the Nurses and Midwives Council and campaigns outside continued throughout that summer and autumn and a settlement package was eventually agreed in December. Although this package included the usual components of an increase in basic salaries and a slight improvement in certain allowances, it also contained two unusual elements. The first was that the agreement covered a much longer period than usual, as it was to continue in force until April 1984 instead of April 1983; the second element was much more significant in that the package included the proposal to establish a Pay Review Body for nursing staff, midwives and health visitors (and the professions allied to medicine), along similar lines to those already in existence for doctor's and dentists, the armed forces and the top salaries group.

In announcing the setting up of the Review Body emphasis was laid on its complete independence and freedom to make whatever recommendations it felt appropriate. It would receive and consider evidence from both sides – the Department of Health and Social Security (as it then was) and unions and professional organisations, both collectively through the Staff Side of the Nurses and Midwives Council, and individually, and would report directly to the Prime Minister. Although recognising the Review Body's independence and freedom to make recommendations and expressing the intention to implement them in full, needless to say the government reserved the right to vary the recommendations if there were clear and compelling reasons for so doing. The award set out in the Report for April 1984 did no more than make good some of the ground lost in the years since 1979, but there was a clear indication that better times were ahead when the Review Body would have a longer timetable for the consideration of the evidence submitted to them and time also to obtain additional information: the 1984 Report had been a 'rush job'. The ensuing years saw a gradual improvement in the relative as well as the absolute levels of nurses' pay, a process brought to an abrupt halt by government policies on public sector pay in 1991/92 and 1992/93.

CLINICAL GRADING STRUCTURE

In their first report the Review Body said that they intended to set in hand various pieces of work to assist in making informed judgements about appropriate levels of nurses' pay. One such piece of work, to which they attached considerable importance, was a complete review and evaluation of the work of nurses, midwives and health visitors in clinical grades and the grading system itself, so that, in future, they might have confidence that the salary recommendations they made were entirely appropriate for the relevant grades. After an unacceptable pilot study carried out by a firm of management consultants, the task was given to the Nurses and Midwives Council. The outcome, a new set of grade definitions relating to a nine-level salary structure, was achieved in 1988 and formed the basis for the Review Body's recommendations for that year. The underlying philosophy of the new structure was that nurses should be paid for the responsibilities they actually carried: if it was thought that a particular job-holder should not carry certain responsibilities, it was the task of management to change the working practices, but while a nurse undertook those responsibilities she should be paid the rate for the job, it being the job that was graded, not the job-holder. The new grading structure also gave recognition to the role of the clinical nurse specialist and laid the foundations of a clinical career ladder. Unfortunately, its implementation was anything but smooth, and appeals against gradings are still being processed.

TRADE UNIONS AND THE GROWTH OF ORGANISATIONS

Laissez-faire was the driving force of the Industrial Revolution and Common Law developed as a response to ensure the free exchange of goods and services; neither the state nor the workers were allowed to interfere with this freedom. After the failure of Robert Owen's Grand National Consolidated Trade Union (1834) and the growth of the large unions for unskilled workers towards the end of the century, workers organised to put pressure on the government to change the law. This gave rise to the series of judgments, such as the *Taff Vale* case of 1901, which made the union responsible for damages, and the Trade Union Act of 1906, which reversed that decision. Since they were weak at that time it is remarkable that the unions gained so many concessions, but Crouch argues that 'the English political system had a long history of dominant élites coming to terms with emerging antagonistic groups, and compromising with them on condition that they accepted the main outlines of the system. This was made possible by the dominant position of Britain in the world'.[7] This accounts for the fact that, by and large the unions worked within the system and that they won concessions, as in the Conspiracy and Protection of Property Act 1875 they were not given a code of rights but merely exemption from certain legal penalties. The unions, drawing strength from their members, organised from the shop floor upwards and, through the Labour Representative Committee, were largely responsible for the founding of the embryonic Labour party. Working at first through the Liberals, then finally replacing them, the new movement placed emphasis on the need for a distinct working-class representation in Parliament. This is in opposition to what happened on the Continent, where labour first organised itself into political parties, socialist or communist, which in their turn created union movements downwards, usually rationalising them to one union for each industry. In Germany there were 17 unions, in England 460 representing 9 million members or about half the work force, and this of course ignored employee organisations that were not certified unions.[8] Membership of TUC-affiliated unions has fallen significantly in recent years and at the end of 1992 stood at 7,301,025 – less than 35 per cent of the workforce.

Another feature of late-nineteenth-century England was the growth of professions which organised in professional associations whose main concern was not the regulation of wages but the protection and advancement of their profession to ensure high levels of competence and standards of conduct. When their members were mostly independent practitioners there was no need for such organisations to concern themselves with pay, although they often recommended a scale of fees; but as more professional people were employed by the growing bureaucracy, some organisations, like the British Medical Association, secured negotiating rights. Apart from the older professional organisations, the recent years have seen a growth of 'white-collar' organisations like the National Union of Bank Employees and the Guild of Insurance Officials, whose concepts of differentials are not necessarily the same as the manual unions and some of which have objectives more akin to professional organisations. Some of these unions are affiliated to the TUC, but many are not; some pay a political levy and some do not; there is therefore a wide spectrum of employee organisations many of which have grown up to meet the needs of the historical past.

INDUSTRIAL RELATIONS

Having won concessions, except for the left wing which wanted more revolutionary change, the unions were happy with free collective bargaining and the *status quo*, but outside the unions there was a growing body of opinion that felt these legal exemptions could no longer be justified because social and economic circumstances had changed. This concern was exacerbated by the case of ballot-rigging by the Electrical Trade Union and in 1965 the government set up a Royal Commission on Trade Unions and Employers' Associations under the chairmanship of Lord Donovan. The Commission, which included Hugh Clegg and W. E. McCarthy – both later to be associated with nurses' pay, did not produce the radical report that was expected but pronounced in favour of 'voluntarism', and made the suggestion that factory or company agreements should replace the usual industry-wide arrangements which had a habit of devolving into uncontrolled shop-floor bargains which often led to unofficial strikes. The Commission did, however, suggest an Industrial Relations Act with an independent Industrial Relations Commission to advise the government.

In 1969 the Labour government established a Commission, but in spite of the findings of the report prepared *In Place of Strife*, which, although it proposed new rights for workers, also recommended measures to limit the power to strike. The TUC refused to consider such legislation and in this they were backed by the union-sponsored members in Parliament, and industrial relations became an election issue. The consensus was crumbling.

The Conservatives returned to power in 1970 on a promise to reform the industrial relations law and to stand firm against excessive wage claims. In 1971 the Industrial Relations Act was introduced, with little consultation with the unions. This Act brought to an end the long association between trade unions and the Registry of Friendly Societies and replaced it with a new Registry and definition of workers and unions. Now, the regulation of wages and relations between employees and employers no longer had to be the principal objective of an organisation but merely one of its objects, a change that cleared the way for professional organisations, which were *bona fide* negotiators and which complied with the new rules, to register. The Act made 'the closed shop' illegal, although registered unions were allowed something similar; but the pill the unions could not swallow was that registered unions had a duty to restrain members from taking action against 'legally binding agreements'; such agreements were hitherto unknown and completely changed the character of the relationship of the unions with employers. Some of the provisions of the Act rendered certain conduct 'unfair industrial practice' – a new offence, which could be tried in the National Industrial Relations Court. As an inducement to register, unregistered unions would lose certain tax concessions, a loss that would affect the less wealthy and leave them open to poaching. This placed many unions in a quandary, and some registered, some did not; on the whole, resistance was passive although there were sporadic political strikes, and towards the end of the year ugly scenes with one incident leading to the jailing of two dockers. The Act which tried to improve industrial relations ended by doing the opposite.

From the point of view of organisations not normally concerned with industrial action there were a number of advantages. Workers now had a *right* to belong to a union, to take part in its activities, not to be unfairly dismissed and to have a contract of service. Hitherto hospital authorities had been free to ignore organisations if they so wished, and, depending on the political leaning of the authority, different organisations could be virtually proscribed. More important was the fact that the Act laid down the reasons for dismissal that could be construed as fair; previously it had been up to organisations representing their members to panels, that were sometimes both judge and jury, to show that the reasons (which the authority might decline to make clear) were unfair. Justice was sometimes not done, but more often, not seen to be done. The other great advantage for nurses was that they now had a clear right to a contract of service; the Contract of Employment Act 1963 was updated with more explicit instructions as to what the contract should contain, and it now applied to workers in the employ of the Crown.

Although the Industrial Relations Act was not a success, and in fact proved the prognostication that it would be a 'martyr's charter', the positive side established a number of new rights for employees which could not subsequently be rescinded.

The Trade Union and Labour Relations Act 1974

During its election campaign in 1974 the Labour party placed great stress on the need to restore the consensus and good relations with the unions. In spite of the fact that, like Mr Heath before, it wished to find ways of limiting industrial action which was now quadrupling the number of days lost compared with the 1960s, it immediately offered the repeal of the Industrial Relations Act as a sop to Cerberus in the hope that unions would accept voluntary pay restraint. The Act of July 1974 repealed the 1971 Act and replaced 'Registration' with a return to voluntary certification with the Registrar of Friendly Societies. All unions registered before 1971 and those on the current Register were entitled to apply and legal immunity returned to the *status quo ante*. The Industrial Relations Commission was abolished and replaced by the Advisory Conciliation and Arbitration Service (ACAS). This body consisted of a chairman and nine members, three appointed after consultation with the Trade Union Congress, three sponsored by the Confederation of British Industries and three to be holders of academic appointments. 'ACAS', as it was known, offered conciliation to both the public and private sector, but it only intervened when all other methods had failed and if necessary it appointed Boards of Arbitration to hear disputes.

The Employment Protection Act 1975

Under the Trade Union and Labour Relations Act the whole body of labour law was re-enacted or amended. The 1975 Act extended the legislation about unfair dismissal to enable the new tribunals to award the reinstatement of a dismissed worker and reduced to 26 weeks the period of completed employment before which a worker could complain of unfair dismissal, was more explicit about the time off for union activities and improved the right to maternity leave. Perhaps the most controversial part of the Act was that concerning the 'closed shop'. Schedule I, para 6[9] laid down that dismissal is fair

> where a union membership agreement is in force, when an employee who is not a member of a specified union or who refuses to join, or who threatens to resign from such a union – except in the case of someone who genuinely objects on grounds of religious belief to joining any union or has reasonable grounds for refusing to belong to a particular union.

It was feared that this clause might lead to a 'closed shop' among journalists and so endanger the freedom of the press, but in fact it did little more than restore the situation that had existed before 1971. The 'closed shop' argument is very complicated, as there are several different kinds of 'closed shop' – one being the 'labour pool shop' which has been useful to both management and workers and is a sensible way of dealing with casual labour. And, as was seen in the Durham dispute, it is sometimes the employing authority which prefers a 'closed shop' – or dealing with one organisation. The Donovan Commission was cautious in its approach to the subject: it noted, contrary to the disarming claim on its behalf, that industries with a closed shop were in fact the most strike-prone, but the Commission thought that the negative aspects could be contained by measures other than by outlawing.

Other provisions under the Act included a new policy on redundancy payments, with the laying down of a sliding scale and the proviso that there must be consultation with the unions before redundancies took place.

Health and Safety at Work etc. Act, 1975 (see also Chapter 18)

The Act, which grew out of the Robens Report, was amended to bring agriculture within its purview and to redefine the regulation of powers so that the appointment of statutory safety representatives was vested solely with the certified unions, and the initiative for requesting the establishment of Safety Committees rested with those representatives who then had the power of inspection and the access to information on health and safety matters. Initially, the setting up of such committees in the health service produced problems while organisations were awaiting certification, and some were excluded. Moreover, in highly technical areas such as laboratory work, such committees may either lack the necessary knowledge, or find themselves in conflict about immediate short-term measures as set against the long-term greater good; no advance was ever made without some risk. Some of the difficulties have been smoothed by the introduction of a *Code of Practice* which offers guidelines on the main content of training courses, the skills members require and the time off necessary for workers to be trained.

The Equal Pay Act 1970 (revised 1976)

Equal pay, which was the subject of an International Labour Organisation convention in 1951, is embodied in Article 119 of the Treaty of Rome 1957, and all Common Market countries are allegedly committed to it. In England it was the last legislation of the Labour government of 1970 but did not become effective until 1975. In that year the Employment Protection Act made provision for the new Central Arbitration Committee to take over functions concerning equal pay. The 1970 Act set out to eliminate discrimination between men and women in regard to their pay, contracts of employment and other entitlements, by establishing

> a woman's right to equal treatment when she is employed on work of the same, or broadly similar, nature to that of a man, or that the job, though different, has been given equal value by job evaluation, and further, by providing for a central committee (now the CAC) to remove discrimination in collective agreement, pay structures and orders which embrace provisions for men, or for women, only.

The Sex Discrimination Act 1975

This Act was complementary to the Equal Pay Act and set out to cover non-contractural discrimination and made it unlawful for an employer to treat a woman, on the grounds of her sex, less favourably than a man, or to treat a married person less favourably than a single one. The Act also provided safeguards, in so far as they are possible, for those who did appeal.

The Equal Opportunities Commission

This Commission was set up by the above Act with the statutory duty of promoting equality of opportunity between men and women generally and by keeping under review all the anti-discrimination laws. Equal pay is useless unless women have greater opportunity. As Ross Davies points out, out of the 9 million working women, only about half do the same jobs as men and as far as the other half is concerned it is easy to circumvent the Act by rigging job evaluation.[10] So long as women are confined to the typewriter, the sewing machine and women's tasks, they will not be equal, and women will not break out of the vicious circle of low pay and unequal opportunity. Equality will only come when attitudes change, when education and training are truly equal and when women themselves want to fulfil their potential rather than their expected role.

To some extent the success of the campaign is predicated on the growth of the economy, for as women's labour becomes more expensive the only thing that will protect them is a wider range of job opportunities. Already men have started applying for, and getting, the top jobs they once would have scorned and that were considered the prerogative of women, such as heads of primary schools and of the nursing service. It will be an irony of history if women lose out on promotion in their traditional fields and fail to break into the wider employment market.[11]

The Race Relations Act 1968

Apart from the legislation under the Trade Union and Labour Relations Act there is the Race Relations Act, which makes it unlawful to discriminate against a person on grounds of colour, race, or ethnic or national origin about recruitment, terms and conditions of employment, training promotion or dismissal. The Act not only sets out to avoid discrimination but also to encourage employers to develop positive attitudes to promote equal opportunity. As in the case of women, mere anti-discrimination legislation will do little until there is true equality in such basic rights as education, housing and environment.

THE EFFECT OF THE LABOUR LAW ON NURSING

The Industrial Relations Act 1971 made a difference to nursing because a high percentage of the organised registered nurses were contained in the professional organisations whose status at times appeared ambiguous. They were now able to claim 'Registration', and, with it, rights on behalf of their members for such things as contracts of service, and of course to benefit from the new provisions relating to dismissal and redundancy. At the same time most of these organisations took the opportunity to set up training schemes for local representatives so that once trained these stewards would be able to undertake the tasks set out in the *Code of Practice* (paragraphs 99–129). Even when the 1971 Act was repealed, this Code remained, and continues to offer sensible guidelines to management and union representatives. This devolution of responsibility helped to educate nurses in industrial relations matters.

After the 1975 Act most organisations who had been on the old Special Register now became 'certified'; that is to say, they were classed as an independent union. However, many trade unions felt that organisations whose primary purpose was not wage regulation should be excluded from wage negotiation, and this they made clear in the evidence they gave to the Review of the Whitley System set up under the chairmanship of Lord McCarthy, where they recommended that 'the staff side should be confined to TUC affiliated unions' – a view held strongly by the Association of Scientific Technical and Managerial Staffs (ASTMS), which campaigned vigorously, and said, 'they would not participate where professional associations *had any rights*'.[12] In the end, the McCarthy recommendations were not specific, and organisations were merely asked to review their ability to represent their members and to do their best to eliminate inter-union competition and to reduce the 'excessive fractionalisation'.

If the union proposals had been accepted, it could have led to an increase in the number of organisations applying to belong to the TUC, and this could have changed the character of the Congress, but it would have been contrary to the need to reduce the number of organisations representing workers. On the other hand, to compel all workers, who then by legal definition included many in various professions, to join one of the existing 117 affiliated unions would have been an infringement of liberty and would have bordered on the philosophy of totalitarianism. In the event, the harsh reality of falling memberships in some unions has brought about a number of mergers between unions recruiting in the health services, thereby reducing the number of organisations. The labour laws gave extended rights to workers and defined them more clearly, particularly the right not to be unfairly dismissed. However, the new legislation created problems for nurse managers, who needed to be aware of the new legal requirements, and this led to the need for nurse personnel officers to look after such matters as advertising, contracts of employment, staff appraisal, training courses and counselling on labour-relations problems.

Legislation has brought more rights to workers, but apparently it has done little to improve industrial relations, although more research needs to be done in this area; it would be wrong to read increased militancy as *post hoc ergo propter hoc*. Many of the reasons for the unrest lie in the historical past traced in this book. Neither the charity system nor the Poor Law were noticeable for worker participation, and the legacy of their authoritarianism remained long after the rest of the world had become democratic. Moreover, once health care was 'national' and paid for out of taxation, it was seen as a right and not as a charity for which the recipient should be humbly grateful, and this perception extended to those who worked in the health service. Furthermore, most people are now aware that care and cure are achieved by the work of a complicated and inter-related team with different skills and not by one spectacular prima donna. Perhaps the hope for the future lies in true worker participation on the lines suggested by the Committee of Inquiry on Industrial Democracy under the chairmanship of Lord Bullock, which involves much more than inviting workers to give an opinion on the colour of the canteen walls but takes them to the heart of the aims of the organisation. Although some attempts have been made at this approach in the health service, there are special difficulties in a service with so many groups of professionals, and by the very nature of the service itself and of course by the fact of its very historical tradition neither workers nor management have much experience upon which to call.

Looking at the economic position of the nurse after 45 years of campaigns, reviews and much struggle, it must be seen in relation to the service as a whole. The NHS is still the largest single employer in the country, and nurses comprise the largest group within that workforce. Although demand may be infinite, resources are very clearly finite, and restraints on the number of nurses now are not due, as they were in the early days of the service, to lack of suitable manpower, but the money to pay for it. What impact the NHS reforms and the introduction of NHS Trusts, with the freedom to negotiate their own rates of pay, will have on the overall position it is too early to say. To date, only a handful of Trusts have set up their own pay scales and their effect is negligible, but in times of recession and high unemployment market forces favour the employer rather than the employee.

REFERENCES

1 Mars, K. (1848) *Das Kapital*, J. M. Dent, London: Everyman Library.
2 Galbraith, K (1969) *The Affluent Society*, London: Hamish Hamilton.
3 Webb, S. and Webb, B. (1894), *The History of Trade Unionism* (re-edited 1921). Longman.
4 Thompson, F. M. L. (1962) *English Landed Society in the Nineteenth Century*, London: Routledge & Kegan Paul, p. 187.
5 Lawrence, D. H. (1915), *The Rainbow*, London: Penguin Books.
6 Woolf, V. (1929) *A Room of One's Own*, London: Penguin Books.
7 Crouch, C. (1979) *The Politics of Industrial Relations*, London: Fontana, p. 189.
8 Central Office of Information (1978) Pamphlet 128, p. 30 and *Guardian* Leader, 2 June 1979.
9 Davies, Ross (1972) *Women at Work*, London: Hutchinson, p. 19.
10 Ibid., ch. 8.
11 HMSO (1977) *Review of the Whitely System* (McCarthy), ch. 9.
12 HMSO (1977) *Committee of Inquiry on Industrial Democracy* (Bullock).

FURTHER READING

Cooper, B. N. and Bartlett, A. F. (1976) *Industrial Relations – a Study in Conflict*, London: Heinemann.
Crouch, Colin (1979) *The Politics of Industrial Relations*, London: Fontana/Collins.
Davies, Ross (1972) *Women and War*, London: Hutchinson.
HMSO (1974) *Report of the Committee of Inquiry into the Pay and Related Conditions of Service of Nurses and Midwives* (the Halsbury Report).
—— (1975) *Trade Unions*, Central Office of Information, Pamphlet 128.
Phelps Brown, E. H. (1959) *The Growth of British Industrial Relations*, London: Macmillan.
Roberts, Ben (1987) *Mr. Hammond's Cherry Tree: the Morphology of Union Survival*, Institute of Economic Affairs
HMSO 1984/90 *Reports of the Review Body for Nursing Staff, Midwives and Health Visitors*.

Chapter 27

The health problems of the world

Muriel Skeet

For the first time ... the world has ... a set of universal principles for health, a social helix whose strands can shape many different health systems in response to different needs and different capacities. In many developing countries these strands are being put together in such a way as to offer a totally new approach to social and economic development. In many industrialised countries they are being put together to attain health targets for improved health through better deployment of existing resources.

> Halfdan Mahler, former Director-General,
> World Health Organisation, 1988

Since those words were spoken at a 'midpoint perspective' conference convened to reaffirm the Declaration of Alma-Ata,[1] the world has been forced to joust continuously and intensely with the four horsemen of the apocalypse – war, pestilence, famine and death. In spite of having that set of universal principles for health, the facts and figures relating to the current state of the world's health make very depressing reading. Even in those regions where some progress has been made, it has not been uniform, either between countries or within them, and in many, health conditions persist at levels which are so limiting and destructive of human potential and so contrary to the principles and interest of Health-for-All as to be unacceptable to the global community. In short, although the majority of nations made a positive start in their quest for Health-for-All after the Alma-Ata Conference on Primary Health Care in 1978, formidable political, economic and social circumstances have meant that in very many instances, the gap between policy-making and policy implementation remains very wide indeed.[2]

Galen defined health as 'a condition of perfect harmony and equilibrium'[3] – an ideal to be striven for, but which few, except in fleeting moments, could attain. To Galen all disequilibrium was 'dis-ease', but he recognised that minor imbalances were so frequent as to be normal and most people lived with them without impairment to life. Galen's view was positive, ill health was something that fell below his apotheosis and related not only to the body but also to the mind and soul. Definitions of health have passed through many vicissitudes since the second century, and in 1948 the World Health Organisation (WHO), stated.

A state of complete physical, mental, and social well-being is a fundamental human right and ... the attainment of the highest possible level of health is an important world-wide social goal, whose realisation requires the action of many social and economic sectors in addition to the health sectors.[4]

THE EFFECTS OF THE DISTURBANCE OF ECOLOGY

Evolution depends on competitive food-gathering: plants manufacture protoplasm from the air and soil, the herbivores live on the plants, the carnivores live on the herbivores, all flesh dies and decomposes and is fed on by bacteria. In an undisturbed state, the number of species remain more or less controlled; high mortality is compensated for by high reproduction – the lemmings, when their numbers become too high for their feeding-grounds, rush to find a new food supply and perish in the attempt until the numbers return to normal. But as man's intellectual powers develop he is able to disturb ecology: he cuts back forests, drains marshes, his flocks denude pasture, and his mines and wells mineral resources, while his technology can alter topography and even the climate. Perhaps most important of all, man has found the means of defeating most of the known bacteria – a disturbance which has added to his comfort but the consequences of which involve many new problems.

Because countries are at varying stages of this disturbance, their health needs as well as their capacities to meet them are varied and complex, as Mahler stated. But the past decade has seen almost all countries of the world facing the pandemic caused by the human immunological virus (HIV), and in recent months the WHO has announced that tuberculosis, poliomyelitis and tetanus are present in every country.

Nutrition

Like many diseases, malnutrition is preventable. Mankind has chosen to not make it so. Reports of famine and starvation appear in our newspapers and on our television screens almost every day. Wars and conflicts rage on all continents, resulting in millions of hungry refugees, hostages and prisoners.

Even among peaceful populations, nutritional status varies markedly, with very significant consequences for health status. Studies undertaken throughout the developing world have found consistently that women's calorie intake, and in particular that of pregnant and lactating women, is often below the minimum daily requirement. As a consequence, poor maternal nutrition in developing countries is a major factor contributing to low birth-weight, which, in turn, influences child survival.

Millions of children suffer from cretinism and other permanent brain damage, because their diets and those of their parents are deficient in iodine. Every year about half a million young people go blind simply because their diets do not contain enough Vitamin A. But blindness is only the first symptom: if the victims do not receive immediate treatment, around two-thirds of them die from nutritional deficiency.

Enough is known about nutrition to be able to correct such deficiencies and also to prevent the development of disorders due to feasting too well. One encouraging sign is that affluent societies are taking more care about what they eat. Many people with hypertension are controlling their condition by diet so that they do not develop heart disease and other related problems. Governments, often urged by pressure groups, are insisting on clear, detailed labelling of the nutritional content of packaged food and drinks and banning the use of potentially harmful pesticides, preservatives and colourants.

Drinking water can also be hazardous. It is reported that one of the greatest health risks world-wide are those directly linked to the ingestion of water contaminated with sewage.[5] WHO has reported that nearly 3,000 million people are still exposed to water containing pathogenic organisms. Cholera, dysentery, guinea-worm infection, hepatitis, schistosomiasis and typhoid are some of the better-known killers in the catalogue of water-borne disease. There are also concerns over pesticides and industrial chemicals contaminating water sources. An example is lead. Lead is toxic to the central and peripheral nervous system. Prolonged exposure may cause serious neurological damage, especially among infants, children and pregnant women. High lead content in drinking water is associated with household plumbing, through piping, solders and other lead-treated materials.

Infection

The constellation of health problems that affect people throughout the world includes infectious and parasitic diseases, non-communicable diseases, mental and neurological problems, injuries and disabilities. These affect populations in varying proportions depending on where they are in the epidemiological transition. Typically, developing countries have a larger proportion of communicable diseases and developed countries a larger proportion of non-communicable diseases.

The infectious and parasitic diseases continue to pose serious risks to adult health in developing countries. Tuberculosis claims around 3 million lives each year, 90 per cent of which are among the adult population. Pneumonia is the cause of 2 million adult deaths each year in developing countries and over another million die from diarrhoeal diseases.[6]

Sexually transmitted diseases continue to be among the most frequent infectious conditions world-wide. Reasons for the high incidence can be found in a number of variables, including urbanisation, unemployment, economic hardship and a loosening of traditional restraints on sexual activity, as well as the emergence of antibiotic-resistant strains of micro-organisms. In addition, the population pyramid is heavy with individuals in the most sexually-active age groups.

While infection rates are similar in men and women, it is women and children who bear the major brunt of complications and serious sequelae of sexually transmitted diseases. A large proportion of infertility and ectopic pregnancy is a consequence of pelvic inflammatory disease, and is preventable. Sexually transmitted diseases in pregnant women can result in prematurity, still-birth and neonatal infections. In many areas 1.5 per cent of newborns are at risk of gonococcal ophthalmia neonatorum – a blinding disease – while in some countries syphilis causes up to 25 per cent of perinatal mortality.

HIV infection and AIDS are pandemic world-wide. But they have not affected the world's population uniformly. In retrospect, the extensive spread appears to have began in the late 1970s primarily in populations of (1) homosexual and bisexual men and injecting drug-users in certain urban areas of the Americas, Australasia and western Europe; and (2) men and women with multiple sexual partners in parts of the Caribbean and eastern and central Africa. The cumulative number of reported AIDS cases in late 1992 was 501,272 from 168 countries. The actual cumulative total of adult AIDS cases in the world at that time, as estimated by the WHO, was approximately 1.7 million. Reasons for the discrepancy include less-than-complete diagnosis and reporting and delays in reporting.[7]

Two viruses are recognised, HIV-1 and HIV-2. Their modes of transmission are similar, and signs and symptoms of AIDS resulting from them are indistinguishable. The predominant virus world-wide, is HIV-1.

In infants born infected with HIV, the progression to AIDS is more rapid than in adults. Virtually all individuals diagnosed as having AIDS die within a few years. The longer survival period of some appears to be directly related to the routine use of antiviral drugs, the use of prophylactic drugs for some opportunistic infections, such as pneumonia due to pneumo-cystis and to a better overall quality of health care.

AIDS has become increasingly a problem of developing countries, accounting for 50 per cent of the global total of HIV infections in 1985, 60 per cent in 1991 and (projected) 75–80 per cent by the year 2000. WHO also projects cumulative totals of 40 million HIV infections (including 10 million children) by the year 2000.

Even as a conservative estimate this will represent a tripling or quadrupling of the present total in just over seven years. If these estimates are accurate, then by the end of the 1990s over a million adult cases and deaths a year can be expected, the majority of them occurring in developing countries – about half a million in Africa and about a quarter of a million in Asia.

Two-thirds or more of all 10–12 million HIV infections in the world today are the result of heterosexual transmission, and this proportion will increase to 75–80 per cent by the year 2000. Approximately one out of three children born to an HIV-infected woman is HIV-infected and dies from AIDS. Thus, almost 1 million infected children have been born to HIV infected women, and over half of them have developed AIDS or died, while almost 2 million uninfected children of HIV-infected women are, or are likely to become, orphans. Most of these children are in sub-Saharan Africa. The demographic consequences of this pandemic are already seen. For example, in sub-Saharan Africa, child mortality rates, substantially reduced during the past decade by successful immunisation and other child survival programmes, are again rising to 1980 levels because of childhood deaths from AIDS.

Tuberculosis is one of the most widespread infections and also causes about 3 million deaths per year in this decade. Approximately 1,700 million people are at risk of developing the disease. The risk is markedly increased in persons with certain conditions such as malnutrition and in those with HIV infection. In 1990 there were 8 million new cases, of which 7.6 million were in developing countries. The high incidence and mortality rates were in the economically most productive age groups (15–59 years) and accounted for over 25 per cent of all preventable deaths in those countries.[8] Tuberculosis is now a problem in European countries, tourism and mass migrations making its control extremely difficult.

In the developing countries most affected by HIV infection, the tuberculosis problem has assumed dramatic dimensions, and in some areas the number of diagnosed cases has doubled over the past five years, causing large demands on diagnostic services, drugs and hospital beds. As the HIV pandemic is still in an ascending phase and tuberculosis does not normally develop until some time after the initial HIV infection, and since the increase in incidence will cause an increase in transmission, the situation is likely to worsen unless drastic control measures are taken.

The malaria situation has deteriorated over the last decade. More than 2,000 million people are now exposed to varying degrees of malaria risk in some 100 countries and areas. African countries, south of the Sahara, see approximately 100 million clinical cases of malaria every year. Despite a biennial budget of over $26 million for WHO's malaria programmes, the disease is still endemic in 93 countries and kills between 1.5 and 3 million people per year.[9]

In other parts of the world, while malaria remains under control in most developed and stable areas, the situation is dramatically worse in all frontier areas of economic development, such as those with intensified exploitation of natural resources, jungle areas with problems of civil war and other man-made conflicts, illegal trading, tourism and mass movement of refugees.

Degenerative change and mental illness

Until recently, among adults world-wide, deaths were due mainly to the chronic diseases. These have also emerged in recent years as leading causes of death in a number of developing countries. Cardiovascular disease claim about 6 million lives every year in the developing world, as many as in the developed countries and eastern Europe combined. Similarly, cancer now claims more victims in developing countries (2.5 million deaths per year) than in the developed world (2.3 million). A similar number die each year in the developing world from the chronic obstructive lung diseases, primarily chronic bronchitis and emphysema.

Today there are at least 300 million people in the world suffering from a mental or neurological disorder or impairment.[10] Over recent decades, society in all parts of our planet has forced rapid social and environmental change. This has had many effects on mental health and development. Some occupational or technical skills, for example, highly valued for generations, have lost their societal significance and formerly respected groups of artisans find themselves unemployed, under-employed or in a situation where they feel no longer needed or considered to be of use to their community.

There are also significant demographic changes. Between 1985 and 1990, the estimated population of the world grew from 4,851 million to 5,292 million. At the turn of the decade, ten countries had a population in excess of 100 million. Globally, world population growth is slowing from an annual rate of increase of 2.1 per cent in the late 1960s to about 1.7 per cent today. Because of increasing life expectancy, the size of the elderly population has grown enormously, especially that of the old-old (over 75). By the year 2000 the number of people aged 65 years and over in developing countries is expected to reach 250 million or about 50 per cent more than the 173 million projected for the developed world. The senile dementias affect 5–8 per cent of the population over the age of 65, or around 30 million old people.[11]

The proportion of women employed outside the home has increased, and the number of people living in urban areas – often without homes – has grown in many countries. High divorce rates and the high numbers of incomplete or broken families has also increased the number of individuals vulnerable to mental, behavioural and psychosocial disorders or to environmental maladaptation. The breakdown of the extended family in many developing countries, often linked to economic development, has also left many people less well able to cope with new problems or situations. World-wide, 15–35 per cent of all first-level consultations are mainly for psychological disorders.

Epilepsy effects around 8 million people in developed countries and more than 35 million in the rest of the world. The global population of mentally retarded people is thought to be 130 million. Schizophrenia and other psychoses affect 55 million, and some other 120 million suffer from affective disorders.[12]

The current high unemployment rates in industrialised countries have created stress by disturbing important psychological elements such as personal identity, time-structuring and a sense of self-esteem. It may also disrupt social support networks through the loss of social relationships at work, the abandonment of hobbies and social life under financial pressure, and withdrawal from social interaction because of the 'stigma' of being jobless.

THE POPULATION PATTERN OF THE WORLD

Variations in the disease pattern produce different demographic structures in different parts of the world. These differences have important social and economic effects and are one of the main reasons for conflict between nations.[13] It is not without significance that the greatest holocaust of all was partly motivated by a population that was expanding beyond its resources and was looking for *Lebensraum*. Countries believe in their own culture and wish to survive, even to dominate, while contracting or stationary populations fear for survival.

Nations go through fairly clearly discernible demographic cycles. First, there is the undisturbed period when high reproduction is cancelled by high mortality and the population is almost stationary. Then, due to chance or man's mastery, the death rate begins to fall but the birth rate continues high, with the population expanding rapidly: this is the Demographic Transition (see Figure 1.1). In the third stage, the birth rate adjusts to the death rate, but the population continues to grow because people live longer. Finally, if the birth rate falls below the death rate the population declines, as was the case with the Romans about the time they left Britain. In modern times France is the only country in Europe to have reached the fourth stage, and promptly took measures to encourage an increase in population.

Technical advance tends to move faster than changes in social patterns, as the resistance to family planning in India has shown; but unless countries in the second stage quickly reduce their birth rate to match the lower death rate, the present world food supplies may well be unequal to their needs. The corollary of infant lives saved from infection may well be starvation among schoolchildren; indeed, concentrating all resources on reducing infection merely exacerbates the problem.

For this reason world health problems are intrinsically linked with the problems of food supply and education, and one of the most important links in the chain is the education and status of women. It is through the mothers that children can be taught to accept new ideas, and it is this area in which nurses working to alleviate world health problems have an important role to play. Teach the mother, teach the child.

The extraordinary increase in the proportion of older people in the world's population over the past few decades has been described as one of man's greatest triumphs. Unfortunately, it is a triumph which has brought with it a great number of diverse and complex problems. One main reason for this is that planners in the 1950s and 1960s did not give adequate attention to the demographic forecasts being made at that time. Consequently, the gain in survival was not planned. If we are to avoid even greater and more widespread age-associated problems in the future, it is essential that all countries, whether developed or developing, take cognisance now of demographic trends. For example, it is expected that by the year 2000 nearly 70 per cent of all older people will be living in developing countries.

In Europe at the present time, approximately 120 million of its population are over the age of 60 years, and it is projected that by 2020 this figure will have doubled and the elderly will form one-quarter of the region's population. The Commonwealth of Independent States (the former USSR) alone is likely to have 72 million – a growth rate of over 100 per cent since 1980. The greatest increase will be in the number of people over the age of 80 years.[14]

The trend in urban–rural distribution is another important consideration. By the year 2000 the proportion of aged people living in urban areas is expected to be 75 per cent in developed countries and 40 per cent in developing nations. In lesser developed countries, especially the People's Republic of China, ancient culture emphasises the honouring of parents and ancestors and this still holds to some extent today. By and large caring for elders is seen as an important duty. But according to experts from the Philippines and Brazil this pattern begins to break down as urbanisation advances.

MEETING WORLD HEALTH PROBLEMS

Attempts to control epidemics go back to the seventh century, but it was the pandemic of bubonic plague in the fourteenth century that led to the idea of quarantine for ships and goods arriving from areas stricken by the plague. The idea originated in the city state of Ragusa (Dubrovnik) and the *quaranta*, or forty days, was probably due to the general faith in Aristotelian astrology rather than any observed incubation period; or, since it put a brake on trade, ulterior motives on the party of wily Renaissance man cannot be overruled.

Until the discovery of the germ theory of infection at the end of the nineteenth century, health was not seen as an international problem, although in 1851 12 European nations met in Paris at a Sanitary Conference with the idea of making quarantine regulations more stringent. Their deliberations do not appear to have been fruitful, and the idea of international public health did not advance until after the First World War, when the Health Organisation of the League of Nations came into being. An office was set up in Geneva, and for the first time data concerning health problems of the world were collected. Work was begun on the standardisation of terminology and the control of drug traffic, but work in the practical field was hampered for lack of money, and as the clouds of war gathered over Europe the work came to a standstill. In 1944 the United Nations Relief and Rehabilitation Assistance Organisation (UNRRAO) was created which, apart from its work in war-stricken Europe and the Middle East, acted as an international health organisation until a new permanent body could take its place. In 1945 the Charter of the United Nations was signed in San Francisco, where it was minuted that an 'international health organisation be set up'.

THE WORLD HEALTH ORGANISATION

Although the constitution of the World Health Organisation adopted when it was set up in 1946 declares that the WHO's objective is 'the attainment by all peoples of the highest possible level of health', it was not until the Thirtieth World Health Assembly in 1977 that a target date was set for meeting that objective. This came with the decision that the main social target of WHO and its member states should be 'the attainment by all citizens of the world, by the year 2000, of a level of health that will permit them to lead a socially and economically productive life'.[15]

At the Alma-Ata Conference one year later, primary health care was identified as the key to attaining this target, and the relevant Declaration of Alma-Ata was signed by all member states. This marked a turning point in the programming for community health, both nationally and internationally. In its report, the Conference gave nurses, as well as other health workers, broad directives for the development of education, practice and research in primary health care.[16]

Each year, at the World Health Assembly, held in Geneva, a report on the world health situation is presented on the basis of evaluation of the implementation of that agreed strategy. The review provides a global perspective of the main achievements of member states. Progress in coverage by primary health care and in quality of care, and developments concerning specific aspects of health status and of major determinants of health, are examined. Achievements are assessed in terms of progress, adequacy and impact of the strategy, and the global socio-economic, environmental and development trends and implications for health are reviewed.

Finally, drawing on major lessons from the evaluation, future trends and challenges to be addressed in accelerating the implementation of the Health-for-All strategy are identified.

To an outsider, the work of any large organisation is something of a mystery. From news reports of isolated activities and occasional policy statements, from pronouncements of the WHO's experts on topical issues, and perhaps from hearsay, it is possible to piece together a picture of the Organisation which is likely to be either unduly glamorised or unduly jaundiced. WHO is perhaps better known than some of the other specialised agencies of the United Nations, yet in many respects its role is widely misunderstood.

The most important fact about the WHO to bear in mind is that its policies are formulated by a supreme body, the World Health Assembly, which is composed of government delegations from 163 member states. Thus its policies represent the collective views on health of the majority of governments of the world. The WHO is in no sense of the term a world health service; it helps governments at their request and in accordance with policies laid down by the Health Assembly. These policies are based upon the much-quoted principle of the Preamble to WHO's Constitution: 'The enjoyment of the highest attainable standard of health is one of the fundamental rights of every human being without distinction of race, religion, political belief, economic or social condition.'

However, the policies are also based on two other, much less often quoted, but equally important principles:

Governments have a responsibility for the health of their peoples which can be fulfilled only by the provision of adequate health and social services,

and:

Informed opinion and active co-operation on the part of the public are of the utmost importance in the improvement of the health of the people.

Nature and structure of the WHO

Role and functions

The WHO's main role, therefore, under its Constitution, is to encourage and assist governments in fulfilling their responsibilities for the health of their peoples and in securing the active participation of the public. Its functions are to promote the development and improvement of health services, to collate and disseminate information on all matters pertaining to the public health, and to further biomedical research and the publication of most recent health-related advances. Perhaps its greatest success in recent years has been to co-ordinate world-wide efforts to eradicate smallpox. Currently, it is collaborating in the monitoring and research programmes related to the AIDS pandemic and other major problems and resurgences, such as tuberculosis and malaria.

Governing bodies

While the WHO, which has its headquarters in Geneva, forms part of what is commonly called the United Nations system, it is in no way subordinate to the UN. It is a 'specialised agency', as provided for in the UN Charter and has been 'brought into relationship' with the UN by a formal agreement, which provides, *inter alia*, for reciprocity between the two organisations, the exchange of information and the adoption of common administrative practices. There are also formal agreements between the WHO and the Pan American Health Organisation (PAHO), the International Labour Organisation (ILO) in Geneva, the Food and Agriculture Organisation (FAO) in Rome and the United Nations Educational, Scientific and Cultural Organisation (UNESCO) in Paris and the International Atomic Energy Agency (IAEA) in Vienna.

The WHO has its own governing bodies, its own membership and its own budget. While most countries of the world are members – of the UN, the WHO and the other specialised agencies – there are some differences in membership. For example, Switzerland is a member of the WHO but not of the UN.

The WHO consists of three organs: the World Health Assembly, the Executive Board and the Secretariat.

Sessions of the Health Assembly usually take place in May in Geneva. Each member state may be represented by not more than three delegates, one of whom must be designated as chief. Delegations may be accompanied by alternates and advisers. The main tasks of the Health Assembly are to approve the programme and the budget proposed for the following year and to decide upon major questions of policy.

The Executive Board consists of persons technically qualified in the field of health, each of whom is appointed by one of 30 members elected by the Health Assembly. The Board must meet at least twice a year, and its members may also be accompanied by alternates and advisers. The main functions of the Board are to act as the executive organ of the Health Assembly, to prepare the agenda for each Session of the Assembly, and to submit to it a general programme of work covering a specific period. The Board acts on behalf of the whole membership of the Organisation and not on behalf only of those countries elected to designate its members.

Plenary meetings of the Health Assembly and of its main committees are open to the public unless the Assembly or the relevant committee decides otherwise. The same applies to meetings of the Executive Board. The Secretariat is the staff of the WHO, and the Director-General is its technical and administrative head. He is appointed by the Health Assembly on the nomination of the Executive Board. A characteristic feature of the WHO is its decentralisation. It has 'regional organisations', of which there are six, each consisting of a regional committee and a regional office. The head of each regional office is a Regional Director, appointed by the Executive Board in agreement with the relevant regional committee. The seats of the regional offices are in Alexandria (Eastern Mediterranean Region). Brazzaville (African Region), Copenhagen (European Region), Manila (Western Pacific Region), New Delhi (South-east Asian Region), and Washington (Region of the Americas). Membership of the regional organisations is mainly, but not necessarily, geographically determined. Ethiopia and Pakistan, for example, belong to the Eastern Mediterranean Region, whilst Algeria, Israel and Morocco belong to the European Region.

NURSING IN DEVELOPING COUNTRIES

In response to an important resolution adopted at the forty-second World Health Assembly in May 1990, on 'Strengthening nursing/midwifery in support of the strategy for Health-for-All',[17] many countries have undertaken reviews of the education and practice of their nurses and midwives. It is obvious from these that nurses have responded well not only to the call for an emphasis to be placed on primary health care, but also to the special demands made by wars, mass displacement of populations and the consequence of the AIDS pandemic.[18]

In some instances national legislation and professional regulations have been revised or amended to facilitate members' involvement in new activities. These include Ethiopia – where nurses have also drawn up a code of ethics – and most other Anglophone countries of Africa. Argentina has drafted a new nursing practice law, while Costa Rica is focusing on incorporating law and ethics into the nursing curriculum. The Philippines has passed a new law to allow for an extended role for nurses, and Nepal is in the process of establishing a national nursing council.

Throughout Africa, it is nurses who supervise the work and training of community health workers. In response to the AIDS pandemic, management of home-based care is being promoted and developed. For example, in Uganda and Zambia nurses make home visits, provide medicines, diagnose and treat opportunistic infections, give council and try to meet the needs of orphans. Public health nurses in Botswana and Zimbabwe provide integrated care, including family planning, ante-natal care, child health maintenance and immunisations. In Malawi and Swaziland, nurses are training traditional birth attendants.

During the cholera epidemic in Ecuador and Peru, nurses were involved not only in the direct care of patients but also in organising other health services, in educating the public and in epidemiological surveillance. Nurses in Brazil, the Caribbean and Colombia have all developed community-based nursing care. Improvements in levels of immunisation and the control of diarrhoeal diseases throughout Latin America are reported to be due largely to collaborative efforts between nurses and others.

The need for supervision and support of those who work in peripheral areas is of vital importance in a number of countries. In Bangladesh, the job descriptions of all categories of nursing personnel have been revised recently, and in Nepal, the Division of Nursing is steadily increasing the number of public health posts in order to provide adequate and proper supervision of auxiliary nurse-midwives, traditional birth attendants and other health workers practising in remote areas. India has adopted a similar approach.

In the Eastern Mediterranean region, nurses have assumed responsibility for emergency care in situations of armed conflict, as well as for health care in refugee camps. Teaching staff ran first aid courses for Arab women during the Gulf War. In Egypt, nurses have organised, with the national television administration, programmes of health promotion for women and their families. In Cambodia, where large numbers of war victims need emergency treatment and rehabilitation, a core of nurse educators have been prepared to train nurses to meet these special needs.

Although a number of new initiatives have not yet revealed their full impact, it is clear from information available from WHO member states that in all regions, professional nursing and midwifery skills are crucial to efficient and effective health-care services in four major areas:

1 *Preventive care* In many countries nurses and individuals are the primary care-givers, especially in relation to health promotion and disease prevention. They work with the most vulnerable populations, such as the urban poor, those living in remote areas, mothers and children, the elderly and people with chronic diseases. Midwives also play a vital role in reducing neonatal and maternal mortality rates and in preventing birth-related complications.

2 *Curative care* As front-line workers in many countries, community or public health nurses or nurse practitioners diagnose and treat a wide range of common health problems. Globally, however, the vast majority of nurses work at the various levels of hospitals, where needs have increased in recent years. Advanced technology at the tertiary level of health care has made highly skilled and specialised nursing care crucial to the recovery and survival of hospital patients.

3 *Chronic and rehabilitative care* Increasingly, nurses see themselves, besides actively meeting the professionally defined needs of passive patients, as facilitators, who enable people to participate in their own health care and maintenance. This is of great importance in work with chronically ill and/or elderly people. They need to learn new ways of self-care in order to be able to control symptoms and manage complex medical regimens. Both teaching and care are needed to ensure optimal quality of life for patients and their families or friends.

Nurses are also assuming major responsibilities in the area of mental health, working in special clinics or schools, caring for elderly disturbed patients, and giving support and guidance to the families of mentally ill patients discharged form hospital.

4 *High dependency care and care of dying people* A growing number of severely physically and/or mentally disabled people survive for many years in a state of complete dependency. The literature describes them as the 'failures of success' of modern medicine. This has led to a rapidly growing need for specialised home care, support to family and informal carers and also institutional long-term nursing care. In addition, the AIDS pandemic has greatly increased the need for nursing care of severely ill and dying young people, and support and care of care-givers and orphans.

As well as providing direct care in these four areas, today's nurse/midwife often acts as the co-ordinator of care provided by colleagues of other professions. Not fully appreciated by many governments is the severe demoralisation of nurses/midwives working in both hospital and community settings. The unresponsiveness of health systems, and the neglect in most developing countries in empowering nursing to fulfil its proper role in the Health-for-All movement, are leading to increasing despondency and a lack of motivation. The gap between what nurses could do in the implementation of health strategies and what nurses are allowed to do and have been prepared to do remains very wide. This large army of health-care personnel could not only invigorate the Health-for-All movement at the periphery; it could also provide quality leadership at all levels of a health-care system. What are needed are better management practices and personnel support systems to encourage initiatives and innovative patterns of practice. These should incorporate supportive policies related to incentives, amenities, continuing education and career development opportunities.

REFERENCES

1 World Health Organisation (1988) *Alma-Ata Reaffirmed at Riga: from Alma-Ata to the Year 2000 – a Midpoint Perspective*, Geneva: WHO.
2 World Health Organisation (1992) *Implementation of the Global Strategy for Health-for-All by the Year 2000, Second Evaluation and Eighth Report on the World Health Situation*, A45/3, Geneva: WHO.

3 Galen, translated by R. M. Green, in *Hygiene (De Sanitate tuenda)*, 1951 edn, Springfield, IL.
4 World Health Organisation (1948) *The Constitution of the World Health Organization*, Geneva: WHO.
5 World Health Organisation (1992) *World Health: Major Health Risks*, Geneva: WHO.
6 World Health Organisation (1992) *Implementation of the Global Strategy for Health-for-All by the Year 2000*.
7 Ibid.
8 Ibid.
9 Ibid.
10 Ibid.
11 Ibid.
12 Ibid.
13 Andreski, S. (1954) *Military Organization and Society*, London: Routledge & Kegan Paul.
14 Hermanova, H. (1993) *Options in Educating Health Professionals in Gerontology/Geriatrics: a European Perspective*. Paper given at a one-day workshop organised by the Educational Centre for Health and Aging, McMaster University, Hamilton, Canada, held in Budapest.
15 World Health Organisation (1977) *Report on the Thirtieth World Health Assembly*, Geneva: WHO.
16 World Health Organisation/United Nations International Children's Emergency Fund (1978) *Primary Health Care*, Report of the International Conference on Primary Health Care, Alma-Ata, USSR, Geneva: WHO.
17 World Health Organisation (1992) *Strengthening Nursing and Midwifery in Support of Strategies for Health-for-All*, Report by the Director General, A/45/4/, Geneva: WHO.
18 Ibid.

FURTHER READING

1 *World Health*. Magazine published six times a year. Contains reports on the world's major health issues designed to increase public awareness of health problems and what can be done to prevent them.
2 *World Health Forum*. A quarterly record of ideas, arguments and experiences contributed by health professionals the world over.
3 *World Health Statistics Quarterly*. Provides fundamental health guidance on what can be learned when statistical data, drawn from global sources, are submitted to appropriate analysis.
4 *Bulletin of the World Health Organisation*. Bi-monthly presentation of original research findings selected on the basis of their immediate or potential relevance to problems of human health.
5 *International Digest of Health Legislation*. A quarterly report on world-wide developments in law and regulations designed to protect public health and the human environment.

Chapter 28

International and inter-regional organisations

Shelagh Murphy

During this century, because of the speed of travel and the interdependence of one area of the world on others, groups of health workers have increasingly thought in terms of international organisations. There are now 125 non-governmental organisations which, because of their world-wide record in the field of health, have a special relationship with the World Health Organisation. Almost all medical specialities have some international touchstone, and organisations like the World Federation for Mental Health or the World Federation of Neurology play an important part in disseminating knowledge and promoting research. Nursing, probably because of its long international history dating back to the early monastic orders of Christendom and the Knights Hospitallers, was early on the modern international scene, with the International Council of Nurses and the nursing arm of the Red Cross movement.

THE RED CROSS ORGANISATION

The Red Cross was founded as a result of the experience of Henri Dunant (1828–1910), a citizen of Geneva, who, travelling to Italy on a business mission in May 1859 reached Solferino in Lombardy where an indecisive battle with heavy casualties had just been fought in the Franco-Piedmontese war against Austria. Deeply distressed at the lack of provision for the sick and wounded of both sides, and having tried to mobilise local help, the scene so haunted him that when he returned to Geneva he published *A Memory of Solferino*.[1] In this he argued the case for organising relief agencies 'who would be in permanent existence and always ready for the possibility of war', and further, 'that a special congress formulate some international principle, with the sanction of an inviolable Convention, which, once accepted, might constitute a basis for Societies for the relief of the wounded in the various countries of Europe'.

In February 1863 the Swiss Committee of Five was formed to give practical effect to the recommendations set out by Dunant, and in October, as a result of Dunant's personal pleadings and visits, 16 nations sent representatives to an international conference in Geneva, the proposals from which formed the basis of the great Red Cross movement and which, among other things, provided for:

- The setting up of a Relief Committee able to assist the army medical services in wartime;
- the training of voluntary male nurses in peacetime;
- the neutralisation of ambulances, military hospitals and medical personnel;
- the adoption of a uniform and distinctive emblem – the white arm band with the red cross, which was of course the Swiss flag with the colours reversed.

In August 1864, the International Conference of the Red Cross initiated the First Geneva Convention, in which the states signing the Convention agreed to give medical attention to friends and enemies alike, to respect human honour, dignity, customs and religious practice, to allow the delegates of the Red Cross to visit prisoner of war and civilian internee camps, and to prohibit cruel or degrading treatment, the taking of hostages, mass extermination, torture, execution without trial, deportations, pillage, acts of violence and wanton distruction of property.[2] This Convention formed the basis of all other Conventions and the various amendments that followed in 1906, 1929 and 1949, the latter being ratified by 141 states.

Today the International Red Cross consists of the International Committee (ICRC) which is the founder body and the promoter of the Conventions. This Committee has 25 members, all of whom are Swiss citizens, and is responsible for disseminating humanitarian law and ensuring that the principles of the Red Cross as a neutral intermediary are observed. Apart from the Committee there is also the International Conference of the Red Cross which meets in principle every four years, and the Standing Commission, which co-ordinates the work between the different international bodies. The international organisations are concerned with intervention during armed conflict on behalf of the sick and wounded and such bodies as the Central Tracing Agency, which deals with both prisoners of war and civilians.

However, more familiar to nurses is the League of Red Cross Societies, which was founded by Henry P. Davidson in 1919, although many of the national societies were founded earlier. Today the League consists of 105 Red Cross Societies, 19 Red Crescent and one Red Lion (Iran), and 19 other societies in formation. Each country has developed its society to meet its own needs, and although the principal aim was the protection of the wounded in wartime and the training of auxiliary medical personnel, the idea was expanded to cater for the fresh needs of peacetime. One of the main reasons for founding a national society was the training of auxiliary medical and nursing personnel, but, in spite of the fact that Henri

Dunant, when he addressed a meeting in London in 1872, claimed that the inspiration of his work had been the achievements of Miss Nightingale in the Crimea, she herself was lukewarm. Asked her opinion about the value of the Geneva Convention, she wrote to the British representative, Sir Thomas Longmore, with characteristic laconism, 'it will be harmless for our government to sign the Convention as it now stands. It amounts to nothing more than a declaration that humanity to the wounded is a good thing.'[3] In this letter Miss Nightingale states starkly the paradox of trying to humanise war, for 'humanity may prolong the agony', or as General Sherman put it in another context in Georgia in 1864, 'war is cruelty – you cannot refine it'. In another part of the letter Miss Nightingale wrote, 'pious vows will be kept by those who need no vows to make them humane', a remark that foreshadowed events to come, for in spite of efforts to humanise war at the end of the nineteenth century, all too soon these were to prove ineffective. All the main participants in the Second World War had been signatories to the Convention.

Although Miss Nightingale was interested in Dunant's work and actually advised him, by the time of the Franco-Prussian War in 1870 when the British Red Cross Society was founded, Miss Nightingale's own scheme for training professional nurses was under way and this particular function was not necessary in England. Also during the African wars the Order of St John of Jerusalem had been reconstituted and had some of the same aims as the Red Cross, with a special emphasis on first aid and the St John Ambulance Brigade. However, the British Red Cross Society did important work in training nursing auxiliaries and by 1909 there were 80,000 ready to work in hospitals. In 1914 the Order of St John claimed equal status with the Red Cross, a situation that was met by the formation of the Joint War Committee, and, in the absence of a Minister of Health, this committee became responsible for the organisation and posting of auxiliary nursing and medical personnel. It must be remembered that, although the advent of the Nightingale training – which spread to the Empire and some other Protestant countries – introduced a new dimension in nursing in England, nursing in Catholic Europe was continuing on the religious order system of the Counter-Reformation, and although nursing was devoted, it was unscientific and lacked professional training. In these countries the national Red Cross Societies, as they developed, were able to add a new professional standard, the Red Cross School of Nursing often being considered the elite and the most advanced school, trainees from which have made a most important contribution to nursing throughout the world.

Now that in most countries the armed services have their own medical and nursing services, with personnel trained for forward relief work – the Royal Air Force, for example, trains sisters to drop from parachutes – the need for auxiliary assistance on the battlefield is no longer urgent. Moreover, the nature of war has changed, the casualties of Hiroshima or jungle guerrilla war are not the same as at Solferino or even the Somme. Today the Red Cross Societies have taken on a new and even more urgent role. First, national societies now aim at promoting activities with an accent on primary health care, the training of health workers and a voluntary membership that can be used in rural areas where medical aid is not available – a programme in line with the philosophy of the World Health Organisation with its emphasis on health education and self-help. Second, there is a new stress on community involvement, which incorporates first aid, social welfare and 'disaster preparedness'. It is in this last field that the Red Cross has made its most spectacular contribution during recent years, for hardly a month goes by without news of the Red Cross being called in on behalf of victims of natural disasters such as floods, typhoons, fires and earthquakes, or of civil war or other disorders. For over six years the League co-ordinated and conducted relief in Vietnam, and in 1976, 72 national societies participated in providing relief for the victims of the earthquake in Guatemala; the League has been concerned with the plight of the Vietnamese 'boat people' and the victims of the war in Nicaragua and, now, in the former Yugoslavia. Because of these activities the Red Cross has built up a vast body of expertise in disaster relief, and, more important, the preparation for disaster. In all these activities nursing plays an important part and in Geneva the Red Cross has its own department of nursing and Nursing Advisory Committee, in which a number of British nurses play leading roles.

THE INTERNATIONAL COUNCIL OF NURSES

The International Council of Nurses, founded in 1899, is a federation of national nurses' associations, and was formed in the belief that nursing practice throughout the world could be developed and improved by sharing the contributions of the various member associations. 'A major function of the International Council of Nurses is to assist national nurses associations to play their part in developing and improving:

- the health service to the public;
- the practice of nursing;
- the social and economic welfare of nurses.[4]

The idea of an international organisation for nurses came to Mrs Bedford Fenwick when she was the treasurer of the International Congress fund for the International Council of Women which met in London in 1899, when Lavina Dock of the United States and several other nurses read papers. A meeting took place in the Bedford Fenwicks' house in Hanover Square and it was agreed that steps be taken to organise an International Council of Nurses. At a second meeting at St Bartholomew's Hospital officers were elected and an embryo constitution drawn up; nursing associations in other countries were approached, and in 1901 the first Congress was held in Buffalo, attended by nurses from the eight founder countries. The constitution laid down that each country be represented by only one national organisation, and Britain overcame this by linking together a number of diverse bodies and leagues in a National Council which continued to represent the United Kingdom until 1962, when it amalgamated with the Royal College of Nursing, and British representation has since been through that body.

The management of the International Council was in the hands of a Grand Council, consisting of an allotted number of representatives from each country. However, the Council was too large for the general running of such an organisation and a Board of Directors was set up as an executive body and headquarters were opened in Oxford Street, London. Congresses were organised quadrennially, and the Council, which grew rapidly at the beginning of the century, met in Berlin, Paris, London, Cologne and San Francisco, with much of the time devoted to the need to improve the standard of nursing education, to the fight for registration, which was going on in a number of countries, and above all, to the problems raised for nursing by the status of women. The First World War brought a hiatus to the work and it was not until 1922 that another Congress was held, and then in 1925 a new headquarters was opened in Geneva and the *International Nursing Review* founded as the Council's official publication.

In 1934 the Florence Nightingale Foundation was established as an educational trust which provided many nurses with bursaries and scholarships, until after the Second World War when this fund was ultimately transferred to the aegis of the Education Committee of the International Council which now controls the income and the way the money is spent.

In 1939 hostilities again brought international communication to a halt, and many wondered whether an organisation founded to meet the needs at the beginning of the century would be viable in the post-war world, especially as the Nursing division of the World Health Organisation and other international agencies were supplying links for nurses. However, a Congress was held in Stockholm in 1949 where nurses from countries that had been former friends or foes were emotionally reunited. The Council found new headquarters in London until it was able to return to Geneva.

Even before the war the Council had links with the International Labour Organisation (founded in 1919), and now it increased its association with other international agencies and became a non-governmental body acting in an advisory capacity to the World Health Organisation, and became increasingly concerned with the social and economic problems confronting nurses, especially in the developing world. Meanwhile, an upsurge of postwar nationalism and the emergence of new countries at a bewildering rate, the Council doubled its membership with groups who had very different aspirations from the organisation founded in 1899. In 1969, reporting on the Montreal Congress, the *Nursing Times* wrote:

> The 74 member nations now have widely disparate problems and are at different stages of their development in their nursing programmes; the emerging countries are struggling, often against odds, to get nursing recognised as a profession; the older countries with a century of professional nursing behind them are developing programmes to deal with the changing health need of Western codification, spiralling costs, and the need to conserve skill.

Written in 1969, these words could have been penned today. The late eighties saw the reunification of Germany, the break-up of the Soviet Union and the collapse of communism in Eastern Europe and the advent of the killer disease AIDS. All countries, rich and poor, are examining their health-care systems and seeking ways to cut costs and obtain better value from increasingly scarce resources. The role of nursing is crucial, and nurses are called upon to demonstrate, as never before, the cost-effectiveness of skilled nursing care and its contribution to the improved quality of health care.

Today the International Council of Nurses provides advice and assistance to 111 member associations; it is in official relationship with the WHO and UNICEF, has consultative status with the Council of Europe and is on the consultative register of the Social and Economic Council of the United Nations, as well as having a working relationship with a number of other international organisations where it represents the interests of nurses world-wide.

'The ICN faces a future of limitless possibilities; this will be the history of the next 65 years. For the end of an era is not only an end – it is also a beginning.' So wrote Daisy Bridges, ICN General Secretary 1948 to 1961 at the end of the last chapter of her book *A History of the International Council of Nurses 1899–1964, the First 65 Years*. As we move towards the end of the first century of ICN we are certainly coming to the end of an era. But what a beginning lies ahead for the International Council of Nurses in the new century.

COMMONWEALTH NURSES FEDERATION

In response to a request from the Executive Director of the International Council of Nurses and from the Canadian Nurses Association, the Commonwealth Foundation in London agreed to make a very substantial grant to enable representatives of nurses' associations in developing countries in the Commonwealth to attend the International Council of Nurses Congress in Montreal in 1969. One of the conditions in making this grant was that a meeting should be convened in Montreal of representatives of all Commonwealth countries attending the Congress to consider the establishment of a Commonwealth Nurses Association. The meeting of representatives of Commonwealth countries took place on Friday, 20 June, before the ICN meeting began. Thirty-three Commonwealth countries were represented.

At an early stage in the discussions it became clear that the representatives of the developing countries were convinced of the need to establish a Commonwealth Nurses Association. In arguing the need, they referred to the fact that the profession in their countries was based on British traditions; help was needed to develop the service and to establish nursing as a profession; this help must come from interchange of knowledge and experience between the countries concerned and from a body outside the countries concerned which had a real understanding of their problems. On the question of finance, while they could not themselves finance the venture, they believed that money would be forthcoming.

A small committee, set up to discuss all the implications of setting up such an organisation, agreed a constitution, which was then circulated to nurses' associations throughout the Commonwealth. The Commonwealth Nurses Federation, as it came to be called, was finally established in 1971.

The first President was Miss Muriel Skeet, and the first Executive Secretary Mrs Margaret Brayton, who was appointed in 1973.

From a modest beginning the Federation grew into an international organisation with 53 members. However, although much good work was done, communication was difficult, and insufficient finance made regular meetings of the Federation and its Board difficult.

In 1989, the Ninth Commonwealth Health Ministers' Meeting, held in Melbourne, Australia, requested the Commonwealth Secretariat to convene a meeting of Commonwealth Chief Nursing Officers to consider the challenges and opportunities affecting the efficient and effective delivery of nursing and midwifery services and, in particular, their leadership, planning and management, regulation, professional education and practice. The aim of the meeting was to produce a succinct report for presentation to the Commonwealth Health Ministers at their Tenth Triennial Meeting in Cyprus in October 1992. The key section of the Summary Report was to be the recommendations. These were to address action required by governments, professional associations, international and regional agencies and non-governmental organisations. All were to be realistic and identifiable to the economic and health status of member countries, and the development of the health service and the health professionals within it.

This unique meeting with its theme, 'Challenges and Opportunities', was held in Malta in September 1992. The agenda was divided into three main topics, Human Resources, Preparation for Practice, and Standards and Accountability for Practice.

The meeting, which included representatives from professional associations, the WHO and the International Council of Nurses, resulted in a unanimous view that nurses and midwives were pivotal in the provision of health care; their role and contribution would become increasingly important in the years ahead. They, more than anyone, were involved in identifying health needs and in the provision of health care to communities. It was recognised that in many parts of the Commonwealth the nurse or midwife was often the only available and acceptable source of health-care provision and advice. It was also recognised that the contribution of nurses and midwives must be exploited to the full, and the challenge was to ensure this contribution to health care. The recommendations and a plan of action were incorporated into a report to the Tenth Commonwealth Health Ministers Meeting in Cyprus, which wholeheartedly endorsed them.

A meeting of the Commonwealth Nurses Federation took place in Malta immediately following this meeting, at which a way forward for the Federation was agreed and a Working Group set up to take this forward. Because of difficulties with the location of the headquarters, the Royal College of Nursing offered to accommodate the office of the Federation for four years and agreed to undertake the administrative function on the retirement of the Executive Secretary until a new Executive Secretary was appointed. A new constitution was drafted and disseminated to all associations within the Commonwealth, and a full meeting of the Federation was scheduled to take place at the time of the International Council of Nurses Congress in 1993 in Madrid.

At that meeting it was agreed that the Recommendations and Action Plan from the Malta meeting would form a firm basis for the future work of the Federation. Elections had taken place, and, with the benefit of generous funding from the Commonwealth Foundation, a residential Board Meeting took place in October 1993 when a new Executive Secretary was to be appointed.

THE EUROPEAN COMMUNITY

Sickened by the magnitude of the Second World War and its aftermath, the post-war generation of Europe joined together in 1949 in the Council of Europe. A headquarters was established in Strasburg, and the delegates of the various countries met monthly. The Council did much useful practical work although its effect on the unity of Europe was slight. On health matters it was in contact with the World Health Committee for the European Region, and was advised on nursing by the Groupement du Nursing l'Ouest Européen of the International Council of Nurses. This group recommended minimum requirements for nursing education in line with those laid down in a World Health Report,[5] which advised that nursing programmes should be concerned with five main categories of care, namely:

- the maintenance of health programmes;
- the protection of groups at increased risk;
- early detection of disease;
- the clinical stage; dealing with patients whose ill health was neither prevented nor detected at an early stage;
- rehabilitation and prevention of disability; and finally assisting patients in those activities that contribute to a peaceful death.

The Council of Europe recommendations were, however, only advisory and its impact was limited; because of this, six of the members – France, Germany, Italy, Holland, Belgium and Luxemburg – formed an inner community with the aim of bringing about greater co-operation. This group was the forerunner of the European Economic Community, which came into being in 1957 with the signing of the Treaty of Rome.

As the European Community approaches its fortieth anniversary, it is interesting to look at the major milestones in its development from a Coal and Steel Community to a Single Market.

1951 Treaty of Paris establishing the European Coal and Steel Community between Belgium, Germany, Italy, France, Luxemburg and the Netherlands;

1957 Treaty of Rome establishing the European Economic Community and the European Atomic Energy Community;

1962 Implementation of the Common Agricultural Policy;

1965 Merger of the three Communities;

1969 First draft text of Directives relating to the nurse responsible for general care submitted by the Commission to the European Parliament;

1973 Denmark, Ireland and the United Kingdom join the European Communities;

1975 First meeting of the EEC Working Party composed of experts from member states on the content of the nursing Directives; meetings continue through 1975 and 1976;

1975 Publication of the *Official Journal of the European Communities of the Medical Directives*; the first profession to agree Sectoral Directives ensuring harmonisation of qualifications and freedom of movement;[6]

1977 Publication in the *Official Journal of the European Communities of the Directives relating to the Nurse Responsible for General Care*;[7]

1979 First direct elections to the European Parliament;

1980 Publication in the *Official Journal of the European Communities of the Directives for Midwives*;[8]

1981 Greece joins the European Communities;

1986 Portugal and Spain join the European Communities;

1987 Entry into force of the Single European Act providing for the completion of the internal market by 1 January 1993.[9]

THE INSTITUTIONS

The Treaty of Rome provided for the establishment of four permanent institutions to ensure that the objectives set out in the Treaty were attained. These institutions, each with its own permanent secretariat or civil service, are:

- the Council, or decision making body;
- The Commission, or policy making body;
- the Court of Justice, to ensure that the interpretation and application of the Treaty complies with the law;
- the Assembly of Parliament, to exercise advisory and supervisory powers.

By the 1970s the initial enthusiasm of the 1950s and 1960s had begun to dim, and progress towards economic and social harmony and integration seemed to lose its relevance and momentum in the face of world depression. Fortunately, the arrival of the 1980s brought about revitalisation and a welcome change in the fortunes of the Community. A Dublin Summit in 1984 brought a new and enthusiastic commitment to the completion of the internal market. This was followed by the Milan Summit in 1985, which instructed the Council of Ministers to put in place the framework and conditions for a single market in the Community by the end of 1992. The means of implementing the Single Market were consolidated in the Single European Act, which became law on 1 July 1987. By the end of December 1992 an area was created 'without internal frontiers within which the freedom of movement of goods, persons, service and capital is ensured' – a true Common Market.

The real significance for the nursing profession of the completion of the Single Market lies in the removal of the final obstacles to free movement for every citizen, whether self-employed or employee. While workers have for some time had the freedom to live and work where they like in the Community, the professions could not do so without harmonisation and recognition of their diplomas. The Treaty of Rome recognised this particular need, and for almost two decades much of the impetus and effort of the Commission and the professions themselves was devoted to the negotiation of separate Directives – the Sectoral Directives. Sectoral Directives were agreed for most of the health professions but the process was lengthy. It is proving extremely complicated to amend the 'Nurse Responsible for General Care' Directive in order to ensure that the text reflects the advances in education and practice, or even to ensure that its fundamental objective applies to all branches of the profession. Despite Directives proposed by the Commission on the basis of recommendations drawn up by the Advisory Committee on Training in Nursing, which would extend the same privileges to paediatric and psychiatric nurses and to those trained in specialist nursing practice as are currently enjoyed by the general care nurse, it has not been possible to reach agreement.[10]

With the advent of the Single Market and the inordinate amount of time taken to process each Sectoral Directive, the Commission decided to move away from harmonisation in favour of recognition. This new approach, enshrined in the so-called 'General Systems' Directives, means that a person recognised as a professional in one member state must be recognised as a professional in all other member states, providing that the profession concerned is a regulated one.[11] The implications for the nursing profession are far-reaching. Unless the profession is able to achieve agreement in the form of a Sectoral Directive or an annexe to the General Care Directives, at least for those specialist nurses whose speciality training has been undertaken after training in general care, there will be a schism between the 'old' and the 'new' approaches. Some areas would then be covered by specific regulations requiring harmonisation, while others would be subject to the equivalency test of one or more 'General Systems' Directives. The profession may not wish to continue with the minutiae of the harmonisation of training programmes in the EC, but it does wish to remain in control of its own education and practice, particularly in the field of specialist training, where experience and training programmes vary so greatly in level and content.

ADVISORY COMMITTEE IN TRAINING IN NURSING

This was set up by decision of the Council of Ministers and published in the same *Official Journal* as the Directives. It is established within the Commission, thus giving it formal status within the EC. Its remit is 'to help to ensure a comparatively high standard of training of the various categories of nursing personnel throughout the Community'. The Committee is also charged to keep under review the need for adaptation of training in the light of developments in nursing and medical science. It is able to make recommendations to the Commission, including amendments to Directives, and is to advise on any matter referred to it by the Commission.

The membership of the Committee is composed of three experts from each member state, one of each from

- the practising profession
- establishments providing nursing education
- the competent authorities of member states.

Each member has a deputy who may attend meetings and may speak but not vote. The Committee has been operating since 1979, and each term lasts for three years. All members are appointed at the beginning of each term, but there is no limit to the number of terms a member may serve.

In considering the size of the Committee – 72 members if all attend, all requiring simultaneous translation – the cost implications are enormous. The economic climate of the Commission has led to changes which inevitably limit the Committee's function. Expenses are now only paid for members, and deputies have to fund themselves. Of more concern, however, is the fact that meetings have been cut from two days twice a year to two days once a year and, in 1993, from two days to one day. There is finance for two working parties to meet twice a year, but the limit on the full meeting makes it difficult to progress major work.

In spite of these drawbacks a considerable amount of work has been carried out. Major work leading to reports adopted by the Committee and formal recommendation to the Commission include:

- Report on the training of nurses responsible for general care, in particular the balance to be found between theoretical and clinical instruction for this category of nurse. (This was undertaken in response to the requirement contained in the remit of the Committee to study the situation and make recommendations to the Commission. The work was carried out by April 1981, and, although accepted by the Commission, the consequent amendment to the Directive was not made until 1986.)
- Report on psychiatric nursing in the European Community[12] and recommendation for a Directive on psychiatric nursing in the EC.[13]
- Report on paediatric nursing in the European Community[14] and recommendation for a Directive on psychiatric nursing in the EC.[15]
- Report and Recommendations on Training in Cancer Nursing.[16]
- Report on Primary Health Content in the Training of Nurses responsible for general care.[17] This was adopted in April 1992 from work carried out in the previous term. Following from the position revealed in the Report, the Committee progressed to *Guidelines for Primary Health Care Instruction on the Training of Nurses Responsible for General Care*.[18]

There is a feeling that time and cost may well lead to less emphasis on the work of the Advisory Committees in general, and there are strong hints that the profession needs to take more responsibility for work in its field. The Advisory Committee is limited by its remit to matters related to training in nursing.

THE STANDING COMMITTEE OF NURSES OF THE EUROPEAN COMMUNITY

The Standing Committee of Nurses, otherwise known as PCN, held its first formal meeting in 1971 following representations by both the European Nursing Group and the International Council of Nurses to the Commission seeking recognition of a formal liaison committee of nurses. Membership consists of one representative from each member state and a deputy. All national associations except one – Denmark – were also members of the European Nursing Group, and Denmark is a member of another regional group, The Northern Nurses Federation. As other countries have become members of the EC, or have declared their intention to seek membership, PCN offers observer status to acceding countries with full membership in due course. In addition, PCN invites representatives of countries in eastern Europe to one meeting per year as observers.

As an official liaison committee, PCN has a formal link with the Commission, which has been freely used. The first major occasion on which it used its privileges was for the presentation of the Memorandum giving views on the shortcomings of the first draft of the Nursing Directives in 1971. When the Advisory Committee was set up, PCN considered the separate remits of both itself and the Advisory Committee, the latter being restricted to training, while PCN is free to agree its own remit. In an endeavour to construct a picture of nursing within the EC, PCN undertook a number of surveys and published the following documents:

- a summary of the educational condition of nurses in nine countries of the EC (1974);
- an examination of the work and conditions of first-level nurses in the public sector of the EC countries and in the four Nordic countries outside the EC (1975, updated 1977);
- a survey of health services and the nursing structure within the health services in the countries affiliated to the EC (1978);
- a survey of basic and post-basic qualifications in primary health care in the countries of the EC (1985);
- a document on the preparation of nurse teachers in ten member states of the EC (1986);
- *The Nurses Contribution to an EC Public Health Policy* (1993);
- *The Nurses Contribution to Care of the Elderly: a European Perspective* (1993).

Two books, *Nursing in the European Community*[19] and *Nursing – the European Dimension*,[20] were both edited by Dame Sheila Quinn in 1980 and 1993, respectively, from material largely supplied by the members of the Committee.

In the early years most attention was given to education. However, when the directives were agreed and the Advisory Committee was set up, although PCN still followed events with great interest and close contacts were maintained between the two committees, PCN began to extend its contacts to the directorates of the Commission where work had relevance to health matters and nursing. Most of the work lay within Directorate General V; Employment, Industrial Relations and Social Affairs, although other Directorates had relevance and importance. This Directorate is responsible for social security, social protection, living conditions, labour law, health and safety at work, public health and strategic planning. It is the home of many of the Directives and Regulations arising out of the Social Charter, the Europe Against Cancer Programme and the European Year of Safety, Hygiene and Health Protection at Work.

The Treaty on European Union, negotiated at Maastricht in December 1991, contains a Public Health Article which provides for general Community competence on health issues. This Article allows for a European Public Health Policy by requiring member states to co-operate in the development of their individual health policies and to take health issues into account when formulating social and environmental policies.

The programme on the elderly is another of great interest to nurses, as are the Social Charter, from which the United Kingdom is excluded at its request, Health and Safety at Work, Medical Research and Assistance to Eastern Europe.

By 1990 PCN felt that, in order best to serve the interests of the profession, an address was needed in Brussels in order to keep close contact and be up to date with events so as to be able to react speedily. In November 1991, a contract was signed for an office in Brussels, and all meetings are now held there.

THE COUNTRIES OF THE EUROPEAN FREE TRADE ASSOCIATION

The European Free Trade Association (EFTA) reached political agreement on the establishment of a European Economic Area in October 1991. This has still to be signed by the European Court of Justice. The member countries of EFTA are Austria, Finland, Iceland, Liechenstein, Norway, Sweden and Switzerland. Part of the delay is due to the fact that, following a referendum, Switzerland has withdrawn from the agreement. It is now hoped that this agreement, which extends to EFTA most of the principles and regulations of the Single Market, will be signed in late 1993 or early 1994. The most significant of these principles for health professionals is the free movement of persons and the recognition of diplomas and other agreed professional qualifications.

HEALTH-CARE SYSTEMS IN EUROPE

Apart from the important reminder that the Reformation influenced the way in which nursing developed in the different countries of Catholic Christendom, nursing has evolved in each country to meet its own particular health system. Each country has a different background, and as always, the position of nurses cannot be separated from the status of women, past and present, in the countries concerned. All over Europe expenditure on health care has risen at an alarming rate, and all countries face the same inexorable problems, the chief of which are the financial implications of an ageing population and the extraordinary but costly development of medical technology combined with the explosive bill for wages. Most countries are evaluating their health-care systems and undergoing significant change, none more so than the United Kingdom.

The Public Health Charter does not mean that all health-care systems must be harmonised throughout the EC. In future, the public health aspects of all Community legislation will be examined but, unlike other more familiar areas of Community activity, harmonisation of national legislation is excluded. Harmonisation, the concept which has so dominated the professional scene in the Community is 'out', and co-operation is 'in', and the formulation of an EC Public Health Policy will, we hope, be free to develop in an imaginative and different way.

REFERENCES

1 Dunant, H. (1864) *A Memory of Solferino*, reissued International Committee of the Red Cross, Geneva.
2 International Committee of the Red Cross (1963) *The Geneva Convention* (handbook containing the main text), Geneva.
3 Nightingale, F. (Aug. 1864) Letter to General Longmore, quoted by Dame Beryl Oliver, *The Red Cross in Action*.
4 ICN Basic Documents; Constitution and Regulations, Article IV 1–6, 37, rue Vermont, Geneva.
5 World Health Organisation (1966) *Report of the Expert Committee on Nursing 1966*, Geneva.
6 Council Directives 75/362/EEC and 75/363/EEC, *Official Journal of the European Communities*, No. L 167, 30 June 1975.
7 Council Directives 77/452/EEC and 77/453/EEC, *Official Journal of the European Communities*, 20 No. L 176, 15 July 1977.
8 Council Directives 80/154/EEC, 80/155/EEC and 80/156/EEC, *Official Journal of the European Communities*, No. L 33, 11 Feb. 1980.
9 Single European Act (1986) *Bulletin of the European Communities*, Office for Official Publications of the EC, Luxemburg.
10 Draft Proposal for a Council Directive supplementing Directives 77/454/EEC and 77/453/EEC as regards specialist nursing, particularly psychiatric and paediatric care (1990), 111/F5385/90, Brussels.
11 Council Directives of 21 Dec. 1988 on a General System for the Recognition of Higher Education Diplomas awarded on completion of professional education

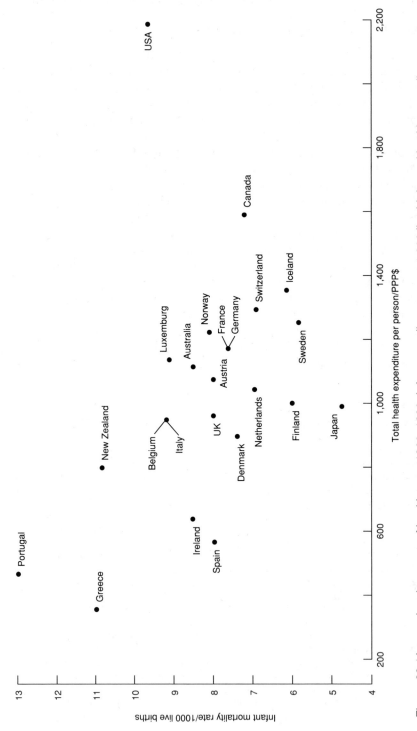

Figure 28.1 International patterns of health care, 1960–1990, Infant mortality rates per 1,000 live births and health expenditure per person (PPS$) in 23 OECD countries, 1988
Source: Data from OECD Health Data, Version 1.01, CREDOC/OECD, Paris

and training of at least three years' duration. EEC/89/48 *Official Journal of the European Communities*, 32 L 19, 24 Jan. 1989.

12 Advisory Committee on Training in Nursing (1984) *Report on Psychiatric Nursing in the European Community* 111/D/7/82, 24 Feb.

13 Advisory Committee on Training in Nursing (1986) *Recommendation for a Directive on Psychiatric Nursing in the European Community*, 11/D/1832/4/85, 21 Oct.

14 Advisory Committee on Training in Nursing (1986) *Report on paediatric Training in the European Community*, 111/D/1027/6/84, 17 April.

15 Advisory Committee on Training in Nursing (1989) *Recommendation for a Directive on Paediatric Nursing in the European Community*, 111/5/5158/4/88, 10 Oct.

16 *Report and Recommendations on Training in Cancer*, 111/D/248/3/88, 20 Dec. 1988.

17 Advisory Committee on Training in Nursing (1989) *Report on Primary Health Care Content in the Training of the Nurse Responsible for General Care*, 111/D/5011/6/89.

18 Advisory Committee on Training in Nursing (1990) *Recommendation for Guidelines for Primary Health Care Instruction in the Training of Nurses Responsible for General Care*, 111/D/5370/3/90.

19 Quinn, S. (ed.) (1980) *Nursing in the European Community*, London: Croom Helm.

20 Quinn, S. and Russell, S. (eds) 1993, *Nursing – the European Dimension*, London: Scutari Press.

FURTHER READING

European Health Services Handbook, European Healthcare Management Association, Institute of Health Service Management and National Association of Health Authorities and Trusts, published by Institute of Health Service Management.

Epilogue

The number of nurses is falling. Slowly the skill mix is changing, but it was never static. In the nineteenth century the number of trained nurses formed but a small proportion of the total nursing force, and it was never envisaged that all the patients should be cared for by fully trained staff. In the 1930s the Lancet Commission complained about the inordinate number of orderlies, auxiliaries and assistants who had undefined roles and a variety of rewards and were often undisclosed in the records. In the 1970s we bemoaned the fact that the number of auxiliaries had risen by 290 per cent since the beginning of the National Health Service.[1] The message of Chapter 18 in the second edition of this book was that the patients of tomorrow would be nursed by auxiliaries and student nurses with a high wastage rate, therefore the present phenomenon and anxiety are not new. However, the present demographic trend and the likely health needs of tomorrow mean that Britain needs all its nurses. Until well into the year 2000, the number of elderly in the population will rise, and an increasing proportion of these will be frail and many will need care in the community. We have learned that a fitter nation in the lower age groups does not mean less demand on the service; we survive to have new health needs.

Apart from the frail elderly, there are those who are the victims of their own life-style who need support and education, and there are the casualties of society. We thought that we had abolished the diseases of poverty, but those sitting on our pavements with 'hungry and homeless' notices, are prone to tuberculosis, bronchitis, skin diseases, not to mention their being prone to the likelihood of drug abuse and AIDs. The old and the poorly housed unable to face their heating costs are liable to hypothermia and all the ills of the cold. Until we readjust resources, we are unlikely to meet these health needs.

As we approach the year 2000 and the World Health target of Health for All, we have to realise that health lies largely outside the medical services, and until we correct the use of scarce resources the achievement of the World Health goal is likely to remain beyond our reach. A start has been made with the government's campaign for a healthier Britain; the hit list of cancer of the lung, cancer of the breast, heart disease and strokes have all decreased between 1986 and 1991, though internationally Britain's rates are comparatively high. However, there has been no reduction in teenage smoking or obesity, and the number of suicides is up by 4 per cent. The lack of health education by school nurses and health visitors, whom some authorities regard as too costly, may have been a factor in teenage smoking and obesity in the young, but the alarming rise in the number of suicides is at least partly due to early discharges from mental hospitals and the lack of adequate care in the community – a reminder, if one were needed, that care in the community is not a cheap option, and that, if not properly planned with adequate trained staff, the results can have disastrous consequences.

If the health needs of the nation are not being met today, does it mean that the health services are under-funded? Internationally Britain is a low spender on health care, though in terms of outcomes it is halfway up the scale. Because there are so many imponderables a precise assessment is difficult, but it does look as if the National Health Service gives good value for money (see Table 25.2). Or, have we spent as much as we can afford on health care and has it to be rationed? If so, what are the criteria for decision-making and who is to make the decisions? Nurses as the patient's advocates, should have a say in this debate. On the other hand, are health budgets arbitrary, and does whether needs are met or not met depend on where you live or whether your doctor is a fund-holder?

On the credit side, wastage from training has fallen to between 6 and 11 per cent.[2] Therefore, we do not need to educate so many nurses to keep up the supply of trained nurses, and there are signs that the intake of student nurses, having been curtailed, is now being raised. Project 2000 will have its teething problems and will be viewed with suspicion by teachers of traditional courses, but this is not new. Miss Nightingale's 'ordinary' probationers were very suspicious of the paying probationers, especially when they did a shorter course. The old-style nurse and many doctors were critical of the newfangled registration, and, at the time of the Platt Report, there was an outcry from doctors and administrators who feared that aiming at recruits with at least five 'Ordinary' levels would deny the service of people with natural aptitudes for nursing. Some, reminiscent of Mr South, who criticised the Nightingale scheme, said that all that was needed from a nurse was a kind heart, cool hands and obedience. This is an ongoing situation as the demand for education rises. Nursing will become more academic, but so will other occupations, and a third of young people will be graduates. Moreover, as technical demands in medicine increase, nursing education needs to improve if nurses are to understand the 'why' as well as the 'how' and to be at ease in explaining treatment to patients.

Although there may be fewer posts in hospitals, the number of practice nurses has doubled and there are signs that the primary health-care teams are growing and care, particularly preventive care, is becoming more efficient. If, however, the number of hospital beds is to be reduced, there must be a switch of funding and resources and it means that there must be more post-registration training for nurses in the community. The art of advising and nursing in the community, with all its calls on multi-disciplinary co-operation, is not naturally acquired with basic training. But these trainings are expensive, and Trusts, looking at their budgets, are loath to fund nurses where no immediate benefit is manifest. Nurses must demonstrate by research and debate that quality nursing pays; they must speak up when they see inadequate care.

Some will argue that we are becoming leaner and fitter, and that it is a waste of nursing skills for expensive trained nurses to do what can be done by untrained staff. In 1985 Sir Roy Griffiths claimed that the National Health Service was under-managed and was not cost-effective; now it looks as if it is over-managed. Figures published by the Health and Social Services Statistics in October 1993 show that the number of service managers rose from 1,200 in 1988 to 13,000 in 1991 and that the salary bill rose from £30 million to £384 million, but the number of nurses fell by 9,000. A note states that 'the sharp jump in figures is due to the extension of the senior management pay scheme to include lower tiers of management and the fact that student nurses no longer work on the wards in the early part of their training'.[3] However, it seems unlikely that this accounts for 9,000 nurses or the sharp increase in management figures.

Florence Nightingale dreamed of making nursing an autonomous profession with nurses teaching hygiene, but the demands of medical science and hospital administration decreed that nursing should become an adjunct to medicine, and the medical model began. Now the wheel is coming full circle; we have largely cured what can be cured and have prevented much of what can be prevented, and what is left is care and the correction of unhealthy life-styles. In this role the nurse must be an educator and develop independent expertise. The nurse of the future has been taught to question what she does and why she does it; she cannot step aside from the many ethical and moral issues that beset medicine today, and she is well placed to be the patient's advocate. However, in welcoming a new role she should look back to the past; much of nursing is changeless, and, in spite of moving from crisis to crisis and reorganisation to reorganisation, the present revolution may turn out to represent an unexpected degree of historical continuity. Those who do not remember the past are condemned to relive it and repeat its mistakes.

REFERENCES

1   See *Nursing and Social Change*, 2nd edn of this book, p. 247.
2   English National Board Training Statistics, July 1993.
3   *The Times*, reporting on the Health and Social Services Statistics, 18 Nov. 1993.

Index